The Boston IVF Handbook of Infertility

This new edition of an established go-to reference provides a structured approach to treating the infertile couple that will be of benefit to the gynecologist, reproductive endocrinologist, and reproductive medicine nurse alike. Both clinical and laboratory techniques are included, with material on preconception care and office management.

- Provides a comprehensive but concise go-to reference for the whole IVF team
- Enables busy clinicians, embryologists, counselors, and staff to access information quickly
- Brings an established resource up to date with current practice

REPRODUCTIVE MEDICINE AND ASSISTED REPRODUCTIVE TECHNIQUES SERIES

David Gardner

University of Melbourne, Australia

Zeev Shoham

Kaplan Hospital, Rehovot, Israel

Kay Elder, Jacques Cohen

Human Preimplantation Embryo Selection, ISBN: 9780415399739

John D Aplin, Asgerally T Fazleabas, Stanley R Glasser, Linda C Giudice

The Endometrium, Second Edition, ISBN: 9780415385831

Nick Macklon, Ian Greer, Eric Steegers

Textbook of Periconceptional Medicine, ISBN: 9780415458924

Andrea Borini, Giovanni Coticchio

Preservation of Human Oocytes, ISBN: 9780415476799

Ben Cohlen, Willem Ombelet

Intra-Uterine Insemination: Evidence Based Guidelines for Daily Practice, ISBN: 9781841849881

Adam H. Balen

Infertility in Practice, Fourth Edition, ISBN: 9781841848495

Nick Macklon

IVF in the Medically Complicated Patient, Second Edition: A Guide to Management, ISBN: 9781482206692

Michael Tucker, Juergen Liebermann

Vitrification in Assisted Reproduction, ISBN: 9780415408820

Ben J Cohlen, Evert J P van Santbrink, Joop S E Laven

Ovulation Induction: Evidence Based Guidelines for Daily Practice, ISBN: 9781498704076

Botros Rizk, Markus Montag

Standard Operational Procedures in Reproductive Medicine: Laboratory and Clinical Practice, ISBN: 9781498719216

Michael M. Alper, Denny Sakkas, Denis Vaughan, Alan S. Penzias

The Boston IVF Handbook of Infertility: A Practical Guide for Practitioners Who Care for Infertile Couples, Fifth Edition, ISBN: 9781032607030

For more information on this book series, please visit https://www.routledge.com/Reproductive-Medicine-and-Assisted-Reproductive-Techniques-Series/book-series/IHCRMEDASREP

The Boston IVF Handbook of Infertility

A Practical Guide for Practitioners Who Care for Infertile Couples

Fifth Edition

Edited by

Michael M. Alper, MD

Medical Director and Reproductive Endocrinologist, Boston IVF;
Associate Clinical Professor, Harvard Medical School, Boston, MA, USA

Denny Sakkas, PhD

Chief Scientific Officer, Boston IVF-IVIRMA North America, Boston, MA;
USA Associate Professor, Obstetrics, Gynecology & Reproductive Sciences, Yale
University School of Medicine, New Haven, CT, USA

Denis Vaughan, MD, FACOG, MRCPI

Reproductive Endocrinology and Infertility
Co-Founder, Terra Fertility, Dedham, MA, USA

Alan S. Penzias, MD

Surgical Director and Reproductive Endocrinologist, Boston IVF;
Director of the fellowship program in Reproductive Endocrinology and Infertility,
Beth Israel Deaconess Medical Center/Harvard Medical School and Associate
Professor of Obstetrics, Gynecology & Reproductive Biology, Harvard Medical
School, Boston, MA, USA

CRC Press
Taylor & Francis Group
Boca Raton London New York

CRC Press is an imprint of the
Taylor & Francis Group, an **informa** business

Fifth edition published 2026
by CRC Press
2385 NW Executive Center Drive, Suite 320, Boca Raton FL 33431

and by CRC Press
4 Park Square, Milton Park, Abingdon, Oxon, OX14 4RN

CRC Press is an imprint of Taylor & Francis Group, LLC

ISBN: 9781032607047 (hbk)
ISBN: 9781032607030 (pbk)
ISBN: 9781003460275 (ebk)
ISBN: 9781041093619 (Indian PB Edition)

DOI: 10.1201/9781003460275

Typeset in Times
by Deanta Global Publishing Services, Chennai, India

Contents

Preface

From its early inception over 35 years ago, the field of assisted reproductive technology (ART) and infertility has been rapidly changing. The field is one of the most innovative and fascinating areas of medicine. In order to keep up with the latest advances, it is critical for any textbook in the field to be up to date. Much has changed since our initial edition 20 years ago. Also, much has changed at Boston IVF as well—our group of fertility specialists has expanded from four to now more than 35, resulting in many more contributors sharing their expertise in this new edition.

In this new edition of the handbook, all of the core topics in the field of infertility have been updated and several new chapters have been added. Genetics is playing a more and more important role in our specialty. The chapter on pre-implantation genetic testing highlights the application of genetics in modern day ART. The ability to screen embryos for their chromosomal status has led to improved implantation rates and efficiency in IVF, and the ability to test for monogenic diseases allows for the elimination of a disease from a family pedigree. The chapter on treatment options for the LGBT community has been updated. Access to effective treatment for same sex couples remains difficult in some areas due to legal, cultural, and logistical reasons. Some treatments for same sex couples are simple (such as donor insemination for same sex female couples) and some may be more involved such as donor egg/gestational surrogacy for same sex male couples. The transgender community also deserves special attention to help these individuals pursue their gender identification and, at the same time, plan for their reproductive options as well. The advent of egg freezing and banking has revolutionized the donor egg field; in fact, vitrification techniques to freeze eggs is one of the most important advances in our field since ICSI was introduced more than 20 years ago. Planned egg freezing has increased severalfold since the last edition, and this is reflected in the chapter on egg freezing. Finally, realizing the role of other key players in the delivery of quality care, we have added chapters highlighting our expertise in the areas of nursing, the IVF laboratory and administration.

This Fifth Edition of *The Boston IVF Handbook* represents the collective efforts of the many professionals at Boston IVF. It represents almost four decades of our company's efforts to improve the care that we provide and help our patients resolve their fertility issues. We hope you enjoy our book and it helps you with the care of your patients.

This edition was produced with collaborators from Eugin Group with several chapters added. Of note, during the production of this text, Boston IVF joined the IVI RMA global group. We look forward to collaborating with them in future editions.

Michael M. Alper, MD
Co-founder & President, Boston IVF

Contributors

Elise Abi Antoun
Resident, Obstetrics and Gynecology
Tufts Medical Center
Boston, MA, USA

Goli Ardestani
IVF Laboratory Director, Boston IVF
Portland, ME, USA
and
Research Embryologist, Boston IVF
Waltham, MA, USA

Sara Arian
Reproductive Endocrinologist, Boston IVF
Beth Israel Deaconess Medical Center
and
Clinical Instructor, Harvard Medical School
Boston, MA, USA

Jill Attaman
Reproductive Endocrinologist, Boston IVF
and
Instructor, Harvard Medical School
Boston, MA, USA

Emelia Bachman
Director of Fertility Preservation, Delaware
Institute for Reproductive Medicine
Newark, DE, USA

C. Brent Barrett
Chief Laboratory Director, Boston IVF
Waltham, MA, USA

Brian M. Berger
Director, Third Party Reproduction, Boston IVF
Clinical Instructor, Harvard Medical School
Boston, MA, USA

Keith Blauer
Medical Director/Partner, Reproductive Care Center
Sandy, UT, USA

Pietro Borteletto
Reproductive Endocrinology and Infertility
Co-Founder, Terra Fertility
Dedham, MA, USA

Naveena Daram
Resident Physician, Obstetrics & Gynecology
Wright State University, Dayton, OH, USA

Valeria Donno
Reproductive Specialist, Dexeus Fertility
Department of Obstetrics, Gynecology and Reproductive Medicine
Dexeus University Hospital
Barcelona, Spain

Sharon Edwards
Chief Operating Officer, Boston IVF
Boston, MA, USA

Sonia Elguero
Chief Reproductive Endocrinologist, Boston IVF
Albany, NY, USA

Marsha Forman
Laboratory Manager and Tissue Bank Director, Boston IVF
Albany, NY, USA

Gary Frishman
Clinical Professor, Obstetrics & Gynecology,
Warren Alpert Medical School, Brown University
Providence, RI, USA

Demián Glujovsky
Scientific Director
Cegyr (Eugin group), Buenos Aires, Argentina

Daniel Griffin
Reproductive Endocrinologist, Boston IVF
The Women's Hospital
Newburgh, IN, USA

Quetrell D. Heyward
Clinical Fellow, Boston IVF
Beth Israel Medical Center
Boston, MA, USA

Alexandra Huttler
Clinical Fellow, Reproductive Endocrinology & Infertility
Beth Israel Deaconess Medical Center/Boston IVF
Boston, MA, USA

Ann Korkidakis
Reproductive Endocrinologist, Boston IVF
Beth Israel Deaconess Medical Center, Harvard Medical School
Waltham, MA, USA

George Kovalevsky
Reproductive Endocrinology & Infertility
Delaware Institute for Reproductive Medicine
Newark, DE, USA

Antonio LaMarca
Director, Gynecology & Obstetrics Clinic
University of Modena and Reggio Emilia
Modena, Italy

Benjamin Lannon
Reproductive Endocrinologist, Boston IVF
Portland, ME, USA

Karina Lattes
Specialist, Reproductive Medicine, and Research Coordinator
CIRH Barcelona, Spain

Stephen Lazarou
Chief, Andrology, Boston IVF
Clinical Instructor at Harvard Medical School
Boston, MA, USA

Carol Lesser
Nurse Practitioner, Boston IVF
Brookline, MA, USA

Sandy Li
Reproductive Endocrinologist
Boston IVF and Beth Israel Deaconess Medical Center
Boston, MA, USA

Theo LoPreste
Director, Marketing, Boston IVF
Boston, MA, USA

Kerri L. Luzzo
Reproductive Endocrinologist, Boston IVF
Providence, RI, USA

Lauren Murphy
Reproductive Endocrinologist, Boston IVF
Beth Israel Deaconess Medical Center
and
Clinical Instructor, Harvard Medical School
Boston, MA, USA

Adrienne B. Neithardt
Delaware Institute for Reproductive Medicine (Boston IVF Network clinic)
Milford, DE, USA

Lynn Nichols
Clinical Social Worker, Boston IVF
Boston, MA, USA

Samuel Pang
Reproductive Endocrinologist (retired), Boston IVF
Waltham, MA, USA

Karishma Patel
Clinical Fellow, Obstetrics, Gynecology, & Reproductive Biology
Boston IVF and Beth Israel Deaconess Medical Center
Harvard Medical School, Boston, MA, USA

Samuel A. Pauli
Reproductive Endocrinologist, Boston IVF
Waltham, MA, USA

Romina Pesce
Head of the Reproduction and ART Unit
Hospital Italiano de Buenos Aires
Buenos Aires, Argentina

Mina Popovic
Scientific Director, Eugin Group
Barcelona, Spain

Nina Resetkova
Reproductive Endocrinologist, Boston IVF
Beth Israel Deaconess Medical Center
and
Clinical Instructor, Harvard Medical School
Boston, MA, USA

Brooke V. Rossi
Reproductive Endocrinologist, Ohio Reproductive Medicine
and
Adjunct Assistant Professor, Obstetrics & Gynecology
Ohio State University Wexner Medical Center
Columbus, OH, USA

Riwa Sabbagh
Reproductive Endocrinologist, Boston IVF and Beth Israel Medical Center
and
Instructor of Obstetrics, Gynecology & Reproductive Biology
Harvard Medical School, Boston, MA, USA

Emily A. Seidler
Reproductive Endocrinologist, Boston IVF
Beth Israel Deaconess Medical Center
and
Clinical Instructor, Harvard Medical School
Boston, MA, USA

Rita M. Sneeringer
Reproductive Endocrinologist, Boston IVF; Beth Israel Deaconess Medical Center
and
Clinical Instructor, Harvard Medical School
Waltham, MA, USA

David L. Stern
CEO, Boston IVF
Boston, MA, USA

Kim Thornton
Reproductive Endocrinologist, Boston IVF
and
Chief, Reproductive Endocrinology & Infertility, Beth Israel Deaconess Medical Center
and
Assistant Professor, Harvard Medical School
Boston, MA, USA

Marc Torra-Massana
Embryologist and Researcher
Clínica Eugin, Barcelona, Spain

Thomas L. Toth
Reproductive Endocrinologist, Boston IVF
and
Associate Professor, Obstetrics, Gynecology, & Reproductive Biology
Harvard Medical School, Boston, MA, USA

Jeanie Ungerleider
Licensed Independent Clinical Social Worker, Boston IVF
Waltham, MA, USA

Marta Venturas
Lab Supervisor, Boston IVF
Waltham, MA, USA

Kristen Page Wright
Reproductive Endocrinologist, Boston IVF
and
Assistant Professor, Dartmouth College's School of Medicine
Hanover, NH, USA

1

Overview of Infertility

Alan S. Penzias

Overview of Infertility

Fertility and treatment to achieve it when unassisted means are not successful or, through biological circumstances, not possible have been the subject of social discourse and scientific study throughout human history. This chapter is meant to provide historical context to the contemporary approach to fertility and treatment of infertility by sharing its history as viewed through the eyes of our predecessors. Historical accounts presented herein are abbreviated and by no means comprehensive. There are numerous other sources covering the approach to fertility across many different cultures and geographic locations spanning millennia. Because of its centrality in society, many peoples and nations rightly can claim advances that have moved our understanding forward. Likewise, the individuals cited for their contributions are just a few of many upon whose shoulders we stand.

A theme that is evident across time is that progress is not linear. Breakthroughs in understanding and disruptive scientific achievements punctuate long intervals of incremental change. From the modern perspective, some dogma that governed treatment in the past, even recent past, seems antithetical to current beliefs; and yet, scientifically sound new discoveries often require a long ramp before they are adopted by the majority and disseminated into practice broadly. One thing is clear: Infertility is not a simple medical problem. There are ethical, legal, religious, and social issues along with economic dimensions to the topic that require exploration in parallel with advances in embryology, cell biology, and genetics.

Infertility in the Bible

The earliest references to reproduction date back to antiquity with the biblical directive to "be fruitful, and multiply." In fact, those words are used three separate times in the book of Genesis. It is no surprise, therefore, that fertility and procreation played a part in a cornerstone of early life and beliefs. A woman was measured by her ability to bear children, and infertility was viewed as a punishment for wrongdoing, with God being the source of fertility. Sarah and Abraham were unable to conceive. Sarah considered the problem and asked Abraham to "go in unto my maid; it may be that I may obtain children by her." Abraham honored Sarah's request and Hagar conceived. We can probably view this as the first recorded test of male infertility but in retrospect confirmed that the infertility perhaps resided with Sarah.

Ancient Greece

Hippocrates (460–380 B.C.) was one of the first authors of various medical works dealing with gynecology. Six treatises which deal with reproduction were attributed to him. The diagnosis of infertility was based on the concept of free passage or continuity of the external genitalia and the vagina with the rest of

DOI: 10.1201/9781003460275-1

the body. In the Aphorisms of Hippocrates he wrote, "If a woman do not conceive, and wish to ascertain whether she can conceive, having wrapped her up in blankets, fumigate below, and if it appear that the scent passes through the body to the nostrils and mouth, know that of herself she is not unfruitful." In the same treatise Hippocrates speculated on the conditions needed to foster pregnancy. "Women who have the uterus cold and dense do not conceive; and those also who have the uterus humid, do not conceive, for the semen is extinguished, and in women whose uterus is very dry, and very hot, the semen is lost from the want of food; but women whose uterus is in an intermediate state between these temperaments prove fertile."

Aristotle of Stagira (384–322 B.C.) was one of the greatest Greek philosophers of his time and was also one of the greatest zoologists and naturalists of antiquity. Although not a physician, he discussed many issues relating to reproduction in his thesis "The Generation of Animals." Aristotle gave to medicine certain fundamentals such as comparative anatomy and embryology. A common ancient method of interfering with male fertility was castration. Aristotle knew that castration makes a male infertile despite his belief that the testes are only weights holding down the spermatic passages and not the source of the seed. "For the testes are no part of the ducts but are only attached to them, as women fasten stones to the loom when weaving." He was probably misled by his observation that a recently castrated bull succeeded in impregnating a cow, "a bull mounting immediately after castration has caused conception in the cow because the ducts had not yet been drawn up."

The Renaissance

Andreas Vesalius (1514–1564), a Belgian physician and anatomist published his revolutionary book *De Humani Corporis Fabrica* (trans. On the Structure of the Human Body) in 1543. Vesalius contributed to an accurate description of the entire female genital system including ligaments, tubes, and blood supply. He was the first to use the terms pelvis and decidua. He also was the first to describe the ovarian follicle.

Gabrielle Fallopio (1523–1562) of Modena was a student of Vesalius. He described the oviducts and wrote further on the morphology of the ovaries. His name has been permanently connected with the oviduct or fallopian tube. He also named the clitoris, the vagina, and the placenta.

Lazzaro Spallanzani (1729–1799), though not a physician, made enormous contributions to our understanding of fertility. In his monograph "Fecondazione Artificiale," he showed that conception was achieved as a result of contact between eggs and sperm. He succeeded in fertilizing frog eggs by placing them in the immediate contact with the secretions expressed from the testicles of the male frog. He also performed some of the first successful artificial insemination experiments on lower animals and on a dog.

John Hunter (1728–1793) made the first attempt at human artificial insemination in 1785. A baby is born that same year.

The 20th Century

Max Huhner (1873–1947), in his 1913 book *Sterility in the Male and Female and Its Treatment*, introduced the Sims–Huhner test (later termed the postcoital test). In this test, sperm survival in the cervical mucus was thought to correlate with fertility.

I.C. Rubin (1883–1958) introduced the first clinical test to determine tubal patency. Initially, he started by using a radioactive material but realized that this approach had its limitations. He then turned to tubal insufflation using oxygen in 1920. This was later changed to carbon dioxide as it was reabsorbed more easily, caused less discomfort, and avoided the danger of embolism. In the test, the insufflation is usually carried out at a gas pressure of less than 120 mm of mercury. The manometer reading decreases to 100 or less if the tubes are clear; if between 120 and 130, there is probably partial stricture; if it rises to 200 and above, it is suggestive that the tubes are obstructed.

In 1935, Stein and Levanthal described a series of patients with amenorrhea, hirsutism, and obesity. They named the condition the Stein–Levanthal Syndrome, later termed Polycystic Ovarian Syndrome.

They noted that several of these women started to menstruate after they underwent an ovarian biopsy. This led to the development of the wedge resection as a treatment for this condition, which proved to be quite effective in the restoration of menstrual function.

The Development of the Radioimmunoassay (RIA)

In the 1950s, the RIA was developed by Solomon Aaron Berson and Rosalyn Sussman Yalow. The RIA allowed the detection and measurement of steroid and peptide hormones that are present in the serum and urine in very low concentrations. As a result of this monumental work, Yalow received the Nobel Prize in Medicine or Physiology in 1977. The introduction of RIA was pivotal and developed the foundation to modern day endocrinology. The information gained helped us to understand the steroid pathways in endocrine organs and also helped with the diagnosis and characterization of endocrine disorders. The RIA also provided an important tool in monitoring the patient undergoing ovulation induction.

The Introduction of Fertility Medications

Clomiphene citrate (CC) was an oral medication first synthesized in 1956 [1]. It was the first medical therapy developed to correct ovulatory dysfunction secondary to anovulation. To this day it continues to be a commonly prescribed medication for the infertile female.

In the 1960s, FSH and LH were extracted from the urine of menopausal women, which gave rise to the development of an injectable human menopausal gonadotropin. This medication was used for ovulatory dysfunction that was refractory to CC. It was a much stronger agent and required closer monitoring of serum estradiol levels, which could now be measured by RIA. In 1962, Dr. Bruno Lunenfeld reported the first pregnancy achieved with the use of human menopausal gonadotropins [2].

Reproductive Surgery

Kurt Semm developed an interest in laparoscopy in the 1960s. In the early 1970s, as chairman of the department of Obstetrics and Gynecology at the University of Kiel, he faced stiff resistance to clinical use of laparoscopy in human patients. Attempts to publish about the technique were rebuffed with laparoscopic surgery deemed an unethical technique. Semm persisted and is credited with numerous inventions including the uterine manipulator, electronic CO_2 insufflator, and a tubal patency testing device [3]. It wasn't until the introduction of the automatic insufflator and the development of a fiber optic light source that laparoscopic surgery became practical. Initially laparoscopy was only a diagnostic tool and the surgeon would have to resort to a laparotomy to correct altered pelvic anatomy.

During the 1980s there was an emphasis on reproductive surgery to correct tubal/peritoneal factors which were causing infertility. Surgery was almost entirely conducted through the open abdomen. In the ensuing years, laparoscopic instrumentation evolved and studies emerged suggesting equivalent or improved outcomes when surgery was performed laparoscopically. Laparoscopy had other advantages from the patient perspective; a lower likelihood of needing a hospital stay, as most cases were performed on an outpatient basis, and overall faster recovery time.

The *In Vitro* Fertilization Revolution

There are a handful of dates in world history, the mere mention of which call to mind a specific event with global implications. July 25, 1978, is such a date as it marks the day on which Louise Joy Brown, the world's first successful "test-tube" baby was born in Great Britain. This marvelous achievement earned Robert Edwards the 2010 Nobel Prize in Physiology or Medicine [4], whereas his partners, Patrick

Steptoe and Jean Purdy, had already passed away and were not eligible by Nobel Prize Award rules to be recognized for their parts in this achievement. The first IVF success was a culmination of decades of work. In 1944, along with Harvard scientist Miriam F. Menkin, John Rock fertilized the first human egg in a test tube. On Feb 6, 1944, they produced the first laboratory-fertilized, two-cell human egg.

Author Martin Hutchinson summarized the chronology of IVF technology when he wrote:

> Rabbits were one thing, but, as scientists were finding out, the secrets of the human reproductive system proved to be hard-won indeed. Professor Edwards said: "By 1965 I'd been trying to mature human eggs for the past five years." There was nobody racing against us—nobody had figured any of the ideas of this concept. It took further years of effort to produce a magical figure—37 hours—the length of time it took for a human egg to become ready for fertilization after a particular point in a woman's cycle [5].

The establishment of the first IVF pregnancy was truly amazing, and the initial birth was detailed in a letter to the editor in *Lancet* by Steptoe and Edwards. The initial cycles involved women who were followed during their natural cycle. The LH surge was identified with 3 hourly LH determinations and the laparoscopic egg retrieval was scheduled accordingly. Numerous attempts over more than a decade were initiated before a success was achieved, which led to the birth of Louise Brown. Since the inception of IVF, many modifications have been instituted in every step of the treatment which has resulted in increased success, including the first frozen pregnancies reported by the group of Alan Trounson [6]. Following this first success, IVF programs were established all throughout the world. Presently, approximately 2.5 million assisted reproductive treatment (ART) cycles are now performed globally each year, producing more than 500,000 babies each year. It is estimated that more than 10,000,000 children have been born through this technique.

Today, advances in IVF technology enable conception and childbirth in couples with conditions that were previously thought to be uncorrectable. Direct aspiration of sperm from the testes, uterine transplant for women born without a uterus, and transplantation of frozen ovarian tissue were beyond anyone's wildest imagination in 1978. Further advances in the field of molecular genetics and the ability to biopsy a blastocyst in the laboratory has created new opportunities for couples who are carriers of genetic conditions as well as those who wish to reduce the risk of miscarriage.

The Definition of Infertility

The American Society for Reproductive Medicine updated the definition of infertility in 2023, defining infertility as "disease, condition, or status characterized by any of the following":

- The inability to achieve a successful pregnancy based on a patient's medical, sexual, and reproductive history, age, physical findings, diagnostic testing, or any combination of those factors.
- The need for medical intervention, including, but not limited to, the use of donor gametes or donor embryos in order to achieve a successful pregnancy either as an individual or with a partner.
- In patients having regular, unprotected intercourse and without any known etiology for either partner suggestive of impaired reproductive ability, evaluation should be initiated at 12 months when the female partner is under 35 years of age and at 6 months when the female partner is 35 years of age or older.

The new ASRM definition concluded by stating that "Nothing in this definition shall be used to deny or delay treatment to any individual, regardless of relationship status or sexual orientation." This represents a major shift in thinking about a problem that left many individuals and couples without access to care or health insurance coverage of treatment.

Access to Care

Through advances in science and technology, the majority of people who are treated for infertility will be successful. But to enjoy the outcomes that are available, you need to have access to care. Inequities in access to and utilization of care are well documented. While insurance coverage does ameliorate some disparities, it does not entirely level the field. Further research is needed to explain why members of certain racial and ethnic groups are consistently under-represented in treatment despite having the same incidence of infertility. Understanding what the barriers are is the first step in developing measures to overcome them.

Evidenced-Based Treatment

In 2008 the United States Congress asked the National Academy of Medicine "to identify the best methods used in developing clinical practice guidelines in order to ensure that organizations developing such guidelines have information on approaches that are objective, scientifically valid, and consistent" [7]. The principles developed by the Academy revolve around TRUST, which stands for Transparency and Rigor Using Standards of Trustworthiness. Organizations that want to meet the rigorous standard for producing a nationally recognized guideline are required to have authorship groups that are multidisciplinary, include a methodologist, and ideally have a patient and a public member. Conflicts of interest must be disclosed and managed. They are required to conduct a systematic literature review, grade the quality of evidence, the strength of the evidence, and when drawing conclusions from the evidence, qualify the strength of recommendation. Before publication the manuscript must be sent for external review. Finally, guidelines must be updated no less frequently than every 5 years, or sooner, if there is a landmark study published that significantly influences practice.

Why, then, do organizations like the American Society for Reproductive Medicine produce committee opinions and guidance documents in addition to guidelines [8]? Not all topics are appropriate for a systematic review. In some cases, the literature is not yet available. Committee opinions use applicable literature without formal assessment of the Quality and Strength of Evidence. Recommendations represent the clinical consensus of subject matter experts on clinical care. Guidance documents, like committee opinions, represent consensus of subject matter experts on best practices.

Guidelines, committee opinions, and guidance documents are meant to be the starting point for busy clinicians. The transparency of methodology, objective interpretation of the available data, and, in the case of guidelines, qualification of the quality and strength of evidence afford the practitioner a comprehensive and balanced view of the literature. This is a stronger basis for formulating patient treatment plans compared to treatment that is based merely on one or two favorite papers. Guidance is also available from the European Society for Human Reproduction and Embryology, the British Fertility Society, and the Endocrine Society.

Medical Ethics in Reproductive Medicine

The Hippocratic Oath is perhaps the world's most widely known statement of medical ethical principles. The oath charges those in the healing arts with the responsibility to practice medicine in an ethical manner. Highlights of what the oath taker swears to uphold include

- I will use those dietary regimens which will benefit my patients according to my greatest ability and judgment, and I will do no harm or injustice to them.
- Into whatever homes I go, I will enter them for the benefit of the sick, avoiding any voluntary act of impropriety or corruption.

- Whatever I see or hear in the lives of my patients, whether in connection with my professional practice or not, which ought not to be spoken of outside, I will keep secret, as considering all such things to be private.

Between 1932 and 1972, the US Public Health Service conducted a study at Tuskegee without the consent of participants in which they followed the natural progression of syphilis without offering treatment even after it became available. When it came to light in 1972, it shocked the nation and led Congress to pass the National Research Act of 1974. The Act called for the formation of a committee to identify the ethical principles for conducting biomedical research. The product of the commission was the now famous Belmont Report on the Ethical Principles and Guidelines for the Protection of Human Subjects of Research [9]. Three overarching principles were defined: respect for persons, beneficence, and justice.

In the first edition of their book *Principles of Biomedical Ethics* published in 1979, Beauchamp and Childress identified four core principles for ethical reasoning in healthcare: respect for autonomy, nonmaleficence, beneficence, and justice.

To cover all of the nuanced aspects of how bioethics is applied in the practice of reproductive medicine in a single chapter is not feasible. Whole books, monthly journals, and quarterly reports of high caliber are available for that task.

How, then, can the average practitioner operate in the current environment with guidance on ethical practices if you're not fortunate enough to have a consulting ethicist for your group? The ASRM has available online, at no charge, a host of well-reasoned and accessible ethics opinions on a wide array of topics that directly address issues we see in practice [10].

Conclusion

The desire to have a child or children is as old as humankind itself. What has changed over millennia is the way we approach diagnosis and treatment. The combination of advances in science and technology, along with methods of aggregating, analyzing, and interpreting data, have led to incredible success for a large number of people who, without application of these advances, would fall short of their reproductive goals. However, access to care is not something enjoyed by all who need it.

Inequities exist in both the availability and utilization of services for a variety of reasons. Economic barriers are insurmountable for some who would otherwise be good candidates for success. Racial and ethnic differences in utilization of services are narrowed when health insurance is available in part or in full but still persist for reasons that remain to be elucidated. Ethical issues in the practice of reproductive medicine are often related to what is technically feasible to do. Practitioners commonly seek guidance on a case-by-case basis but can be heartened to know that there are ethical frameworks and rubrics available to help.

New analytics, therapeutics, and scientific advances are perpetually on the horizon. With knowledge of our past, understanding of how to incorporate these advances guided by use of data, ethical principles, and with a goal of expanding access to care for all who need and want it, the future of our field is indeed bright.

Key Points

1. Infertility is the subject of concern, study, and treatment through recorded human history.
2. Key advances in diagnosis and treatment advanced dramatically in the 20th century and continue to the present.
3. Guidelines, committee opinions, and guidance documents from professional societies, developed using reproducible, consistent methodologies, are excellent aids to practitioners.
4. Principles of ethics and frameworks are available to assist practitioners analyze clinical situations where ethical issues are raised in practice.

REFERENCES

1. Adashi EY. Clomiphene citrate at 50: The dawning of assisted reproduction. *Fertil Steril* 2017;108:592–3.
2. Rabau E et al. Human menopausal gonadotropins for anovulation and sterility. Results of 7 years of treatment. *Am J Obstet Gynecol* 1967;98:92–8.
3. Bhattacharya K. Kurt Semm: A laparoscopic crusader. *J Minim Access Surg* 2007;3:35–6.
4. The Nobel Prize in Physiology or Medicine 2010 [internet], 2010: www.nobelprize.org/uploads/2018/06/press-8.pdf.
5. Martin Hutchinson. Edwards: The IVF pioneer. *BBC News* [internet], 2003: http://news.bbc.co.uk/2/hi/health/3093429.stm.
6. Trounson A, Mohr L. Human pregnancy following cryopreservation, thawing and transfer of an eight-cell embryo. *Nature* 1983;305:707–9.
7. National Academies Sciences, Engineering, Medicine [internet], 2011: https://nap.nationalacademies.org/catalog/13058/clinical-practice-guidelines-we-can-trust.
8. American Society for Reproductive Medicine. Definition of infertility: A committee opinion. *Fertil Steril* 2023;120:1170.
9. The Belmont Report [internet], 1979: www.hhs.gov/ohrp/regulations-and-policy/belmont-report/index.html.
10. American Society for Reproductive Medicine. Ethics Committee Opinions [internet]: www.asrm.org/practice-guidance/ethics-opinions/.

2

Factors Affecting Fertility

Riwa Sabbagh and Denis Vaughan

Any medical visit with an individual of reproductive age is an opportunity to counsel them on their fertility and habits to optimize their reproductive outcomes. It is important to be familiar with the different factors that can affect an individual's fertility and incorporate that during counseling. Of these factors, some can be modifiable while others are non-modifiable factors.

Non-modifiable Factors

Age

Fertility declines with age, but the decline is more pronounced and occurs earlier in oocytes than it does in sperm.

Ovarian Age

The single-most important factor that influences an individual or couple's chance of conceiving with or without assistance is ovarian age. Advanced ovarian age has become more of an issue over the last 10–15 years with the increased prevalence of delayed childbearing. There are several contributing factors to this trend. Pursuing a higher level of education and career, the desire for smaller families, achieving financial stability prior to having children, the availability of assisted reproductive technology, as well as better awareness and access to contraception particularly for adolescents, all play a role in the decision to delay childbearing. In the light of these trends, patients should be appropriately counseled and made aware of the age-related decline in fertility.

Fertility generally begins to decline after the age of 24, and there is an acceleration of the decline after the age of 37. This decline stems from several factors including reduced oocyte quality and quantity, age-related uterine dysfunction with the former being the most causal one.

In fact, every person with ovaries has the highest number of oocytes (6–7 million) *in utero* at 20 weeks of gestation. The eggs are present in the primordial follicles and arrested in prophase of meiosis I. From this time forward, atresia sets in and the number of oocytes is reduced to 2 million at birth and 600,000–700,000 at puberty. At age 37 a person with ovaries has approximately 25,000 eggs—just over 1% of the eggs that they were born with. There is data that suggests that the process of atresia is accelerated after the age of 37 [1]. Up until the time of menopause, follicular development is a continuum. The only chance that any follicle will progress to ovulation is that it must be at a critical stage of maturation and rescued by rising FSH levels that only occur for a short period of time during the early follicular phase.

In addition to the reduced quantity of eggs that occur with aging, there is reduced quality of the eggs as well. With aging there is a greater chance that the egg released at ovulation has an abnormal chromosomal complement that results from errors in meiosis. The actual cause of the aneuploidy is poorly understood but could be the result of dysfunction with the mitotic spindles and/or a loss of adhesion between

DOI: 10.1201/9781003460275-2

sister chromosomes, which would interfere with their alignment during meiosis. These chromosomal imbalances can prevent normal fertilization and/or halt early embryonic development. Embryonic chromosomal aneuploidy explains between 70–80% of first trimester losses. Studies performed on embryos resulting from *in vitro* fertilization have confirmed an increased incidence of aneuploidy in embryos arising from older persons. In a previous study, utilizing trophectoderm biopsy and pre-implantation genetic testing for aneuploidy (PGT-A), the rate of aneuploidy in embryos from ages 30, 35, 40, and 45 was 23%, 34%, 58%, and 84%, respectively [2]. The increased chance of chromosomal errors with advanced ovarian age is further supported by the increased rate of spontaneous abortions and chromosomal anomalies in babies born to older individuals with ovaries. Additionally, some studies have shown the impact of uterine aging on pregnancy outcomes and pregnancy rates appeared lower in patients >40 years of age despite the use of donor oocytes [3]. Moreover, adverse pregnancy outcomes are also known to be more prevalent with advanced ovarian age.

Testicular Age

Similarly, persons with testes are also experiencing delayed family building. They experience decreased gonadal function with advancing age. Testosterone production begins to decrease around the age of 40. At age 75, a person with testes has about half of the circulating free testosterone as someone in his 20s. Semen parameters also change with increasing age; there is a decrease in the semen volume, sperm motility, normal morphology, and an increase in DNA fragmentation. In review of prior studies, it has been suggested that the aging individual with testes has reduced fertility that begins in the late 30s and early 40s. Despite these changes, the reduction in fertility is subtle and in some may be insignificant. A systematic review that evaluated the impact of testicular age on ART outcome concluded that it still remains unclear and that there was insufficient data to suggest that testicular age altered outcome of IVF treatment [4].

The rate of aneuploidy in oocytes increases with age and is the cause of most pregnancy losses. Aneuploidy or disomy in sperm may explain some pregnancy losses. The rate of aneuploidy in sperm is 2%, and there is no evidence to support an increased rate of aneuploidy involving autosomes with advanced testicular age. However, there is data to support that with advanced testicular age, there is an increased risk of disomy involving the sex chromosomes.

Owing to the effect of aging in both persons with ovaries and testes, a discussion should be had surrounding reproductive plans and referral to a reproductive endocrinology and infertility specialist should be made to have a more comprehensive discussion, particularly surrounding the option of fertility preservation of oocytes, sperm, and/or embryos.

Modifiable Factors

Timing and Frequency of Intercourse

The establishment of pregnancy is dependent on properly timed intercourse around the time of ovulation. The fertile window is defined as a 6-day interval ending on the day of ovulation [5]. In a study by Wilcox et al., the investigators followed 221 women who were attempting pregnancy [6]. All women kept track of the days they had intercourse and collected daily urine samples which were then analyzed to determine the day of ovulation. Conception only occurred when intercourse occurred in a 6-day window that ended with the day of ovulation. The investigators confirmed that the greatest chance of pregnancy was when intercourse occurred beginning 2 days prior to ovulation (Figure 2.1). No pregnancies were achieved if intercourse only took place after ovulation occurred.

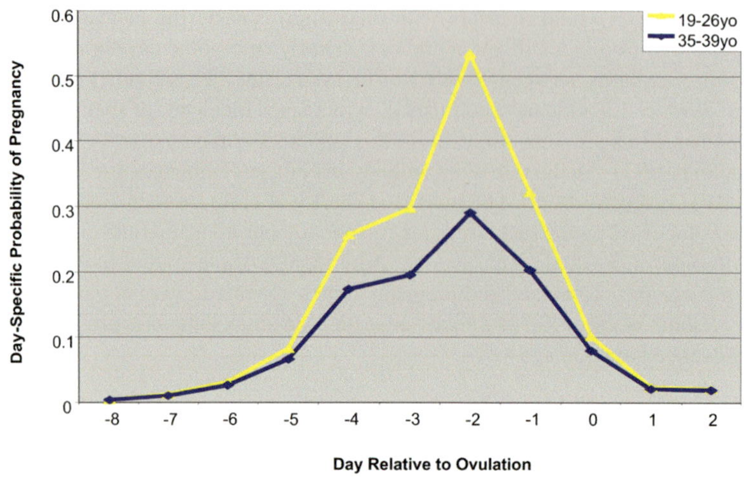

FIGURE 2.1 Probability of pregnancy resulting from recurrent intercourse by persons with ovaries' age and cycle day [from ref 5 with permission].

Diet and Lifestyle

Diet

There has been an expansion in the available literature on diet and fertility. Folic acid supplementation has been shown to have reproductive benefits beyond the prevention of neural tube defects. Vitamin D, on the other hand, has not shown to improve fertility in absence of deficiency.

Moreover, there is no data to suggest that any particular diet per se can impact fertility. However, fertility rates are decreased in persons with ovaries in the extremes of body weight primarily due to ovulatory dysfunction. Persons who are underweight are at risk for hypothalamic dysfunction affecting ovulation and those who are overweight or obese may have ovulatory dysfunction with or without the presence of concurrent polycystic ovarian syndrome. In addition, obesity is known to decrease implantation rates and increase miscarriage rates in euploid embryo transfers, suggesting that obesity creates a negative intrauterine environment also. The Nurses' Health Study II evaluated the impact of a "fertility diet" which favors monounsaturated rather than trans fats, vegetables rather than animal protein sources, low-glycemic carbohydrates, high-fat dairy, multivitamins, and iron from plants on fertility. They found a lower risk of infertility in persons with ovaries who have ovulatory dysfunction; however, there is no difference in live birth rates in persons undergoing ART. Some studies have also found that adopting a Mediterranean diet (high intakes of vegetables, fruits, low-fat dairy, olive oil, fish, and poultry) or Dutch diet (high intakes of whole grains, monounsaturated or polyunsaturated oils, vegetables, fruits, meat or meat replacements, and fish) was associated with higher live birth rates following IVF; however, data is conflicting. Similarly, studies evaluating the effect of a low-processed diet with higher intake of fruits, vegetables, whole grains, and fish did not find an association with improved IVF outcomes [5].

The diet of persons with testes has also been evaluated: Healthy diets such as the Mediterranean diet has been associated with improved semen parameters; however, how this translates to fertility is unknown.

It is important to note that though the data has been inconclusive and mixed on the effects of diet on natural fertility and ART outcomes, adhering to a healthy diet and maintaining a target BMI between 20 and 25 is beneficial for overall health.

In addition, there is promising emerging data on the potential beneficial effect of glucagon-like peptide-1 (GLP-1) agonists, aiding in weight loss and improving fertility outcomes, although more research needs to be done on this drug group before formal recommendations can be made.

Smoking

Smoking is a confirmed reproductive toxin. The deleterious effects of smoking during pregnancy are well established. Several published studies have demonstrated that smoking in persons with ovaries is associated with decreased fertility. Smoking reduces the chances of unassisted conception by almost 50%. Smoking can alter ovarian function in a number of ways. The chemicals in smoke stimulate the hepatic metabolism of steroid hormones, thereby reducing their levels in the blood stream. *In vitro* studies have demonstrated that the chemicals in tobacco alter the enzymes that are necessary for ovarian hormone production. Finally, persons who smoke generally go through menopause 1–4 years earlier than their non-smoking counterparts, suggesting that the chemicals in tobacco may be directly toxic to the ovaries. It is not known whether this is due to a direct action on the ovaries or indirect through an alteration of the blood flow to the ovary. In addition, there is strong data to suggest smoking of tobacco negatively impacts sperm quality. The published data is compelling enough to advise anyone who smokes to stop to improve their fertility and overall health [5].

Caffeine

The impact of caffeine on fertility and pregnancy outcome has been subject to debate.

Daily intake of caffeine at high doses (>500 mg; >5 cups of coffee/day) has been associated with reduced fertility. During pregnancy, moderate caffeine intake (<200–300 mg/day or 1–2 cups of coffee) does not have any apparent adverse pregnancy outcomes or impacts on fertility. However, a consumption of greater than 200–300 mg/day may be associated with a higher risk of miscarriage. Caffeine consumption has not been shown to have any effects on semen parameters [5].

Alcohol

The negative effects of alcohol on pregnancy are well documented. However, the influence of alcohol on fertility has not been well established. In 1998, two separate studies were published that examined the impact of alcohol on the establishment of pregnancy [7, 8]. Both studies arrived at the same conclusion, that alcohol, in a dose-dependent fashion, reduced the chance of a conception in the study populations. There is no evidence linking mild or moderate alcohol consumption with infertility; however, chronic overconsumption (>2 drinks per day) may lead to a decrease in ovarian reserve and fecundability.

Nonetheless, persons undergoing fertility treatment should avoid alcohol once the treatment cycle has begun.

Chronic alcohol consumption has been associated with lower semen parameters and testosterone levels. However, there is a lack of evidence suggesting any effect of moderate alcohol consumption on the fertility of persons with testes.

Recreational Drugs

The use of recreational drugs in a couple attempting pregnancy should be discouraged given obstetrical and perinatal complications.

Studies have been done to evaluate the effect of cannabis on fertility given the increase in its use in the general population. National cross-sectional survey data has not shown a change in the time to pregnancy for couples using marijuana [9]. However, smoking marijuana has been shown to lead to a decrease in total sperm count. Until more data emerges, its use should generally be discouraged in individuals/couples actively trying to conceive.

Environmental Exposures

There has been an increased interest in evaluating the effect of different environmental toxins on fertility. Of particular interest are the endocrine disrupting chemicals (EDCs) that derive from various sources including soy products, industrial chemicals, and household products (such as bisphenol A, phthalate).

Higher serum BPA concentrations were seen in patients with PCOS. However, a systemic review of 12 articles on the impact of EDC exposure and time to pregnancy did not find a significant association [10].

Air pollution's impact on fertility has also been an area of interest. High exposure to air pollution has been linked to lower fertility rates in the United States as well as impaired semen parameters including lower motility, lower normal morphology, and higher DNA fragmentation.

Occupational Hazards

The Occupational Safety and Health Administration (OSHA) is a regulatory agency in the United States that is responsible for ensuring the safety of employees in the workplace. Their primary focus is on potential chemical exposures, and they have identified a number of agents that can impact reproductive health. Of the countless chemical exposures present in the workplace, about 1,000 chemicals have been evaluated for their reproductive toxicities. It is well established that exposure to nitrous oxide (N_20) is associated with reduced fertility and spontaneous abortion [11], and dental hygienists may be at particular risk. Exposure to other work-related chemicals (i.e. cadmium, mercury and dry-cleaning chemicals) has also been reported to decrease fertility in persons with ovaries.

Sperm parameters are more susceptible to environmental toxins since spermatogenesis is an ongoing and dynamic process. The first report of an occupationally related spermatotoxin appeared in the mid-1970s [12] and showed that those who worked at factories which produced DBCP (a pesticide) had an increased incidence of infertility—the severity being dependent on the dose and length of exposure. Since this report was released, other spermatotoxins have been identified and are listed in Table 2.1.

A list of potential environmental toxins and their association with infertility are shown in Tables 2.1 and 2.2 [13].

OSHA requires that all employers must have Material Safety Data Sheets (MSDS) available at all potential workplace exposures and to detail all known risks of the exposure on general health and reproductive health.

Stress

The effect of stress on fertility has been subject to debate. Stress can arise from infertility, but the impact of stress on fertility remains unclear. Some studies did not find an association between the two [14],

TABLE 2.1

Environmental Toxins and Their Association with Aspects of Infertility in Persons with Testes [from ref 13 with permission]

Bisphenol A	
	Reduced sperm concentration, motility, and normal morphology
Phthalates	
	Reduced fertility and semen quality parameters, but results are equivocal
Air pollutants	
	Reduced sperm motility
Dioxins	
	Reduced normal sperm morphology
Pesticides	
	Reduced sperm concentration, motility, and normal morphology
Fracking chemicals	
	Reduced sperm concentration and motility
Triclosan	
	No definitive associations; further research is necessary
Parabens	
	Poorer fertility treatment outcomes in couples

TABLE 2.2

Environmental Toxins and Their Association with Aspects of Infertility in Persons with Ovaries [from ref 13 with permission]

Bisphenol A	
	Disrupted cyclicity, fewer antral follicles
	Miscarriage, shortened gestation, preterm birth
	Poor fertility treatment outcomes
	PCOS, endometriosis, uterine fibroids
Phthalates	
	Fewer antral follicles
	Shortened gestation, preterm birth
	PCOS
Air pollutants	
	Preterm birth
Dioxins	
	Reduced fetal growth
Pesticides	
	Disrupted cyclicity
	Miscarriage, preterm birth
	PCOS, endometriosis, uterine fibroids
Fracking chemicals	
	Reduced fecundity
	Miscarriage, preterm birth
Triclosan	
	No definitive associations; further research is necessary
Parabens	
	No definitive associations; further research is necessary

but others did show that stress can impact IVF outcomes. There are different interventions that can be offered to patients undergoing fertility treatment such as psychological counseling, cognitive behavioral therapy, or acupuncture [15]. Even if the impact of interventions on live birth outcomes is unclear, it may be helpful from a stress management perspective, which is one of the leading causes of patient dropout in treatment.

Conclusions

There are many factors that ultimately impact an individual's or couple's chances of conceiving unassisted or with assisted reproductive technology. While some factors are modifiable and efforts can be made to minimize their exposure, others are not. The single most important factor that impacts a couple's chance of conceiving is ovarian age; however, several other factors come into play, and it is important to counsel patients on each of these factors to help improve their chances of building their family.

Key Points

- There are modifiable and non-modifiable factors that can affect fertility.
- Ovarian aging is the single-most important factor that can affect the chance of conception.
- It is important to counsel patients on both the modifiable and non-modifiable factors to help improve their chances of family building.

REFERENCES

1. Faddy, M.J., et al., Accelerated disappearance of ovarian follicles in mid-life: implications for forecasting menopause. *Hum Reprod*, 1992. 7(10): 1342–6.
2. Franasiak, J.M., et al., The nature of aneuploidy with increasing age of the female partner: a review of 15,169 consecutive trophectoderm biopsies evaluated with comprehensive chromosomal screening. *Fertil Steril*, 2014. 101(3): 656–63.
3. Cano, F., et al., Effect of aging on the female reproductive system: evidence for a role of uterine senescence in the decline in female fecundity. *Fertil Steril*, 1995. 64(3): 584–9.
4. Jimbo, M., et al., Fertility in the aging male: a systematic review. *Fertil Steril*, 2022. 118(6): 1022–34.
5. Practice Committee of American Society for Reproductive Medicine in collaboration with Society for Reproductive, Endocrinol, and Infertility. Optimizing natural fertility: a committee opinion. *Fertil Steril*, 2013. 100(3): 631–7.
6. Wilcox, A.J., et al., Timing of sexual intercourse in relation to ovulation. Effects on the probability of conception, survival of the pregnancy, and sex of the baby. *N Engl J Med*, 1995. 333(23): 1517–21.
7. Jensen, T.K., et al., Does moderate alcohol consumption affect fertility? Follow up study among couples planning first pregnancy. *BMJ*, 1998. 317(7157): 505–10.
8. Hakim, R.B., et al., Alcohol and caffeine consumption and decreased fertility. *Fertil Steril*, 1998. 70(4): 632–7.
9. Kasman, A.M., et al., Association between use of marijuana and time to pregnancy in men and women: findings from the National Survey of Family Growth. *Fertil Steril*, 2018. 109(5): 866–71.
10. Hipwell, A.E., et al., Exposure to non-persistent chemicals in consumer products and fecundability: a systematic review. *Hum Reprod Update*, 2019. 25(1): 51–71.
11. Cohen, E.N., et al., Occupational disease in dentistry and chronic exposure to trace anesthetic gases. *J Am Dent Assoc*, 1980. 101(1): 21–31.
12. Cohen, E.N., et al., Anesthesia, pregnancy, and miscarriage: a study of operating room nurses and anesthetists. *Anesthesiology*, 1971. 35(4): 343–7.
13. Chiang, C., et al., Environmental contaminants affecting fertility and somatic health. *Semin Reprod Med*, 2017. 35(3): 241–9.
14. Slade, P., et al., A prospective, longitudinal study of emotions and relationships in in-vitro fertilization treatment. *Hum Reprod*, 1997. 12(1): 183–90.
15. Domar, A.D., et al., The impact of group psychological interventions on distress in infertile women. *Health Psychol*, 2000. 19(6): 568–75.

3

Lifestyle in Infertility

Brooke V. Rossi

Introduction

Key factors influencing fertility and the success of infertility treatment, such as age, ovarian reserve, and to some degree, weight, are non-modifiable. However, patients are interested in factors that they *can* control. In fact, many patients believe diet, including vitamins, alcohol, exercise, and caffeine use affects *in vitro* fertilization (IVF) success.

Exercise

Many people use exercise and physical activity to regulate their weight, reduce stress, and for quality of life. As patients face infertility, some wonder if they should do more or less exercise. In general, exercise is beneficial for fertility.

Population studies demonstrate that frequency, duration, and intensity of exercise can be associated with subfertility and childlessness. For example, five hours of exercise per week had a negative impact on fecundability, but only for women with body mass index (BMI) <25 (1). There are positive associations for overweight and obese women. In fact, moderate physical activity demonstrates a modest increase in fecundability in all women.

The benefit of physical activity is likely positive up to a certain threshold, and only for some women, beyond which would be detrimental. High amounts of activity may affect the hypothalamic-pituitary-ovarian axis and inhibit ovulation, leading to infertility. However, it is important to note that with rates of obesity steadily increasing in the population, most patients would benefit, not be harmed, by increasing exercise.

Sperm quality is not greatly affected by exercise. In studies of men presenting for IVF, the amount of exercise is not associated with any differences in semen volume or sperm concentration, motility, or morphology. Only in men who bicycle more than 5 hours per week is a decrease in concentration appreciated.

In vitro fertilization appears to be positively impacted by moderate exercise during the cycle, especially among obese women. However, women with histories of strenuous activity may have a lower chance of live birth.

Sleep

Sleep disturbances, such as short duration and poor quality, are increasing, with at least one-third of adults not achieving the recommended duration of sleep. Kloss et al. propose 3 ways that poor sleep may alter fertility: Hypothalamic-pituitary-adrenal (HPA) activation that is related to sleep disturbance may affect the reproductive axis; abnormal sleep duration or disturbance may interfere with reproduction or

DOI: 10.1201/9781003460275-3

further increase the HPA activation; or circadian dysrhythmia itself may result in infertility (2). Circadian rhythms may be affected by reproductive hormones, and the reverse may be true as well, as sleep may impact reproductive physiology through impact on circadian genes. Cycle regulation may be affected by the differences in circadian rhythms related to shift or night work. Some speculate that these cycle differences may be related to reduced fecundability seen among women with poor sleep. Menstrual cycle irregularity and higher rates of infertility can also be seen when women shift work and sleep schedules. Furthermore, some IVF outcomes, such as total oocytes retrieved, are less among women working nights or shift work.

Regarding polycystic ovary syndrome (PCOS) patients, there are greater rates of snoring, short sleep duration, obstructive sleep apnea, and daytime sleepiness. In patients with unexplained infertility and PCOS, snoring is associated with insulin resistance and elevated BMI. Despite significant differences in sleep characteristics, there are no differences in conception and live birth rates during ovarian stimulation treatment in women with PCOS or unexplained infertility.

Some patients may choose to use melatonin for sleep disturbance. Melatonin does not have any negative impact on fertility or infertility treatment. In fact, there is a body of literature evaluating the benefit of melatonin on infertility treatment due to its anti-oxidative properties. In general, melatonin does not seem to have a significant impact on clinical pregnancy rate or other treatment outcomes (3). More extensive research on the impact of melatonin on IVF has been conducted, specifically on egg quality. Some studies suggest an increase in mature eggs, but no increase in pregnancy rate. If patients need melatonin to facilitate sleep during infertility treatment, they can rest assured that the supplement will not negatively impact treatment. However, melatonin use, for the sole purpose of treatment or IVF improvement, is still unclear.

Alcohol

Most patients are aware that alcohol consumption is not acceptable during pregnancy. However, the amount and type of alcohol that is detrimental to fertility is less understood. Subject reporting bias is a significant limitation with alcohol studies. Also, heavy alcohol use is difficult to assess, as most subjects report either abstinence or moderate (7 drinks per week) use.

A prospective cohort of Danish women did not find a negative impact on fecundability with up to 14 drinks of alcohol per week, and there was no difference in types of alcohol. It is notable that the median amount of use in the study was 2 drinks per week (4).

When patients undergo infertility treatment, it appears that the chance of success is unrelated to mild to moderate alcohol use. Specifically, intrauterine insemination, IVF, and frozen embryo transfer (FET) live birth rates are similar among women drinking up to 7 drinks per week compared to non-users. Regarding IVF specifically, studies have been variable. Virrup et al. found a 22% rate of live birth among IVF cycles in abstinent women and a 20% rate of live birth in cycles in which women drank >14 drinks per week (5). In general, both male and female use was not associated with a lower odd of live birth. In contrast, other large prospective studies find lower likelihood of live birth when women or both partners drink several drinks per week at the start of the IVF cycle.

Tobacco

Tobacco use is one of the first and most studied lifestyle factors. In general, tobacco has a negative impact on male and female infertility. Several epidemiologic studies demonstrate reduced fecundability among women and men smokers. More recent large population studies show that time to pregnancy is longer for women who are active or passive smokers and for men who are heavy smokers. There also appears to be a dose-dependent impact.

Mechanisms for the negative impact on fertility may involve dysfunctional tubal or cervical function based on the infertility diagnoses of women smokers. A higher rate of ectopic pregnancy among women smokers also supports the theory of adverse tubal changes. Furthermore, active tobacco use may lead to ovarian follicular depletion, as anti-Müllerian hormone (AMH) levels are significantly lower among women smokers over 37 years old.

The association with smoking and men's fertility has been more difficult to establish. Several studies have demonstrated a negative impact on sperm parameters among male smokers. However, a larger prospective study did not demonstrate a significant reduction in fecundability among male past, current, or passive smokers (6). Among infertile men, smokers were found to have a lower sperm concentration compared to non-smokers. However, as in many studies, the sperm results are still in a normal range.

The impact of tobacco use is more evident among patients undergoing IVF. Studies have shown that several factors may contribute to the detriment of tobacco use, including altered folliculogenesis and implantation, a lower number of eggs retrieved, and abnormal steroidogenesis. Women smokers appear to have lower odds of pregnancy and live birth, while having greater odds of miscarriage and ectopic. Cotinine, a metabolite of nicotine and biomarker for cigarette use, is found in the serum and follicular fluid among women smokers completing IVF. In fact, cotinine levels are highly correlated with the number of cigarettes used, and there is an inverse association between cotinine levels and the number of eggs retrieved.

The impact of smoking on IVF success may also be related to the uterus and implantation. Among women utilizing egg donor IVF cycles, even after controlling for partner and donor smoking status, recipients of the donor eggs who smoke more than 10 cigarettes/day have a significantly lower pregnancy rate. The way in which smoking affects sperm and IVF outcomes has been questioned. Studies of smokers using conventional insemination during IVF or intracytoplasmic sperm injection (ICSI) show lower pregnancy rates among male smokers whether conventional insemination or ICSI were used. This may suggest that the deleterious impact of smoking and increased DNA fragmentation is not only related to fertilization but also to embryo growth, implantation, and early fetal growth.

Electronic Nicotine Delivery System

Electronic Nicotine Delivery Systems (ENDS) or vaping are growing in prevalence. In addition to nicotine, ENDS contain flavoring, metal nanoparticles such as lead, nickel, chromium, aluminum, iron, copper, silver, zinc, tin, manganese, ceramic, and silica (for the heating process), and vapor containing formaldehyde and volatile organic compounds. Some well-intentioned patients may use ENDS as a "healthy alternative" to combustible cigarettes but need to be educated about the potential reproductive risks.

There are limited data regarding how ENDS affects human reproduction, as most studies have been completed on animals. Male rats exposed to the components of ENDS are found to have abnormalities in their testosterone levels, enzymes involved in spermatogenesis, and sperm cells. In female mice, it takes longer to achieve their first litter and a concern for implantation disruption. In humans, a web-based prospective preconception study cohort of nearly 5000 reproductive-aged women evaluated fecundability and ENDS use (7). Seventeen percent of women had ever used e-cigarettes, and 4% were current users. Users of ENDS had a slightly longer time to pregnancy compared to non-users.

There is no data regarding IVF outcomes and ENDS. However, considering many of the detrimental components in combustible cigarettes are also in ENDS, patients should be counseled that the impact is likely negative.

Marijuana

In 2021, approximately 20% of people over 26 stated that they had used marijuana in the last year. However, many of the studies evaluating the impact of marijuana on reproductive outcomes show much lower rates of marijuana use (approximately 5% among women and 10% of men). The conclusions of many prospective or cohort studies are limited by the relatively low rates of exposure. In addition, the mechanism of impact is not clear. Thus, despite an expected increase due to legalization in several states, there is limited data regarding the impact of marijuana on fertility.

The impact of marijuana has been evaluated, mostly with inconsistent results. Cohort studies of patients using variable amounts of male or female marijuana use did not demonstrate any impact on fecundability. One of the largest studies of men's use and semen outcomes was conducted on over 1200 healthy men (8). Sperm concentration, total sperm count, percentage of motile sperm, and percentage of morphologically normal forms were all lower among men smoking marijuana more than once per week.

However, different effects are seen when couples attempting pregnancy or with infertility are studied. Of women actively trying to conceive with a history of pregnancy loss, preconception cannabis use leads to decreased fecundability, despite a higher frequency of intercourse. They also have elevated luteinizing hormone levels throughout the cycle, but no other hormonal differences. Of note, there is no increase in rate of pregnancy loss. Regarding men's use, longitudinal studies on men presenting for infertility treatment find that past or current marijuana users do not have any negative impact on sperm concentration, DNA fragmentation, or reproductive hormone levels (aside from an isolated report associated with follicle stimulating hormone among past users). Often, overall sperm parameters and testosterone levels are normal.

In regard to IVF, prospective and retrospective studies of patients smoking marijuana at the start of the IVF cycle demonstrate a higher probability of pregnancy loss, while those with partners that smoked marijuana have a greater chance of live birth. In these studies, the authors were concerned that self-reporting and a low number of exposure cases may not make the results generalizable. A retrospective cohort study of over 700 patients was also completed in one center and demonstrated similar results (9). The rate of marijuana use was about 9% and mostly considered light. Most notable, there was a similar implantation rate and on-going pregnancy rate between users and non-users. Similarly, there were no differences with oocyte, sperm, or embryo parameters.

In sum, there are not clear data to suggest definitive harm of marijuana use on fertility or IVF outcomes. However, larger, prospective studies are needed. Due to limited information, the most recent guidelines from reproductive health organizations recommend discontinuing marijuana in people who are pregnant or contemplating pregnancy.

Environment and Occupational Exposure

The relationship between air pollution and IVF failure was evaluated by specifically looking at nitrogen dioxide (NO_2), ozone (O_3), particulate matter, and black carbon (10). The subjects had overall low exposure to air pollution prior to and during the IVF cycle. Women with greater exposure had higher odds of cycle cancellation or early IVF failure. They speculated that the main cause of the negative effects was traffic-related combustion products (diesel). Adverse effects of traffic-related pollutants on follicular and embryo development have also been documented.

There are emerging data on sperm quality and occupational risk. Among men presenting for care to an infertility clinic, those with impaired sperm quality were more frequently exposed to solvents, fumes, or polycyclic aromatic hydrocarbons.

Key Points

- Providers and patients should recognize lifestyle factors that may optimize natural fertility or promote infertility treatment success.
- Diurnal, regular sleep, and moderate exercise supports fertility.
- No more than moderate alcohol or marijuana, and cessation of tobacco and ENDS are beneficial.
- Patients should limit exposure to occupational and environmental pollutants.

REFERENCES

1. Wise L et al. A prospective cohort study of physical activity and time to pregnancy. *Fertil Steril.* 2012;97(5):1136–4.
2. Kloss JD et al. Sleep, sleep disturbance, and fertility in women. *Sleep Med Rev.* 2015;22:78–87.
3. Showell MG et al. Antioxidants for female subfertility. *Cochrane Database Syst Rev.* 2020;8(8):CD007807.
4. Mikkelsen EM et al. Alcohol consumption and fecundability: prospective Danish cohort study. *BMJ (Online).* 2016;354:i4262.
5. Vittrup I et al. Male and female alcohol consumption and live birth after assisted reproductive technology treatment: a nationwide register-based cohort study. *Reprod Biomed.* 2017;35(2):152–60.
6. Wesselink AK et al. Prospective study of cigarette smoking and fecundability. *Human Reprod (Oxford).* 2019;34(3):558–67.
7. Harlow AF et al. Electronic cigarettes and fecundability: results from a prospective preconception cohort study. *Am J Epidemiol.* 2021;190(3):353–61.
8. Gundersen TD et al. Association between use of marijuana and male reproductive hormones and semen quality: a study among 1,215 healthy young men. *Am J Epidemiol.* 2015;182(6):473–81.
9. Har-Gil E et al. The relationship between cannabis use and IVF outcome—a cohort study. *J Cannabis Res.* 2021;3(1):42–5.
10. Gaskins AJet al. Time-varying exposure to air pollution and outcomes of in vitro fertilization among couples from a fertility clinic. *Environmental Health Perspectives.* 2019;127(7):77002.

4

Preconceptional Counseling

Jill Attaman and Emelia Bachman

The goal of prepregnancy counseling includes the opportunity to optimize health, educate on modifiable risk factors, and plan for the healthiest future family. This will contribute to well-being throughout the reproductive lifespan.

Preconception Visit

Prepregnancy care allows for providers to assist in optimization of general health and reproductive health, enhancing pregnancy, and neonatal outcomes. There is an opportunity to make plans for family building, not only for any upcoming pregnancy but for longitudinal family building. One may also consider discussion regarding fertility preservation options. If a pregnancy planner is considering using donor gametes, a gestational carrier, or undergoing reciprocal *in vitro* fertilization, this provides time to educate and discuss options. If a reproductive partner is present, partner counseling for enhancing general and reproductive health may also occur.

Individuals planning pregnancy should be up to date with annual wellness examinations, recommended vaccines, assessment of immunity, infectious disease screening, and additional preconception testing. Review of medical, surgical, family, and genetic history is a key component of the preconception visit. Medications and substance use should be reviewed in addition to assessment of general well-being.

The American College of Obstetricians and Gynecologists (ACOG) Committee on Gynecologic Practice and the American Society of Reproductive Medicine (ASRM) published a joint opinion outlining key components [1].

Annual Wellness Evaluation

An annual comprehensive wellness visit, including a history and physical examination and review of recommended preventive services with an obstetrician-gynecologist or primary care provider, is recommended. Cervical cancer and breast screening guidelines should be followed and results reviewed in efforts to maximize opportunity for health interventions, if needed, prior to pregnancy. Sources for recommended preventative services are available in the ACOG Committee Opinion 755 [2]. For patients planning pregnancy at advanced reproductive age of 45 years or older, comprehensive metabolic and electrolyte testing, and cardiac screening should be considered based on medical history.

Immunizations

Those of reproductive age are recommended to have immunization status assessed for tetanus-diphtheria-acellular pertussis (Tdap), measles-mumps-rubella (MMR), hepatitis B surface antigen (HBsAg), and varicella and human papillomavirus (HPV). Live vaccinations, including MMR and

DOI: 10.1201/9781003460275-4

varicella, should be avoided during pregnancy and thus immunity assessment prior to pregnancy allows for safe administration. Pregnancy should be delayed for one month after receiving a live vaccine. Adults who do not have presumptive evidence of rubella immunity should receive at least one dose of the MMR vaccine. Prenatal assessment for evidence of varicella immunity is recommended by the CDC and Advisory Committee on Immunization Practices (ACIP) as nonpregnant people of childbearing age receive special consideration for vaccine if serologic evidence of varicella is not documented [3]. If the HPV vaccination series is incomplete, vaccination should not be delayed and can be administered preconceptionally. If pregnancy occurs during the series, completion of vaccination should be delayed until postpartum and not given while pregnant. Review of rubeola immunity can also be considered, especially if in the midst of an active community outbreak. Additionally, those age 50 years and older may receive vaccination against herpes zoster prior to pregnancy.

Hepatitis B surface antigen (HBsAg) should be evaluated for all people planning pregnancy or during pregnancy. If immunity is not documented, the vaccination series can be initiated. In addition, a triple panel screen (HBsAg, anti-HBs, and total anti-HBC) is recommended to be performed once for individuals $\geq$18 years of age. The results of testing will determine if vaccination is necessary. This testing and vaccine can be administered prepregnancy or incorporated into routine antepartum care [4].

Influenza vaccinations are recommended annually. Vaccination against SARS-CoV-2 virus in pregnancy planners, pregnancy, and during lactation has been endorsed by multiple governing organizations [5]. For current information, refer to the Centers for Disease Control (CDC) [3].

An up-to-date immunization schedule can be found on the CDC website [3].

Infectious Disease Screening

Sexually transmitted disease screening is recommended at the time of counseling. Gonorrhea, chlamydia, human immunodeficiency virus (HIV), hepatitis C, hepatitis B, and syphilis screening should be performed. Patients screening positive for a curable infectious disease, including hepatitis C virus, ideally should complete treatment before pregnancy [4]. Individuals with HIV infection should receive prepregnancy counseling with discussion of risk reduction for perinatal transmission, long-term health optimization, and neonatal health. Antiretrovirals are currently offered after consultation with a subspecialist working toward the goal of reducing HIV viral load to undetectable levels prior to pregnancy. If gonorrhea or chlamydia infection is detected and the person is presenting with a reproductive partner, personal treatment is prescribed and expedited partner treatment can be considered [1]. If a recipient is using donor gametes for pregnancy, cytomegalovirus (CMV) immunoglobulin M (IgM), CMV immunoglobulin G (IgG) antibody is recommended, and human T-cell lymphotropic virus (HTLV) types I and II may also be evaluated. Please refer to the chapter on third-party reproduction for detailed recommendations.

Preconception Laboratory Testing

(See **Table 4.1**)

In addition to immunity and infectious disease screening, a blood type and screen and complete blood count (CBC) is recommended. Thyroid-stimulating hormone (TSH) screening should be considered in pregnancy planners with risk factors [1]. Thyroid disease is covered in further detail in a later chapter of this handbook.

Vitamin Supplementation, Folic Acid, and Nutrition

A daily multivitamin or prenatal vitamin is recommended. All individuals of reproductive age who plan to or could become pregnant should use daily folic acid supplementation to reduce risk for neural tube

TABLE 4.1

Prepregnancy Laboratory Testing

Blood type and screen
CBC
HIV
HBsAg (consider triple panel: HBsAg, anti-HBs, and total anti-HBC)
Hepatitis C antibody
Syphilis
TSH*
Gonorrhea
Chlamydia
Genetic screening
Rubella titer
Varicella titer
Routine health maintenance screening
CMV IgM and IgG**
HTLV I and II**

*Selective screening recommended.
**May be considered in third-party reproduction.

defects (NTDs). Ideally, supplementation use begins prior to pregnancy as the neural tube develops very early in pregnancy, beginning prior to a first missed menses. This is in addition to dietary intake from foods such as dark-green vegetables, beans, peas, lentils, and fortified grains. Most prenatal vitamins in the United States contain folic acid.

Clinical practice guidelines further stratify recommended folic acid dosing based on risk factors. For those at average risk for NTDs (Table 4.2), 400 micrograms (mcg) per day beginning at least one month prior to conception and continued until 12 weeks of gestation age is advised. Individuals at increased risk for pregnancies with NTDs may require 1–4 mg of folic acid daily. This dosing is inclusive of the folic acid already in a multivitamin. Higher doses of folic acid should not be achieved by using additional multivitamins as this results in unsafe levels of other vitamins such as vitamin A, which can be teratogenic. Folic acid supplementation will not prevent all NTDs, such as those at increased risk from chromosomal abnormalities [6].

The U.S. Departments of Health and Human Services (HHS) and the U.S. Department of Agriculture (USDA) provide dietary guidelines for individuals planning pregnancy and pregnant. This can be used as a valuable resource with the goal of meeting nutritional needs [7].

TABLE 4.2

Risk Factors for NTS (See Further Ref. 6)

Risk Factor for NTDs	Risk Stratification	Daily Dose of Folic Acid	Timing of Initiation Prior to Pregnancy
Reproductive age	Average	0.4 mg	At least one month
Personal history of NTD, prior pregnancy with NTD, first degree relative with NTD*	Increased	4.0 mg	3 months
Anti-seizure medication use±	Moderate – Increased	1.0 mg – 4.0 mg	3 months

*The same dosing is recommended if these risks are present in a reproductive partner.
±4.0 mg of folic acid is recommended with high risk antiseizure medications such as carbamazepine or valproate. The following may be considered moderate risk: second- or third-degree relative with NTD, history of certain conditions, such as bariatric surgery, inflammatory bowel disease, celiac disease, sickle cell with chronic hemolytic anemia.

Reproductive History

The reproductive history of a patient should be reviewed in detail. Anyone with a history of prior pregnancy complications should be counseled on risk of recurrence in pregnancy. Often, measures can be taken to reduce future risk and these should be discussed.

For individuals with a history of recurrent pregnancy loss, defined as two or more miscarriages, a recurrent pregnancy loss workup should be performed. See the associated chapter on recurrent pregnancy loss.

People planning pregnancy with a history of prior stillbirth or an infant born with chromosomal abnormalities, severe preeclampsia, preterm birth, gestational diabetes, or a person with obesity should be referred to maternal fetal medicine for a preconception consult.

This is also an optimal time to discuss ideal interpregnancy interval, or the time interval between delivery and conception of the following pregnancy. The recommended interpregnancy interval is at least 18 months. One should be counseled about the risks and benefits of conceiving if proceeding with shorter intervals. For individuals of advanced reproductive age or infertility, a pregnancy interval less than 18 months but greater than 6 months can be considered. An interpregnancy interval of less than 6 months is not recommended. Risks to shorter pregnancy spacing intervals include, but are not limited to, preterm birth, low birth weight, small for gestational age, and perinatal death [1].

Medical History, Surgical History, and Medication Review

A thorough medical and surgical history is recommended at the preconception visit. All medical conditions should be optimized to reduce health risks during pregnancy and enhance fetal outcome. Additionally, some medical conditions may worsen in pregnancy and affect health. Pregnancy planners should have a recent evaluation with a primary care provider or specialist. A preconception consult with maternal fetal medicine may also be advised for counseling on essential preconception evaluation, risks in pregnancy, and how a pregnancy will be monitored. Conditions such as hypertension, diabetes mellitus, heart disease, renal disease, asthma, thyroid disease, obesity, psychiatric illness, and autoimmune diseases should be addressed as they may affect pregnancy outcome.

If pregnancy is deemed unsafe and pregnancy is contraindicated, then alternate family building options such as use of a gestational carrier, adoption, foster-parenthood, or not pursuing pregnancy should be recommended. See the chapter on third-party reproduction for further information.

This is an appropriate time to review the medications needed for medical conditions. Current prescription and nonprescription medications as well as supplements and herbal preparations should be reviewed. Many have the potential to affect reproduction, health during pregnancy, or are known teratogens. If a medication or product is deemed to be teratogenic, specific counseling is required to discuss risk and assessment for safe discontinuation of the medication.

It should be determined if an alternate medication without known teratogenicity or an alternate therapeutic option is available. Often this will involve a multispecialty approach. Based on a medication's mechanism of action and half-life, there may also be a duration of time in which prevention of pregnancy is recommended to minimize teratogenic potential. For medications without clear contraindications to use during pregnancy but some potential for risk, benefits must be weighed against adverse effects. Alternate medications or health interventions may be available with an enhanced safety profile. If this is not an option and the medication is needed to remain healthy during pregnancy, the lowest effective dose of medicine is recommended.

Lifestyle, Body Weight, Substance Use, Exposures, and Safety

General wellness with a self-care regimen focused on an adequate sleep pattern, movement and exercise, balanced nutrition, substance avoidance, environmental health, and general mindfulness is

TABLE 4.3

Preconception Visit Key Points

A preconception visit allows for counseling regarding optimization of general health, pregnancy outcomes, and neonatal health.
Reproductive health generally follows good general health.
Providers have a unique opportunity to promote healthy lifestyle habits.
Vaccinations should be recommended to optimize health of pregnancy and reduce risk to offspring.
Daily folic acid supplementation is recommended for all individuals planning or capable of conceiving to reduce risk of neural tube defects.
Preconception infectious disease screening offers a chance to cure disease and enhance pregnancy outcomes.

recommended. Modest exercise for at least 30 minutes for 5 days a week or a minimum of 150 minutes of similar exercise per week is advised [1]. Recommendations and support to maintain a healthy body weight, as reviewed in the previous chapters, are reinforced during preconception care. A substance use assessment and screen, including use of opioids and marijuana, should be routinely performed. Preconception discontinuation or reduction of substances as delineated in the previous chapter are endorsed during preconception care. Briefly, these include cessation of alcohol, all drug use, nicotine, and a reduction in caffeinated substances.

An environmental health history with review of known or suspected exposures should be assessed. Exposures are generally grouped into toxic chemicals (many of which are endocrine disrupters), air pollution, and climate-related exposures. Elimination of exposures known to be associated with adverse reproductive potential, pregnancy outcomes, and developmental health of offspring is recommended. If avoidance is not possible, reduction and use of protective equipment when exposure is encountered can confer benefit [8]. Further knowledge in this area is emerging.

It is also advocated to screen for personal safety, such as intimate partner violence and reproductive coercion, during the preconception visit (Table 4.3). Self-administered questionnaires are promoted as useful tools. Providers should be familiar with and understand reporting requirements under state and federal regulations [9]. Patient resources include the national hotlines (National Domestic Violence Hotline 1-800-799-SAFE [7233]; Rape Abuse and Incest National Network [RAINN] Hotline 1-800-656-HOPE [4673]).

Travel History

If a person is planning to travel, it is recommended that vaccinations are up to date. Furthermore, there may be risks endemic to a travel location which would require additional vaccination. The risks of a disease should be weighed against the risks for vaccination in pregnancy [3].

For individuals traveling internationally, the Advisory Committee on Immunization Practices (ACIP) recommends Hepatitis A vaccination for nonimmune individuals. Although the safety of Hepatitis A vaccination has not been established, it is an inactivated virus and fetal risk is estimated to be low.

While most live-virus vaccines are contraindicated in pregnancy, yellow fever vaccine is an exception. If travel is necessary and the risk of yellow fever exposure outweighs the risk of vaccination, then the vaccine should be administered.

Malaria poses serious illness in pregnant people and is associated with high risks including heavy parasitemia, severe anemia, hypoglycemia, cerebral malaria, and acute respiratory distress syndrome. Fetal loss due to miscarriage, abruption, or premature labor is due to sequestration of parasites in the placenta. Preferably, travel is avoided or delayed to these areas as prophylactic regimens do not confer complete protection. If travel is necessary, then the pregnant person should use an effective prophylactic regimen and protect against mosquito bites.

Pregnancy planners should be aware if they are traveling to an area with active Zika virus. Zika infection in pregnancy can cause miscarriage, preterm birth, microcephaly, and congenital Zika syndrome, which includes limb contractures, high muscle tone, hearing loss, and eye abnormalities. Counseling should include strategies to prevent infection, symptoms, and the limitations of Zika testing. Pregnant people should protect against mosquito bites and sexual transmission and should be counseled on appropriate waiting time to attempt conception [1].

Refer to the most updated CDC Yellow Book guidelines for a complete list of travel guidelines.

Genetic Counseling and Screening

Preconception is the ideal time to perform reproductive genetic counseling. Counseling should include discussion of genetic carrier screening options as well as a review of family history to ascertain genetic ancestry, known consanguinity, and heritable disease risk (including known autosomal dominant disorders).

Genetic Carrier Screening

Genetic carrier screening refers to testing individuals who do not have disease or a known family history of genetic disease but may be heterozygous for a variant of an autosomal recessive or X-linked pathogenic condition. Ancestry-based screening for high prevalence conditions has been offered for years based on self-reported familial countries of origin; however, stigmatization and risk bias in self-reported ancestry exists. In addition, self-reported ancestry is often not highly accurate beyond 1–2 generations. Pan-ethnic carrier screening then followed. Now in an ever-evolving field of genetics with improving variant detection and gene sequencing technology, population-neutral expanded screening options are available. Care options will continue to rapidly evolve over time.

While there is no single consensus or standardized testing paradigm, Committee Opinions and practice resources have been published by the American College of Obstetricians and Gynecologists (ACOG) [10, 11] and the American College of Medical Genetics and Genomics (ACMG) [12]. See also Table 4.4.

Reproductive decision-making has expanded with availability of additional carrier screening. All testing is associated with benefits and limitations. Preconception testing offers the opportunity to learn risk

TABLE 4.4

Screening Recommendations by Consensus Group (See Further Ref. 12)

Consensus Group	Recommended Carrier Screening
ACMG and ACOG	Cystic fibrosis Spinal muscular atrophy Risk-based screening* Personal medical and family history
ACOG	As above in addition to: ≥1/100 carrier frequency
ACMG (Tier 3)	As above in addition to: ≥1/200 carrier frequency including X-linked conditions
Expanded molecular carrier Screening (Tier 4) Laboratories and ACMG±	As above in addition to: <1/200 carrier frequency (Will vary by laboratory)

*ACOG lists the following: Hemoglobinopathies (African, Mediterranean, Middle Eastern, Southeast Asian, or West Indian decent); Fragile X Syndrome (family history of X-related disorders or intellectual disability, unexplained ovarian insufficiency before 40 years of age); Tay–Sachs (Ashkenazi Jewish, French–Canadian or Cajun decent); Canavan disease and Familial dysautonomia (Ashkenazi Jewish); Bloom syndrome; familial hyperinsulinism; Fanconi anemia; Gaucher; Glycogen storage disease type I; Joubert syndrome; Maple syrup urine disease; Mucolipidosis type IV; Niemann–Pick disease; Usher syndrome (to be considered if Ashkenazi decent)

±considered by ACMG if consanguinity or when family and based medical history prior to pregnancy, receive detailed counseling to provide prenatal and newborn care, undergo diagnostic testing during pregnancy, make informed decisions regarding availability of preimplantation genetic testing (PGT), select the use of donated gametes or adoption, or opt to decline family building. Carrier screening can be associated with a financial cost, and obtaining genetic information may produce uncertainty and necessitate management of complex information. One may encounter unexpected identification of variants with personal health risks for the carrier, disclosure of unexpected information, as well as challenges in understanding residual risk assessment. Importantly, carrier screening does not test for all possible causes of genetic disease, and variant classification can change over time. Ideally, pretest counseling can be individualized with expectation setting to best manage results prior to testing; however, implementation of such may be challenging. Post-test counseling remains essential. Once positive carrier status is noted, detailed counseling should occur, and individuals may be counseled regarding sharing information with relevant family members. Importantly, the baseline risk of birth defects, estimated to be 3–4% in the general population, continues to exist in individuals with negative carrier screening results. Further counseling resources can be found at the National Society of Genetic Counselors (NSGC) [13].

Concurrent or sequential screening are both options if an individual presents with a reproductive partner. Concurrent screening with the same laboratory can assist in reducing time restraints and test anxiety but may add additional financial cost. Panel composition varies markedly among laboratories, and conditions being tested may not all overlap. This is specifically considered if using donor gametes for pregnancy as donor testing for a specific condition may not be available.

In our practice, molecular screening for conditions recommended by ACMG as well as more rare conditions (ACMG Tier 4) is most performed for patients who are not making use of donor gametes, and concurrent carrier screening is performed if applicable. Pretest counseling is provided by the practitioner at an initial consultation, and post-test counseling is provided by both the practitioner and an experienced genetic counselor.

Chromosomal Testing

Karyotype testing is recommended if a patient has a history of recurrent pregnancy loss, history of prior stillbirth, prior pregnancy with congenital anomalies, or a history of a child or first degree relative with trisomy 21. Karyotype testing is also recommended in cases of severe sperm factor infertility such as azoospermia and severe oligospermia (less than 5 million total motile count). In these patients, there is a 5–15% chance of chromosomal abnormalities. These patients should also have Y-chromosome microdeletion testing. Karyotype and fragile X testing should also be performed in patients with premature ovarian insufficiency.

Genetic Counseling and Screening Key Points

Ancestry-based genetic carrier screening is influenced by accuracy of self-reporting. Expanded screening/pan-ethnic panels are now considered standard of care.

Reproductive decision-making regarding genetic issues can be complex.

Pretest counseling by providers offering carrier screening is important to set expectations, and post-test genetic counseling is strongly recommended.

Practical Pitfalls for Practitioners

Neglecting to inquire about potential future pregnancy

Overlooking the importance of a preconception consult with maternal fetal medicine

Inadequate pre- and post-test counseling regarding genetic screening

Key Points

Preconception care should involve the following:

- Comprehensive Preconception Assessment: Including a full review of medical, surgical, reproductive, family, and genetic history, alongside wellness exams, lifestyle evaluation, and counseling.
- Immunizations and Infectious Disease Screening: Immunization status should be reviewed and updated, especially for MMR, varicella, Tdap, hepatitis B, and HPV.
- Genetic Counseling and Carrier Screening: Genetic counseling before conception allows for informed decisions regarding reproductive risks, especially using expanded pan-ethnic carrier screening. Karyotyping and specific genetic tests (e.g., fragile X, Y-chromosome microdeletions) are recommended in certain histories (e.g., infertility, recurrent pregnancy loss).
- Vitamin Supplementation and Nutrition: All individuals capable of pregnancy should begin daily folic acid (400 mcg) at least one month before conception to prevent neural tube defects.
- Lifestyle Optimization and Environmental Safety: A healthy body weight, regular exercise, cessation of alcohol, tobacco and drug use, and minimizing harmful environmental exposures (e.g., endocrine disruptors, pollutants) are crucial.

REFERENCES

1. ACOG and ASRM, Prepregnancy Counseling. ACOG Committee on Gynecologic Practice and ASRM Committee Opinion 762. *Obstet Gynecol.* 2019;133:e78–89.
2. ACOG, Well-woman Visit. ACOG Committee Opinion 755. *Obstet Gynecol.* 2018;132:e181–6.
3. Centers for Disease Control and Prevention. Vaccines and Preventable Diseases [internet], 2022: www.cdc.gov/vaccines/vpd/vaccines-diseases.html (accessed Nov 2023).
4. ACOG, Viral Hepatitis in Pregnancy. ACOG Clinical Practice Guideline 6. *Obstet Gynecol.* 2023;1;142:745–59.
5. ACOG, COVID-19 Vaccination Considerations for Obstetric-Gynecologic Care. ACOG Practice Advisory [internet], 2020, updated 2023: www.acog.org/clinical/clinical-guidance/practice-advisory/articles/2020/12/covid-19-vaccination-considerations-for-obstetric-gynecologic-care (accessed Nov 2023).
6. ACOG, Neural Tube Defects. ACOG Practice Bulletin 187. *Obstet Gynecol.* 2017;130:e279–90.
7. Office of Disease Prevention and Health Promotion. Dietary guidelines [internet], 2024: https://health.gov/our-work/nutrition-physical-activity/dietary-guidelines.
8. ACOG, Reducing Prenatal Exposure to Toxic Environmental Agents. ACOG Committee Opinion 832. *Obstet Gynecol.* 2021;137:177–97.
9. Lizdas K et al. Compendium of state and U.S. Territory statutes and policies on domestic violence and health care. Futures Without Violence, 2019: www.futureswithoutviolence.org/compendium-of-state-statutes-and-policies-on-domestic-violence-and-health-care/ (accessed Nov 2023).
10. ACOG, Carrier Screening in the Age of Genomic Medicine. ACOG Committee Opinion 690. *Obstet Gynecol.* 2017;129:e35–40.
11. ACOG, Carrier Screening for Genetic Conditions. ACOG Committee Opinion 691. *Obstet Gynecol.* 2017;129:e41–55.
12. ACMG, Screening for Autosomal Recessive and X-Linked Conditions During Pregnancy and Preconception. *Genet Med.* 2021;23:1793–806.
13. National Society of Genetic Counselors [internet]: www.nsgc.org.

5

The Infertility Workup

Sandy Li and Adrienne B. Neithardt

Introduction

The definition of infertility has recently been changed by the American Society of Reproductive Medicine (ASRM) to be more inclusive and to prevent delay or denial of services to any individual regardless of relationship status or sexual orientation (1). Thus, infertility is now classified as a disease or condition characterized by the inability to achieve a successful pregnancy based on any combination of a patient's medical, sexual, and reproductive history, age, physical findings, or diagnostic testing. This includes the need for medical intervention utilizing donor gametes or embryos either as an individual or as a couple.

Women thirty-five years and younger who fail to achieve pregnancy within one year of regular unprotected intercourse or therapeutic donor insemination, without any other suggestion of impaired fertility in them or their partner, should be offered an evaluation. However, this threshold is lowered to only six months of unprotected intercourse or therapeutic donor insemination for women over the age of thirty-five. Urgent attention is advised for women over the age of forty who deserve immediate evaluation and treatment regardless of the duration of unprotected intercourse or use of donor insemination (2).

The recommendation for evaluation and treatment earlier based on female age is due to the change in fecundity. Fecundity is the monthly pregnancy or fertility rate. In humans, this rate declines with advancing female age. For women under the age of thirty-five, a monthly fecundity of 25% to 30% is expected within the first six months of trying to conceive, but women forty years of age will expect only a 5% to 10% monthly pregnancy rate during this same time frame. The fecundity rate declines at an accelerated rate with each year of life beyond age forty and will be 1% or less by age forty-five.

Not only does age impact fertility rates but so does the duration of failed conception. It is known that the monthly fecundity and probability of pregnancy are greatest within the first three months of coitus or insemination and decline precipitously with the increased duration of failed conception (3). For young women, this translates into an 80–90% chance of pregnancy within one year of unprotected intercourse with only an additional 5% to 15% chance of conceiving within the next 12 months of unprotected intercourse or donor insemination (4). It is estimated that nearly 11% of all women aged 15–44 in the United States have impaired fecundity and less than half ever seek out care and treatment (4).

Therefore, it is critical to understand that the guidelines do not justify withholding needed care to those patients who may require earlier evaluation and treatment when physical findings and medical history warrant it.

Causes of Infertility

It has been estimated that one-third of all causes of infertility originate in the female, one-third in the male, and the remaining one-third are due to combined female and male factors. For the woman, contributing aspects include diminished ovarian reserve, endometriosis, disorders of ovulation, uterine

DOI: 10.1201/9781003460275-5

abnormalities, tubal disease, as well as unexplained infertility. Men may experience spermatogenic problems related to both hypothalamic-pituitary impairment as well as anatomic testicular abnormalities and dysfunction. The role of the physician is to carefully assess the couple to determine which of any of the possible reasons are relevant and then target treatment to the identified impairment.

Initial Consultation and Physical Exam

The initial consultation between the physician and the patient is the crucial first step in understanding the needs of the individual seeking your advice and care. An extensive history and physical examination for both the patient and her partner are necessary. A detailed history and focused review of systems should take between 30 to 60 minutes. Findings suggestive of an endocrine disorder should be sought. Screening for thyroid disease, hyperprolactinemia, galactorrhea, and hirsutism should be scrutinized and addressed in all patients. During the initial consultation, the clinician should attempt to define if the patient suffers from pelvic pain, dysmenorrhea, dyspareunia, or vaginismus since they all may have an impact on the likelihood of conception. It is for this reason that even women who desire to achieve pregnancy using donor sperm deserve a detailed evaluation prior to treatment.

A relevant history should contain information regarding all known medical problems including current and past medication usage, drug, latex, and food allergies as well as prior screening or treatment for a suspected clotting or thromboembolic disorder. Chemotherapy and/or radiation exposure for the treatment of a known malignancy can affect the ovaries and should also be addressed at this time.

A gynecologic history encompassing the timing of puberty, menstrual cycle frequency with length and amount of flow are essential components to identify. Details regarding ovulatory dysfunction, polycystic ovarian syndrome (PCOS), endometriosis, uterine leiomyomas, tubal disease, pelvic infection as well as information pertaining to past abdominal, pelvic, and uterine surgeries should be documented. Although it may be intuitive to the clinician, coital frequency, number of prior sexual partners, and details pertaining to past fertility testing and treatments are all essential components to the infertility workup.

Obstetrical information regarding all prior pregnancies with known complications should be recorded. Details such as cervical incompetence, preterm labor and/or delivery, preeclampsia, gestational diabetes, ectopic pregnancy, multiple gestation, and prior miscarriages are also important facets to help the clinician determine relevant testing and treatment options of care.

A comprehensive family history should detail information regarding known cancers or inheritable malignancies. Family members with mental retardation, autism, or other known genetic, congenital, or inheritable conditions should be identified. Social and dietary habits including alcohol and caffeine consumption, cigarette and illicit drug use, body mass index (BMI) calculations along with exercise and lifestyle choices all impact on a patient's fertility and ability to conceive. The psychological wellbeing of the patient is critical to a successful outcome. Thus, risk factors including stress, depression, and anxiety should be evaluated and addressed prior to pregnancy.

When applicable, all male partners should be questioned to determine their ability to achieve a successful erection with ejaculation during coitus. Information pertaining to prior exposure to mumps as well as sexually transmitted diseases should be established. The use of specific medications known to interfere with male fertility including testosterone, 5-α reductase inhibitors, β-blockers and phosphodiesterase inhibitors should be documented and possibly discontinued when appropriate (5). Prior testicular and pelvic surgeries as well as chemotherapy and radiation exposure are critical pieces of information to obtain during the history. All prior sperm tests or relationships resulting in pregnancy should be divulged.

A complete physical and gynecologic examination should be performed following the initial consultation. The exam should contain a complete set of vital signs including blood pressure, pulse, and respiratory rate as well as measurements of both weight and height to calculate BMI. The clinician should describe all thyroid, breast, cardiac, and respiratory abnormalities. When nipple discharge is present, simple microscopy may help determine if it is galactorrhea. Nearly 70% of women with galactorrhea will have hyperprolactinemia which can affect ovulation. Conversely, only 30% to 40% of women with hyperprolactinemia will have galactorrhea (6). Vaginal and cervical discharge as well as uterine size, shape, and position should be noted when abnormal. If possible, adnexal tenderness, masses, and pelvic or vaginal nodules should be identified since these may be signs of underlying endometriosis.

Patients with complaints of hirsutism and ovulatory dysfunction should have a thorough exam to describe the extent of their androgen excess. The clinician should focus attention to findings such as hair coarseness, distribution and density pertaining to patient's face, body, and extremities, and document symptoms of male pattern hair loss on the head when present. Signs of virilization include increased muscle mass and cliteromegaly. For those patients suspected of excess cortisol, denote the color, size, and location of abdominal striae; indicate if fat disposition around the neck, face, and extremities has changed.

Men suspected of having spermatogenic, urogenital, or pelvic problems should have their examination performed by an experienced clinician. An individual with expertise in urology should perform the exam and focus on the presence or absence of varicoceles, document testicular location and size using an orchidometer, and identify congenital malformations of the epididymus, vas deferens, phallus, and meatal opening. A prostate examination may also be necessary for men with low or absent ejaculate.

Overall, the infertility evaluation can be initiated by a less experienced provider, but once an abnormal test is identified, the referral to a specialist with an infertility background is strongly recommended. It is known that the immediate referral of these patients to a physician with infertility training and expertise can reduce the overall emotional stress, cost, and time to conception (7). The physical, psychological, and emotional wellbeing of both the patient and partner are all essential parts of the infertility process, and the practitioner should be cognizant of these factors when creating an appropriate plan of care.

Testing

Testing for both the patient and partner should be focused and streamlined to identify only the relevant factors necessary to render treatment. The practitioner should refrain from ordering redundant and superfluous tests and should make every effort to reduce both the emotional and financial burdens associated with this phase of the evaluation. For the female partner, a multitude of testing is performed during specific intervals of the menstrual cycle. Testing often begins with the onset of menses and usually takes one full menstrual cycle to complete. Once completed, the patient and her partner should return for a consultation to discuss realistic goals and expectations regarding their overall chance of pregnancy and delivery. After all options of care are reviewed, a treatment plan should be created and enacted in both a judicious and expedited manner.

It is critical to understand that test results do not predict outcome. Regardless of a test's sensitivity or specificity or how encouraging or discouraging a result may be, the chance of delivering a live born child cannot be determined by any single test or combination of tests. Testing can only determine what therapeutic options the patient or couple has (all options vs. limited or no options) and if the patient has an average or less than average probability of conception compared to age-matched peers. Religious, ethical, psychological, and physiologic factors are all important aspects in the decision-making process. It is for this reason that test results should not be used in a punitive manner to deny patients the opportunity to undergo treatment when deemed applicable and medically appropriate. Rather, study results should be used to inform patients of their treatment options and inform them when a lower than predicted chance of success is anticipated, and what, if anything, could be done to improve the outcome.

Ovarian Function

Ovarian function and ovarian reserve testing are each performed at specific intervals during the menstrual cycle. Ovarian function tests are used to determine if and when ovulation occurs, and ovarian reserve testing is used to determine the density of remaining oocytes available to compete for ovulation.

A variety of methods are available to assess the timing of ovulation. Low-tech methods include daily basal body temperature (BBT) charting or midcycle luteinizing hormone (LH) urinary predictor kit

(UPK) testing. A more sophisticated, higher-cost strategy involves both blood work and pelvic ultrasound to evaluate follicular growth and function. A day 16 to 24 progesterone level can also be obtained to confirm that ovulation occurred. This last step is valuable for patients with irregular menstrual cycles and chronic anovulation. However, ovulation can be inferred to occur in women who have regular menstrual cycles, with lengths ranging from 21 to 35 days, and who have intercycle variability of less than five days between menses.

BBT Charting: This is the simplest and least expensive method to evaluate and determine if ovulation has occurred. However, as noted earlier, regular cycles indicate regular ovulation, negating the need for BBT recording. For consistency, temperature measurements are recorded daily, upon awakening and prior to any physical activity, eating, or drinking. These temperature determinations can be recorded at other times during the day, but they need to be obtained at the same time daily. The follicular or pre-ovulatory phase of the menstrual cycle can vary in length from one menstrual cycle to the next. However, the luteal phase should constantly last 14 days from the time of ovulation to menses (assuming that pregnancy has not been achieved). Following ovulation, the patient's body temperature will be between 0.4 to 1.1°F higher than what was recorded prior to ovulation. This phenomenon in temperature change is directly related to the secretion of progesterone from the corpus luteum. Progesterone acts directly on the temperature regulating neurons within the hypothalamus and CNS to increase thermogenesis and increase body temperature (8). In ovulatory women, this post-ovulation spike in temperature will persist until menses and forms what is called a "biphasic" pattern in the patient's temperature log. Anovulatory women will not see this biphasic pattern in temperature change nor will they report any significant change in daily temperature throughout their observations. BBT charting requires a minimum of three to four months of measurements to determine a patient's fertile period and only retrospectively predicts ovulation within a three-day window (9).

Home Ovulation Predictor Kits: Most home ovulation predictor kits measure urinary concentrations of LH only. The LH surge is necessary to induce ovulation and usually occurs 24 to 36 hours prior to ovulation (10). However, the timing of the LH surge and measurement of peak values vary based on assay quality and are often difficult to interpret and, unfortunately, inaccurate in their predictive usefulness. In an effort to improve the accuracy of these home tests, some predictor kits measure other hormones such as estrone-3-glucuronide (E3G) in addition to peak LH levels. E3G is a metabolite of estrogen formed following oxidation within the liver and peaks 12 to 24 hours prior to ovulation. This weak form of estrogen begins to rise approximately three days prior to ovulation but then declines to negligible levels five days later (11). The hypothalamic-pituitary-ovarian axis is tonically under negative feedback control. Just prior to ovulation, a transformation occurs inducing a positive feedback system. This phenomenon transpires when 17β-estradiol (E2) levels are sustained for at least 36 hours with peak values ranging from 150 pg/mL or greater. Once released from its follicle, the oocyte has only 12 to 24 hours to be fertilized. If fertilization does not occur, then the process of apoptosis will begin and the demise of the egg will be inevitable (12). It is for this reason that the home ovulation predictor kit accuracy is essential to help predict the appropriate time for fertilization following ovulation.

Pelvic Ultrasound and Blood Work: A more precise predictor of ovulation can be achieved with the use of both blood work and a pelvic ultrasound. Unlike LH urinary predictor kits, blood measurements of E2, LH, and progesterone can be compared with findings observed on a pelvic ultrasound to best predict the occurrence of ovulation. Patients who have an ovarian follicle with a diameter greater than 18 mm associated with an E2 level over 150 pg/mL and LH level over 15 mIU/mL with a progesterone value of under 2.0 ng/mL have a high probability of ovulation within 24 to 48 hours following the documentation of those observations. This method of testing is expensive but useful for patients with PCOS and chronic anovulation. These patients typically have LH values near or at the pre-ovulatory range but without meeting any of the other findings typical of the midcycle.

Day 16–24 Progesterone Levels: Prior to ovulation, the ovary secretes primarily estrogen in the form of estradiol. Following ovulation, the secretory environment of the ovary changes from that of estrogen to one dominated by the secretion of progesterone. This change is due to a loss in the population of cells during ovulation, which contain the enzyme necessary for estradiol production. Progesterone levels above 3 ng/mL are most commonly associated with ovulation and then progressively increase to peak seven days later (13). Following the peak, progesterone levels continually decline over the next seven days until levels again fall to pre-ovulatory values and menses ensues.

Endometrial Biopsy (EMB): A simple and minimally-invasive office procedure used to evaluate the endometrial cavity for both histologic and pathologic changes. Women experiencing abnormal vaginal bleeding often undergo this procedure to determine if an underlying infectious, premalignant, or malignant process is occurring. Dating of the endometrium has long been the gold standard in evaluating infertile women for a suspected luteal phase defect (14). More recently, this process has been replaced by the Endometrial Receptivity Array (ERA) test. This is because histologic dating lacks the ability to distinguish fertile from infertile women and has wide interoperator variability (15). The ERA test can more precisely determine an individual's window of implantation (16). The ERA test accomplishes this by evaluating the mRNA levels within endometrial tissue to identify a specific molecular profile known as a "transcriptomic signature" (17). Overall, 25% of patients undergoing IVF with recurrent failed embryo transfers will have an endometrium deemed "out of phase" when compared to the exact day of progesterone exposure. To improve pregnancy rates, the ERA test evaluates endometrial transcriptomic signatures and then recommends a new personalized change in the day of embryo transfer in relation to the day of progesterone exposure. A recent randomized, controlled trial failed to find that ERA-timed embryo transfers achieved superior implantation rates over embryo transfers utilizing standard timing. This calls into question under what circumstances an ERA would be beneficial (18).

Ovarian Reserve Testing

Ovarian reserve is an attempt to assess the residual pool of follicles in the ovaries. The assessment of ovarian reserve begins with the onset of menses and is generally performed during day two to four of menses. Reserve testing usually entails both blood work and a pelvic ultrasound. Hormonal levels from the pituitary gland and ovary are evaluated and correlated with the total antral follicle count (AFC) obtained during the pelvic ultrasound. Collectively, an estimate of the patient's reproductive potential can be made (19). A patient's ovarian reserve best describes oocyte quantity, and a patient's age best depicts oocyte quality. For young women under the age of thirty-five, each oocyte has roughly a 10% probability of pregnancy and live birth. However, this rate declines rapidly with advancing age with pregnancy and delivery rates declining to 5% per oocyte by age forty and to 1% or less by age forty-five (20). It is for this reason that young patients with diminished ovarian reserve have a better chance of pregnancy and live birth compared to women with advanced maternal age and a robust ovarian reserve (21).

Antral Follicle Count (AFC): The AFC is determined at the time of the initial pelvic ultrasound, and every follicle with a diameter between 2 to 10 mm is counted. Each ovary should contain at least five to 11 follicles. Young patients and patients with PCOS typically have high antral follicle counts, with a minimum of 12 or more follicles per ovary. Women with diminished ovarian reserve usually have four or fewer antral follicles visualized per ovary. Some studies suggest that the AFC is the best predictor of an age-related decline in ovarian reserve and overall oocyte production during an IVF cycle (22, 23).

Day 3 Hormone Testing: Another strategy regularly used to predict ovarian reserve is the serum measurement of specific pituitary and ovarian hormones on day two to four of the menstrual cycle. Hormones commonly measured include anti-Müllerian hormone (AMH), follicle stimulating hormone (FSH), estradiol (E2), and (less commonly) inhibin-B. All four of these hormones independently reflect the follicular pool and can predict ovarian response to gonadotropins better than age alone.

AMH is a dimeric glycoprotein and a member of transforming growth factor-β (TGF-β) superfamily. It is directly secreted from ovarian granulosa cells located on preantral and antral follicles. AMH levels tend to be more consistent between menstrual cycles and is independent of the cycle day obtained. In young women, AMH values are normally above 2 ng/mL but over time progressively decline to become undetectable approximately five years prior to menopause (Figure 5.1). Values of less than 1 ng/mL indicate a diminished ovarian reserve and is associated with both a poor response to ovarian stimulation and a lower likelihood of pregnancy following oocyte retrieval and embryo transfer (24).

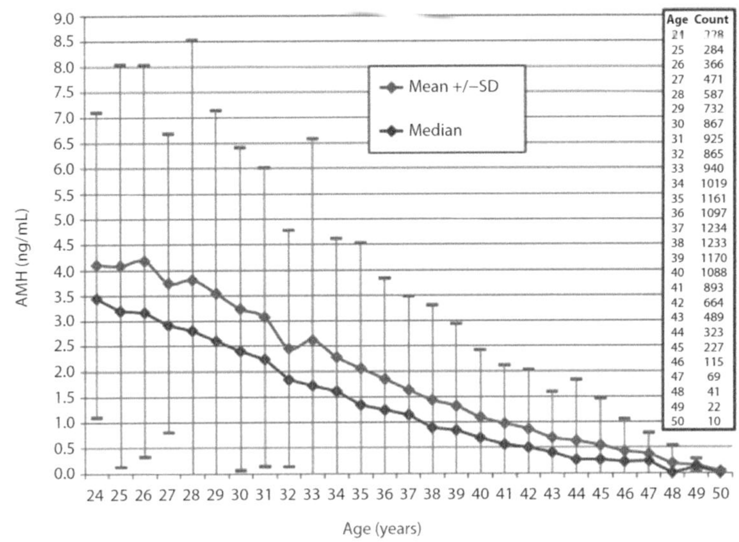

FIGURE 5.1 Age versus AMH levels. AMH, anti-Müllerian hormone. (From Seifer DB et al. Age-specific serum anti-Müllerian hormone values for 17,120 women presenting to fertility centers within the United States. Fertil Steril 2011;95:747–50, with permission.)

Factors known to have a detrimental effect on ovarian reserve include chemotherapeutic drugs, ionizing radiation, and endometriosis (25). Operative procedures involving the ovary or its blood supply can also impact and lower reserve. The surgical resection of an ovarian endometrioma permanently results in a post-procedural decrease in ovarian reserve with up to a 66% drop in serum AMH levels following the procedure. However, other surgeries including bilateral salpingectomy or routine ovarian cystectomy (for a cyst other than an endometrioma) have no lasting effect on AMH values after the procedure (26). Paradoxically, low AMH values can be observed in some women with a normal ovarian reserve. The clinician should be aware that obesity, hypothalamic failure, use of oral contraceptive pills, and prolonged exposure to gonadotropin releasing hormone agonists (GnRH-agonist) all artificially lower serum AMH levels (27, 28). For these women, AMH alone does not accurately reflect ovarian reserve, and actions should be taken to either correct the underlying pathophysiologic problem or discontinue the offending medical therapy, prior to retesting or starting treatment.

Other common endocrine markers used to assess ovarian reserve includes a day 3 serum FSH and an estradiol level. Despite their capricious cycle-to-cycle variability, these two hormones when measured together are useful prognostic indicators of low ovarian reserve and reduced response to ovarian stimulation (29). Single measurements of either FSH or E2 alone are unreliable and not predictive and should not be routinely obtained. Women with a normal ovarian reserve demonstrate FSH levels below 10 mIU/mL and E2 levels below 60 pg/mL during the early follicular phase of the menstrual cycle. As women age and ovarian reserve diminishes, the mechanism controlling the communication and regulation of ovulation breaks down. As a result, an acceleration of follicular development during the late luteal into the early follicular phase of the succeeding menstrual cycle occurs. Eventually, the hypothalamus and pituitary gland become insensitive to rising E2 levels, and the pituitary gland becomes uninhibited and releases increasing amounts of FSH into the circulation. Day 3 FSH levels will often rise above 10 mIU/mL despite having E2 levels greater than 70 pg/mL. This lack of negative feedback control of E2 on the release of FSH from the pituitary gland is an impending sign of low ovarian reserve and a lower reproductive potential.

Overall, AMH appears to be the best endocrine marker for assessing an age-related decline in ovarian reserve and can strongly predict a poor response to ovarian stimulation (30). However, nearly 20% of women who have a reassuring day 3 FSH value under 10 mIU/mL will have a worrying AMH value below 1 ng/mL. Conversely, 5% of women with a normal AMH value will have an elevated and concerning day 3 FSH level. This discordance in values between a day 3 FSH and AMH clearly justifies measuring both day 3 FSH and E2 in addition to a serum AMH level to better predict and detect patients with a diminished ovarian reserve (31).

See the chapter on ovarian reserve testing for more information.

Clomiphene Citrate Challenge Test (CCCT): Clomiphene citrate (CC) is a selective estrogen receptor modulator (SERM) and is composed of a mixture of the two geometric isomers, En-clomiphene (trans-isomer) and Zuclomiphene (cis-isomer). Since both isomers have different half-lifes and affinities for the various estrogen receptors within the tissues of the body, a mixed estrogenic and antiestrogenic reaction is often observed. CC exerts its functions through competitive inhibition of estrogen for its receptor. When administered, CC blocks the negative feedback effect of estrogen on both the hypothalamus and pituitary gland, which in turn increases the secretion of LH and FSH.

The CCCT utilizes this inhibitory effect of CC to identify women at risk of having a low ovarian reserve. A day 3 serum FSH is obtained prior to the administration of 100 mg of oral CC on menstrual cycle days 5-9. A second FSH level is obtained on cycle day 10 following the completion of the medication. An elevated FSH value above 10 mIU/mL obtained on either cycle day 3 or 10 indicates a diminished ovarian reserve. Women with abnormally elevated FSH values demonstrate a dramatically lower ovarian response to medical stimulation and a lower pregnancy and live birth rate when compared to women with a normal FSH following the CCCT (32). However, fewer physicians use this test to predict ovarian reserve and now increasingly rely on serum AMH and ovarian AFCs to manage patient expectations, as it does not provide additional useful information and patients may experience side effects with clomiphene citrate.

Testing for Uterine and Fallopian Tube Abnormalities

Collectively, uterine and fallopian tubal problems comprise 25% of all causes of infertility with the majority of these cases being tubal in origin (33). Anatomic, congenital, pathologic, and infectious abnormalities can impact conception by altering the normal interaction between the sperm and oocyte. Basic screening tests include a vaginal pelvic ultrasound and a hystero-salpingogram (HSG) or Saline Infusion Sonohysterogram (SIS). Abnormal findings are often too unreliable to predict a negative outcome and consideration to perform a more definitive diagnostic test should be made.

Pelvic Ultrasound (US): The safest, least invasive, and inexpensive imaging modality routinely used to visualize and examine the pelvic anatomy is vaginal ultrasonography (US). Both 2-D and occasionally 3-D images are required to evaluate for suspected abnormalities within the uterus and ovaries. Uterine leiomyomas and polyps as well as ovarian cysts and masses can be easily observed, characterized, and even followed over time. Although uterine anomalies account for only 5% of all causes of infertility, they are more often associated with recurrent pregnancy loss and miscarriage. The best time to perform the vaginal ultrasound is during the first four days of the menstrual cycle. At this time, the endometrium is thin and both ovaries are resting and no cysts or follicles larger than 10 mm in diameter should be noticed. Any variation from normal should prompt an investigation to identify the underlying pathologic process and determine if treatment is required.

Hysterosalpingogram (HSG): The HSG is the best test to evaluate the constitution of the endometrial cavity and patency of both fallopian tubes. It can reveal anatomic distortions created by submucous leiomyomas, uterine synechia, and endometrial polyps. Congenital malformations including septate, bicornuate, and unicornuate uteri are easily discerned but often require a pelvic MRI or even laparoscopy to confirm the diagnosis. To identify a tubal anomaly, the HSG has a sensitivity and specificity of 65% and 83%, respectively, and surprisingly, only a 30% positive predictive value to correctly identify pathologies of the endometrial cavity (34, 35).

Fallopian tube abnormalities account for 20% of all infertility-related issues. As a screening test, the HSG is invaluable and can eliminate tubal disease as the root cause of infertility. It can distinguish proximal from distal tubal disease as well as identify infectious and inflammatory etiologies such as hydrosalpinx, peri-tubal adhesions, and fimbria occlusion when present. The HSG requires an iodide-based radiopaque contrast as the infusion media. This contrast media can be oil-soluble (OSCM) or water-soluble (WSCM) in nature. Nearly all procedures performed today use WSCM rather than OSCM. WSCM is less expensive, has better imaging resolution, and harbors less risk of complication. Problems including allergic reactions, anaphylactic shock, and pelvic lipogranuloma formations are more common with OSCM because of its higher viscosity and slower reabsorption rate (36). The most dangerous risk associated with OSCM occurs when the contrast intravasates into the pelvic vasculature leading to fat embolism formation, circulatory collapse, and eventually death. Women with occluded fallopian tubes and submucous myomas are at greatest risk of this problem (Figures 5.2, 5.3, 5.4, 5.5, 5.6, 5.7, 5.8, 5.9, 5.10).

Multiple studies suggest that pregnancy rates increase immediately following the HSG. This increase in pregnancy rate is highest within the first four months following the HSG and then progressively declines over time, to have no impact by eight months later (37). Interestingly, this effect on pregnancy rate is only observed in patients who receive OSCM but not for those who receive WSCM (38, 39). One possible explanation as to how OSCM improves pregnancy rates is through its ability to dislodge and clear mucous plugs formed within the fallopian tubes (40). However, a more likely explanation lies with oil's ability to alter the local pelvic immunity to primarily reduce inflammatory and autoimmune reactions which impact sperm, egg, and embryo survival (41). This phenomenon is best observed in patients diagnosed with endometriosis, unexplained fertility, and male factor infertility. For this reason, some authorities advocate that once tubal patency is established, 3 mL of OSCM should be injected into the endometrial cavity and fallopian tubes as a means to increase fertility rates in subsequent cycles (42).

See Figure 5.11.

Saline Infusion Sonohysterogram (SIS): Saline Infusion Sonohysterogram (SIS) is a valuable diagnostic tool used to evaluate women with infertility and abnormal vaginal bleeding. It is commonly performed on patients with an iodine sensitivity or allergy, who would otherwise undergo an HSG procedure. The SIS is safer and has less patient discomfort compared to the HSG. Sterile normal saline (NS) is used as the infusion media. NS is better tolerated than iodine because of its neutral pH with the tissues of the body. Ultrasound waves are used to evaluate the pelvic anatomy, thus reducing the patient's exposure to the effects of harmful radiation.

The SIS can reveal detailed information regarding the endometrial cavity as well as determine fallopian tube patency. However, unlike the HSG, the SIS is highly sensitive for detecting endometrial cavity abnormalities and has a positive predictive value of >90% for detecting pathologies such as submucous leiomyomas, polyps, and synechia (43). Traditionally, the SIS was considered less helpful in documenting fallopian tube patency. However, newer techniques using Femvue (Femasys Inc.) employ a simultaneous

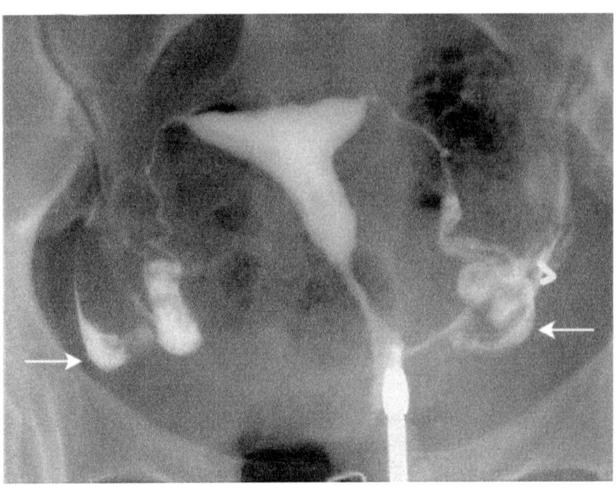

FIGURE 5.2 Normal HSG. This HSG demonstrates a uterine cavity that has a normal shape, and there are no filling defects noted within the cavity. Both fallopian tubes have filled, and the arrows point to the dye that has exited the ends of both tubes into the abdominal cavity. (*Abbreviation:* HSG, hysterosalpingogram.)

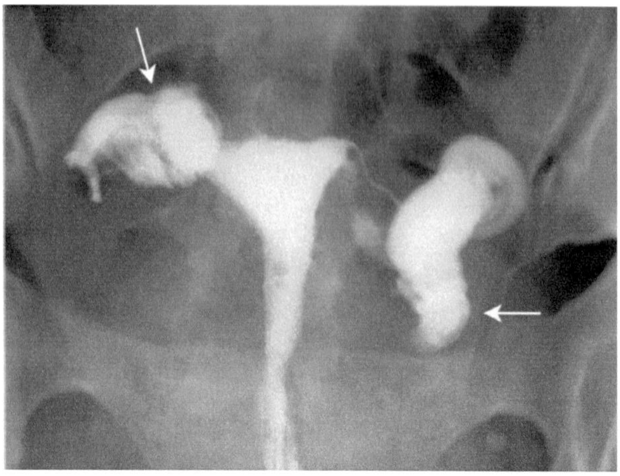

FIGURE 5.3 Distal tubal obstruction. In this x-ray, both fallopian tubes are filled, but their distal ends are dilated and no dye is seen escaping into the abdominal cavity. The ends of the tubes are indicated by the arrows. This finding is most likely the result of a pelvic infection.

mixture of air and saline to create a bubble mixture. On ultrasound, these air bubbles can be visualized traveling through the fallopian tubes to demonstrate areas of patency and occlusion. See Figure 5.12.

Hysteroscopy and Laparoscopy: Hysteroscopy and laparoscopy are the gold standard diagnostic procedures performed following an abnormal screening or imaging test. These procedures allow the physician to correct underlying uterine and pelvic pathologies as well as visualize congenital and acquired anatomic abnormalities. Factors which contribute to infertility include endometriosis, peritoneal adhesions, and congenital tubal and uterine malformations. All of these disease processes can contribute to anatomic tubal distortions and even complete obstruction. When tubal patency is unclearly documented following an HSG or SIS procedure, laparoscopy with chromopertubation can discern fallopian tube patency from proximal and distal occlusion. Hysteroscopy with polypectomy, myomectomy, metroplasty, and resection of intrauterine adhesions can quickly and easily restore the anatomy back to normal and improve implantation, pregnancy, and live birth rates (44).

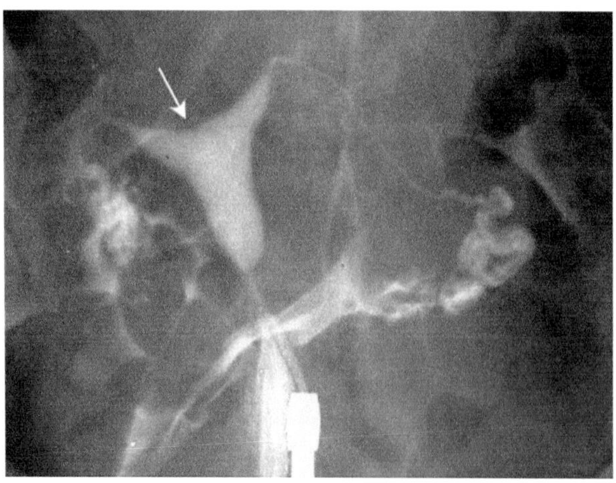

FIGURE 5.4 Arcuate uterus. In this otherwise normal study, a depression can be seen indenting the superior aspect of the uterine cavity (arrow). This is compatible with an arcuate uterus and is considered a normal variant. No additional workup is indicated. For comparison, a normal uterine cavity can be seen in Figures 5.2 and 5.3.

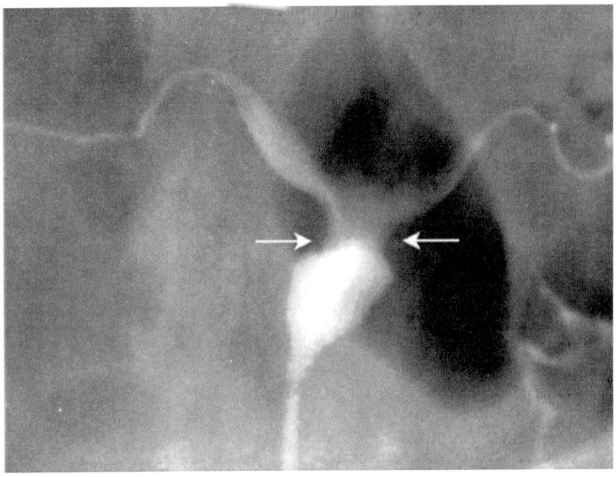

FIGURE 5.5 A DES uterus. The shape of this uterine cavity is compatible with previous DES exposure that causes impingement of the lateral walls as indicated by the arrows. The prominent uterine horns create a bicornuate shape as well. Overall, the uterine cavity has a "T shape" that is classic for previous DES exposure. (*Abbreviation:* DES, diethylstilbestrol.)

Evaluating Male Fertility

The evaluation of the male begins with the semen analysis. This analysis identifies problems pertaining to the ejaculate and details findings regarding sperm count, movement, and shape. Anatomic, hormonal, genetic, and lifestyle factors all can contribute to a male's fertility. Overall, 40% of couples will have a male component contributing to their infertility; for 20%, it will be the sole cause (45). The male fertility evaluation is important as this may often be a male's first encounter with a health provider outside of their pediatrician, and thus the REI provider may play an important role in helping them establish care with a primary care provider who can address any detrimental health behaviors or needs (46). Almost

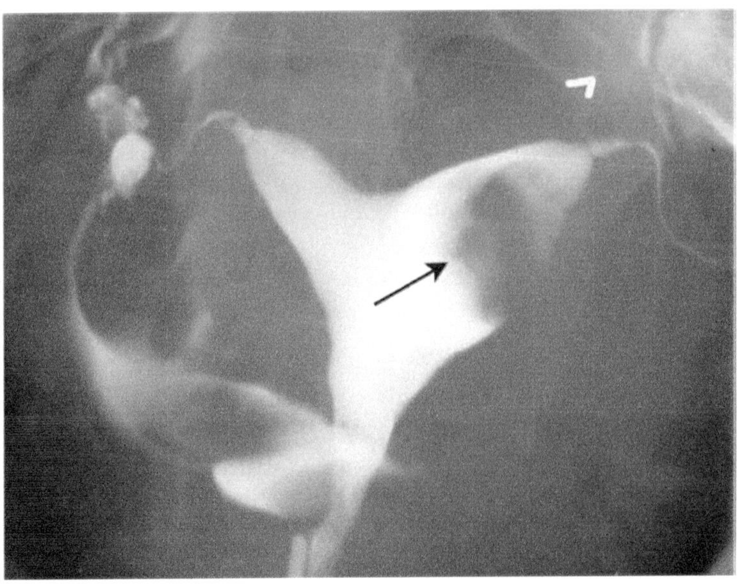

FIGURE 5.6 Submucosal fibroid. This hysterosalpingogram demonstrates a large filling defect in the left uterine horn, which was later found to be a submucosal fibroid. Also note the depression in the superior aspect of the cavity, which is an arcuate deformity.

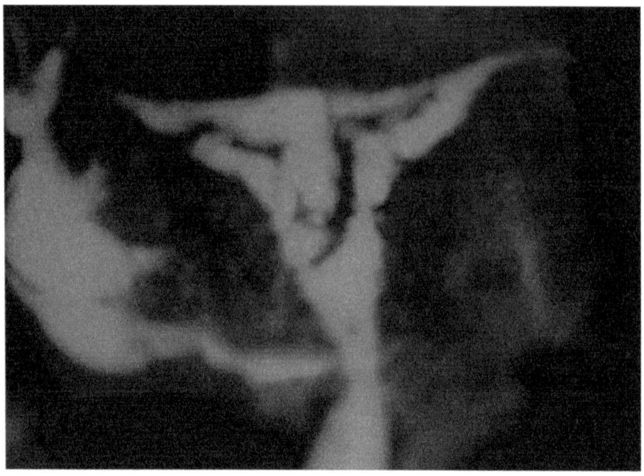

FIGURE 5.7 Asherman's syndrome. This HSG demonstrates multiple filling defects compatible with Asherman's syndrome. The patient is dilation and curettage (D&C) and underwent hysteroscopic lysis of adhesions with restoration of the uterine cavity. (*Abbreviation:* HSG, hysterosalpingogram.)

1 in 10 men assessed for infertility may have important medical conditions, ranging from hormonal, cardiovascular, to malignancies detected during their assessment (47).

Semen Analysis (SA): The semen analysis is a simple and relatively inexpensive gold standard test used to evaluate for male infertility. Although tests with abnormal findings clearly lead to failed fertilization and conception, male infertility can still be found in some men with completely normal sperm parameters. The semen analysis is a standardized test and requires that the patient abstain from ejaculation between two to four days prior to collection. The sperm sample should be produced in the facility processing and performing the analysis, but it can also be transported by the patient to that facility under proper conditions and within 60 to 90 minutes following home collection. Most patients produce samples for testing through masturbation. However, for those men who cannot masturbate, the option of collecting a sample via intercourse can be offered. Special condoms, designed specifically for collecting sperm for analysis, must be purchased and used by the patient. These collection condoms are formulated differently than traditional condoms and do not disrupt or kill the sperm following ejaculation.

Once the sperm sample is collected and analyzed, the provider can determine if further testing or treatment is required. Most authorities use the World Health Organization's (WHO) reference for defining

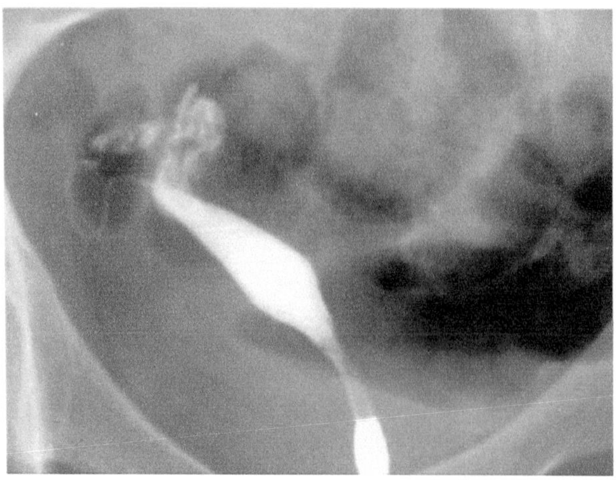

FIGURE 5.8 Unicornuate uterus. During this x-ray, only the right horn of the uterine cavity filled. This is compatible with a unicornuate uterus. A unicornuate uterus increases the risk of premature labor and fetal malpresentations. It can be accompanied by renal abnormalities.

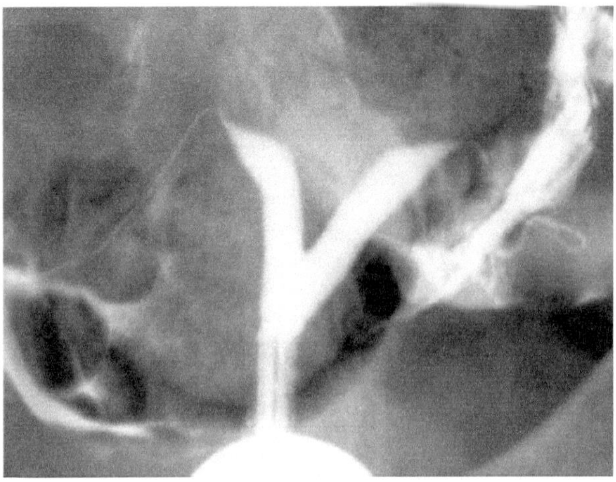

FIGURE 5.9 Uterine septum. This x-ray demonstrates a division in the uterine cavity, which was confirmed to be a uterine septum.

the lower limits of the parameters of a normal semen analysis (48). (Table 5.1, Figure 5.13). The sixth edition of guidelines was released in 2021 and contain several important updates (reviewed in Esteves et al 2022) (49). The guidelines continue to contain the traditional semen analysis parameters for semen volume, sperm concentration, sperm motility, and sperm morphology. Compared to the previous 2010 edition, the data was pooled from nearly twice as many fertile men (defined as natural conception in 12 months or less without fertility treatment/assessment) and drew patients from a broader geographic range. While there are benefits to inclusivity, there may also be variations across populations by race, region, or sociodemographic aspects that are poorly understood and lost when pooled into a larger data-set (50). The normal ranges established for the various parameters are somewhat arbitrary, and a previous study confirmed overlap between the semen parameters in a fertile and infertile population (51).

Spermatogenesis occurs in the testicular tubules and requires a normal secretion of the hormone testosterone for maximum productivity. Varicoceles are dilated veins within the pampiniform plexus and internal spermatic veins located within the spermatic cord. They are the most common anatomic abnormality associated with male subfertility. Over 40% of all men with abnormal semen samples will have at least one varicocele identified on exam. Varicoceles exert their effect by raising testicular temperature,

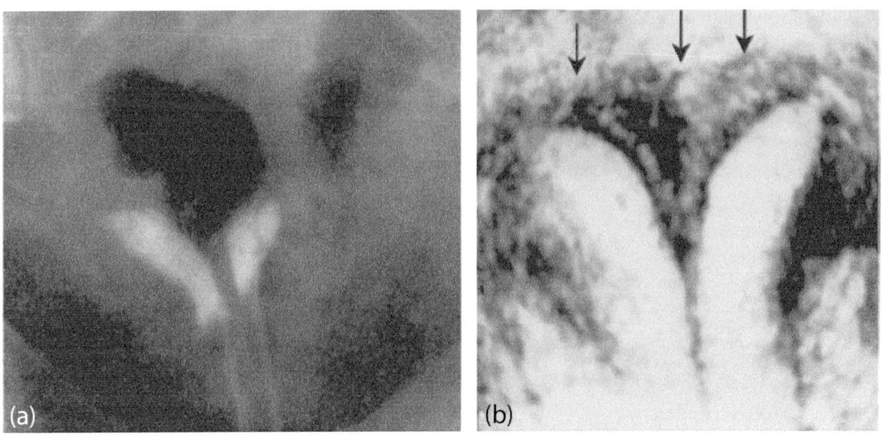

FIGURE 5.10 Is this uterine anomaly a septate or bicornuate uterus? (a) A uterine duplication anomaly confirmed by an HSG. Two separate cervices were cannulated and two separate uterine horns were noted. (b) A three-dimensional ultrasound image of the uterus of the same patient. The black arrows note the border of the outer extent of the myometrium of the uterine fundus. Conclusion: The anomaly is a uterine septum. (*Abbreviation:* HSG, hysterosalpingogram.)

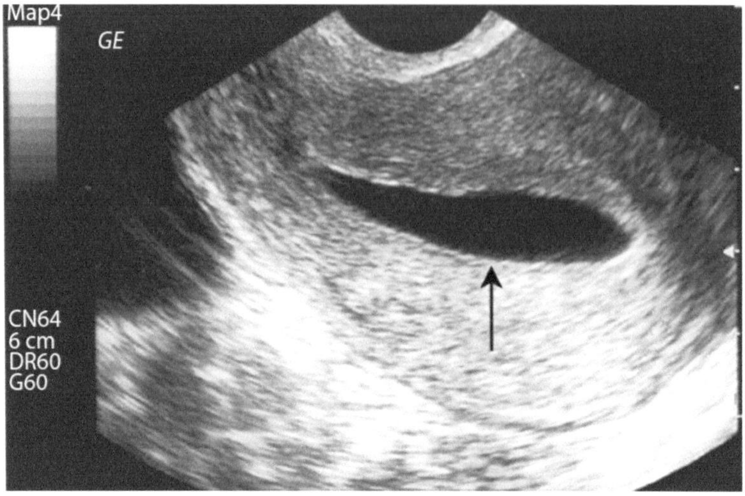

FIGURE 5.11 Sonohysterogram (normal cavity). This is a longitudinal image of the uterus taken at the time of a sonohysterogram. The black area (arrow) is the image of the saline that has been injected into the uterine cavity. Note that the borders of the uterine cavity are sharp and no masses are noted to be entering into the cavity. This study confirms a normal uterine cavity.

which then alters the production and quality of sperm. Eventually all parameters including movement, shape, count, and function are affected. Evaluation by a trained urologist is needed to determine whether surgery or angiographic embolization to treat varicoceles may be indicated (52).

Azoospermia is the term given to samples lacking any visible sperm. Both obstructive and non-obstructive causes can be implicated. Obstructive azoospermia commonly results from a blockage or congenital absence of the vas deferens. The vas deferens connects the testes with the urethra and is easily palpable during the physical exam or observed during a pelvic and testicular ultrasound. Between 1% to 2% of men have a congenital bilateral absence of the vas deferens (CBAVD), and they account for almost 25% of all patients with obstructive azoospermia (53). These men likely have a cystic fibrosis transmembrane receptor mutation (CFTR) which leads to defective Wölffian duct formation. This causes a failure of the vas deferens to connect the testes to the urethra, ultimately preventing the delivery of sperm into the ejaculate.

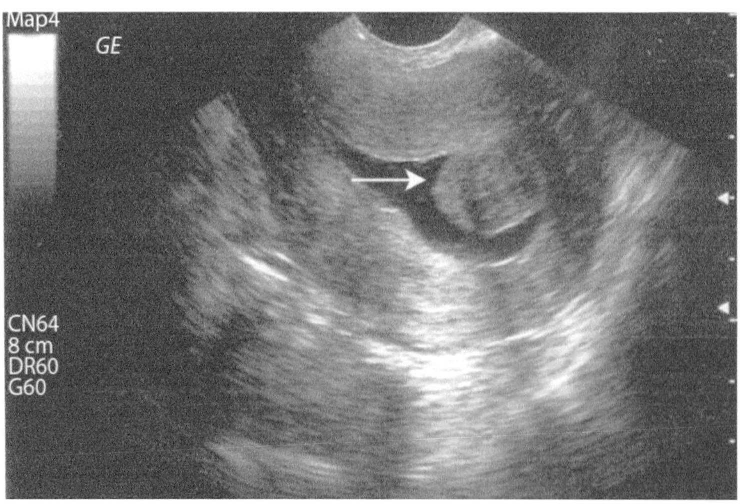

FIGURE 5.12 Sonohysterogram (abnormal cavity). In this image, the injected fluid in the cavity (appearing black) outlines an intracavitary mass, which was later confirmed to be a uterine fibroid.

TABLE 5.1

Normal Sperm Parameters of Semen Analysis (see further ref 48)

Liquefaction Time	15 to 30 minutes
Ejaculate Volume	>1.4 mL
Sperm Concentration	>16 x10^6 spermatozoa/mL
Total Sperm Count	>39 million sperm
Motility	>42% total motility >30% progressive motility
Morphology	>4% normal forms

Non-obstructive azoospermia is caused by either an extremely low level or complete lack of sperm production by the testes. These men typically have low levels of circulating testosterone and are thus unable to achieve normal spermatogenesis. Regardless if the insult is hyper, eu, or hypo gonadotropic in origin, the end result of impaired spermatogenesis is the same. However, the treatment to correct the underlying disorder will be altered.

Hypergonadotropic hypogonadism results from overt testicular failure. This is often associated with either acquired or congenital anatomic defects of the testicles or from chromosomal abnormalities and rearrangements found during Karyotype testing. Genetic deletions within specific regions of the Y-chromosome is another common cause of failed spermatogenesis in the presence of normal testosterone levels. As a result, all men with sperm counts of under 5 million should undergo both Karyotype and Y-chromosome micro-deletion testing. Conversely, hypogonadotropic hypogonadism is common among men with eating and body dysmorphic disorders. Men who routinely overexert themselves with strenuous exercise or those who have central nervous system tumors affecting hypothalamic and pituitary function may have a reversible cause of their azoospermia. Abuse and use of specific medications known to impact spermatogenesis include anabolic steroids, chronic opioid exposure, as well as past or present use of certain chemotherapeutic agents. Eighty percent of all men treated for testicular cancer will resume spermatogenesis within five years following completion of chemotherapy, and only 20% will have permanent azoospermia.

Other diseases and injuries to the testicles which can compromise testicular function include mumps orchitis, testicular torsion, cancer, and uncontrolled long-standing diabetes. The latter is more often

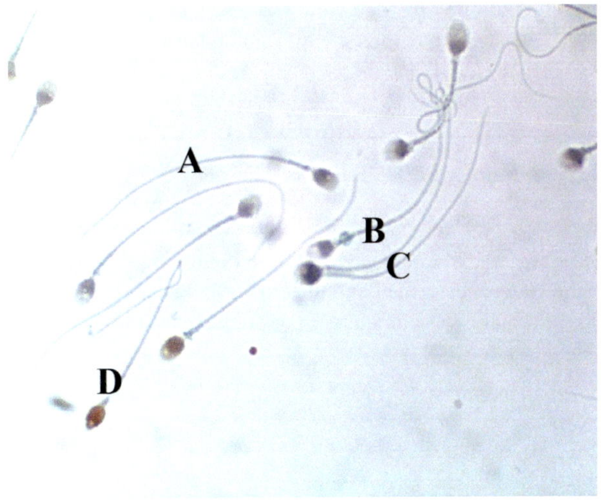

FIGURE 5.13 Examples of varied sperm morphology: (a) normal, (b) midpiece defect, (c) tail defect, and (d) tapered head.

associated with retrograde ejaculation rather than a reduction in spermatogenesis, and sperm can often be retrieved from the bladder during a post-void collection. Testicular Sperm Aspiration (TESA) and Testicular Sperm Extraction (TESE) are two common methods employed to retrieve sperm for men with azoospermia. Even men with overt testicular failure have a 50% chance of retrieving viable sperm for use during an IVF cycle.

All men found to have an abnormal semen analysis should have a repeat semen analysis to confirm the finding. Men with repeatedly abnormal semen samples should undergo hormonal evaluation for FSH, LH, TSH, PRL, Total Testosterone, and estradiol. When sperm counts are continuously below 5 million, genetic testing including a Karyotype, CF with 5T-allele polymorphism analysis, and Y-chromosome micro-deletion testing should also be offered.

One significant addition to the WHO 2021 semen analysis manual is a significant reclassification of several sperm functional assays from "research" to "advanced examinations." These include sperm DNA fragmentation (SDF), sperm aneuploidy, seminal oxidative stress, and reactive oxygen species. Mechanistically, loss of integrity of sperm DNA can significantly reduce sperm's function and potential for fertilization. Oxidative stress sufficient to cause chromatin damage can also significantly reduce a sperm's ability to successfully fertilize an egg. If a sperm with DNA lesions does fertilize, then the chance of a successful offspring depends on whether the oocyte can repair the damage. On a clinical level, SDF has a strong association with infertility; SDF appears to be higher in the semen of infertile men and is associated with both patient conditions (such as varicocele, advanced paternal age, lifestyle, obesity) and environmental factors (radiation exposure). SDF is assessed by several different commercially available tests that evaluate for DNA breaks associated with chromatin damage. The top four tests (TUNEL, SCSA, SCD, and Comet) appear to have good correlation (54). SDF values of thresholds of 20% seem to be able to differentiate between fertile and infertile men, and thresholds between 20–30% have been shown to be able to identify couples requiring a prolonged time to natural pregnancy, lower pregnancy rates by ART, and increased miscarriage.

Although SDF has a high association with infertility, it was not always tested for because the thought was that it could not be treated. However, this is beginning to change. A recent publication by Sperm DNA Fragmentation Study Group reviewed the available evidence to SDF and developed evidence-based guidelines for the application of SDF (55). Data on SDF is growing, although many of the recommendations are still based on Grade B and C evidence. SDF testing is recommended for explanatory purposes in unexplained fertility and for informing couples seeking ART that this may be a limiting factor in their attempts to achieve birth. Varicocele repair can improve SDF, and testing may identify patients who might not otherwise fit the standard indications of varicocele repair (56). Furthermore, it has been found that sperm below threshold could be obtained from the testes of men whose ejaculated sperm is above threshold for SDF (57). SDF testing may thus identify patients for whom ICSI would be an appropriate strategy, potentially over conventional IVF (57).

Conclusion

The causes of infertility can be varied and the infertility evaluation will provide a better understanding of the potential causes. Up to 25% of couples will have a combination of factors. Therefore, it is important that a complete evaluation is performed and the evaluation is not halted after a single abnormal test is encountered. After the evaluation is completed, the couple should be seen in consultation to discuss the results and formulate a treatment plan.

Key Points

- Infertility is a condition characterized by the inability to conceive. Evaluation and treatment can be time-sensitive due to a decline in fecundity with age greater than thirty-five years.
- Ovarian reserve testing comprised of bloodwork and a pelvic ultrasound gives an estimate of oocyte quantity.

- Uterine and fallopian tube assessment is an integral part of infertility evaluation.
- A couple's infertility evaluation should include male fertility evaluation, beginning with a semen analysis.

REFERENCES

1. Practice Committee of the ASRM. Electronic address aao. Definition of infertility: a committee opinion, [internet], 2023: www.asrm.org/practice-guidance/practice-committee-documents/denitions-of-infertility/.
2. ACOG Committee on Gynecologic Practice. Female age-related fertility decline. Committee Opinion 589. *Fertil Steril.* 2014;101(3):633–4.
3. Gnoth C et al. Time to pregnancy: results of the German prospective study and impact on the management of infertility. *Hum Reprod.* 2003;18(9):1959–66.
4. Slama R et al. Estimation of the frequency of involuntary infertility on a nation-wide basis. *Hum Reprod.* 2012;27(5):1489–98.
5. Samplaski MK, Nangia AK. Adverse effects of common medications on male fertility. *Nat Rev Urol.* 2015;12(7):401–13.
6. Romero Gutierrez G, et al. Correlations between hyperprolactinemia and galactorrhea. *Ginecol Obstet Mex.* 1989;57:294–7.
7. VanderLaan B et al. Cost considerations with infertility therapy: outcome and cost comparison between health maintenance organization and preferred provider organization care based on physician and facility cost. *Hum Reprod.* 1998;13(5):1200–5.
8. Charkoudian N, Stachenfeld NS. Reproductive hormone influences on thermoregulation in women. *Compr Physiol.* 2014;4(2):793–804.
9. Kippley J, and Kippley S. The art of natural family planning. *CCL.* 1996;77:298–9.
10. Ferreira-Poblete A. The probability of conception on different days of the cycle with respect to ovulation: an overview. *Adv Contracept.* 1997;13(2–3):83–95.
11. Johnson S et al. Development of the first urinary reproductive hormone ranges referenced to independently determined ovulation day. *Clin Chem Lab Med.* 2015;53(7):1099–108.
12. Miao YL et al. Oocyte aging: cellular and molecular changes, developmental potential and reversal possibility. *Hum Reprod Update.* 2009;15(5):573–85.
13. Wathen NC et al. Interpretation of single progesterone measurement in diagnosis of anovulation and defective luteal phase: observations on analysis of the normal range. *Br Med J (Clin Res Ed).* 1984;288(6410):7–9.
14. Noyes RW et al. Dating the endometrial biopsy. *Am J Obstet Gynecol.* 1975;122(2):262–3.
15. Murray MJ et al. A critical analysis of the accuracy, reproducibility, and clinical utility of histologic endometrial dating in fertile women. *Fertil Steril.* 2004;81(5):1333–43.
16. Mahajan N. Endometrial receptivity array: clinical application. *J Hum Reprod Sci.* 2015;8(3):121–9.
17. Nevins JR, Potti A. Mining gene expression profiles: expression signatures as cancer phenotypes. *Nat Rev Genet.* 2007;8(8):601–9.
18. Doyle N et al. Effect of timing by endometrial receptivity testing vs standard timing of frozen embryo transfer on live birth in patients undergoing in vitro fertilization: a randomized clinical trial. *JAMA.* 2022;328(21):2117–25.
19. Practice Committee of the ASRM. Testing and interpreting measures of ovarian reserve: a committee opinion. *Fertil Steril.* 2015;103(3):e9–17.
20. Lemmen JG et al. The total pregnancy potential per oocyte aspiration after assisted reproduction—in how many cycles are biologically competent oocytes available? *J Assist Reprod Genet.* 2016;33(7):849–54.
21. Demko ZP et al. Effects of maternal age on euploidy rates in a large cohort of embryos analyzed with 24-chromosome single-nucleotide polymorphism-based preimplantation genetic screening. *Fertil Steril.* 2016;105(5):1307–13.
22. Bozkurt B et al. Comparison of age-related changes in anti-Mullerian hormone levels and other ovarian reserve tests between healthy fertile and infertile population. *Hum Fertil (Camb).* 2016;19(3):192–8.

23. Kotanidis L et al. The use of serum anti-Mullerian hormone (AMH) levels and antral follicle count (AFC) to predict the number of oocytes collected and availability of embryos for cryopreservation in IVF. *J Endocrinol Invest.* 2016;39(12):1459–64.
24. Ebner T et al. Basal level of anti-Mullerian hormone is associated with oocyte quality in stimulated cycles. *Hum Reprod.* 2006;21(8):2022–6.
25. Gracia CR et al. Impact of cancer therapies on ovarian reserve. *Fertil Steril.* 2012;97(1):134–40.e1.
26. Rustamov O et al. Effect of salpingectomy, ovarian cystectomy and unilateral salpingo-oopherectomy on ovarian reserve. *Gynecol Surg.* 2016;13:173–8.
27. Kallio S et al. Antimullerian hormone levels decrease in women using combined contraception independently of administration route. *Fertil Steril.* 2013;99(5):1305–10.
28. Chan C, Liu K. Clinical pregnancy in a woman with idiopathic hypogonadotropic hypogonadism and low AMH: utility of ovarian reserve markers in IHH. *J Assist Reprod Genet.* 2014;31(10):1317–21.
29. Jirge PR. Ovarian reserve tests. *J Hum Reprod Sci.* 2011;4(3):108–13.
30. Meczekalski B et al. Fertility in women of late reproductive age: the role of serum anti-Mullerian hormone (AMH) levels in its assessment. *J Endocrinol Invest.* 2016;39(11):1259–65.
31. Ruchelman MW. Solubility studies of estrone in organic solvents using gas-liquid chromatography. *Anal Biochem.* 1967;19(1):98–108.
32. Csemiczky G et al. Predictive power of clomiphene citrate challenge test for failure of in vitro fertilization treatment. *Acta Obstet Gynecol Scand.* 2002;81(10):954–61.
33. Yen S et al., eds. *Reproductive Endocrinology.* W.B. Saunders; 1999.
34. Broeze KA et al. Are patient characteristics associated with the accuracy of hysterosalpingography in diagnosing tubal pathology? An individual patient data meta-analysis. *Hum Reprod Update.* 2011;17(3):293–300.
35. Soares SR et al. Diagnostic accuracy of sonohysterography, transvaginal sonography, and hysterosalpingography in patients with uterine cavity diseases. *Fertil Steril.* 2000;73(2):406–11.
36. Johnson NP et al. The FLUSH trial–flushing with lipiodol for unexplained (and endometriosis-related) subfertility by hysterosalpingography: a randomized trial. *Hum Reprod.* 2004;19(9):2043–51.
37. Steiner AZ et al. Oil-soluble contrast during hysterosalpingography in women with proven tubal patency. *Obstet Gynecol.* 2003;101(1):109–13.
38. Rasmussen F et al. Therapeutic effect of hysterosalpingography: oil- versus water-soluble contrast media—a randomized prospective study. *Radiology.* 1991;179(1):75–8.
39. Watson A et al. A meta-analysis of the therapeutic role of oil soluble contrast media at hysterosalpingography: a surprising result? *Fertil Steril.* 1994;61(3):470–7.
40. Vandekerckhove P et al. Oil-soluble versus water-soluble media for assessing tubal patency with hysterosalpingography or laparoscopy in subfertile women. *Cochrane Database Syst Rev.* 2000;1996(2):CD000092.
41. de Pablo MA, Alvarez de Cienfuegos G. Modulatory effects of dietary lipids on immune system functions. *Immunol Cell Biol.* 2000;78(1):31–9.
42. DeCherney AH et al. Increased pregnancy rate with oil-soluble hysterosalpingography dye. *Fertil Steril.* 1980;33(4):407–10.
43. Seshadri S et al. Diagnostic accuracy of saline infusion sonography in the evaluation of uterine cavity abnormalities prior to assisted reproductive techniques: a systematic review and meta-analyses. *Hum Reprod Update.* 2015;21(2):262–74.
44. Bosteels J et al. The effectiveness of hysteroscopy in improving pregnancy rates in subfertile women without other gynaecological symptoms: a systematic review. *Hum Reprod Update.* 2010;16(1):1–11.
45. Thonneau P et al. Incidence and main causes of infertility in a resident population (1,850,000) of three French regions (1988–1989). *Hum Reprod.* 1991;6(6):811–6.
46. Calvert JK et al. The male infertility evaluation still matters in the era of high efficacy assisted reproductive technology. *Fertil Steril.* 2022;118(1):34–46.
47. Kolettis PN, Sabanegh ES. Significant medical pathology discovered during a male infertility evaluation. *J Urol.* 2001;166(1):178–80.
48. WHO. *WHO Laboratory Manual for the Examination of Human Semen and Sperm-Cervical Mucus Interaction*, 6th edn. Geneva: World Health Organization; 2021.
49. Esteves SC. Evolution of the World Health Organization semen analysis manual: where are we? *Nat Rev Urol.* 2022;19(7):439–46.

50. Glazer CH et al. Racial and sociodemographic differences of semen parameters among US men undergoing a semen analysis. *Urology.* 2019;123:126–32.
51. Guzick DS et al. Sperm morphology, motility, and concentration in fertile and infertile men. *N Engl J Med* 2001;345:1388–93.
52. Nieschlag E et al. Surgical ligation vs. angiographic embolization of the vena spermatica: a prospective randomized study for the treatment of varicocele-related infertility. *Andrologia.* 1993;25(5):233–7.
53. Oates RD, Amos JA. The genetic basis of congenital bilateral absence of the vas deferens and cystic fibrosis. *J Androl.* 1994;15(1):1–8.
54. Javed A et al. Evaluation of sperm DNA fragmentation using multiple methods: a comparison of their predictive power for male infertility. *Clin Exp Reprod Med.* 2019;46(1):14–21.
55. Esteves SC et al. Sperm DNA fragmentation testing: summary evidence and clinical practice recommendations. *Andrologia.* 2021;53(2):e13874.
56. Lara-Cerrillo S et al. Microsurgical varicocelectomy effect on sperm telomere length, DNA fragmentation and seminal parameters. *Hum Fertil (Camb).* 2022;25(1):135–41.
57. Zhao J et al. Whether sperm deoxyribonucleic acid fragmentation has an effect on pregnancy and miscarriage after in vitro fertilization/intracytoplasmic sperm injection: a systematic review and meta-analysis. *Fertil Steril.* 2014;102(4):998–1005.e8.

6

Ovarian Reserve Testing

Antonio La Marca and Valeria Donno

Introduction

Female fertility undergoes a gradual and inexorable decline with advancing chronological age. Studies based on the fertility of different populations and the success of *in vitro* fertilization techniques across various age groups leave no room for doubt. The natural aging process of the reproductive system varies significantly from woman to woman and appears to be largely linked to changes in ovarian function.

The function of the ovaries is, in fact, dependent on the activity of the follicles contained within the ovarian cortex. Ovarian follicles form during embryonic life and remain quiescent in the form of primordial follicles until puberty. After puberty, a small number of primordial follicles resume the process of oogenesis each day, transforming into preantral follicles. Under the influence of pituitary FSH, a portion of these follicles cyclically progresses to the antral phase. Among them, a dominant follicle grows and matures, leading to the release of a mature oocyte (ovulation) and the formation of the corpus luteum. Meanwhile, the remaining follicles that initiated the maturation process undergo degeneration (atresia). Before and after ovulation, the follicle's maturing cells surrounding the oocyte (granulosa cells and theca cells) are responsible for the cyclic production of estrogen and progesterone, which characterize the menstrual cycle during a woman's reproductive years.

The number of primordial follicles in a woman's ovaries at a given time is referred to as "ovarian reserve," as it effectively represents the functional reserve of the organ. This number progressively decreases with age until reaching menopause, marking the point in life when the ovaries cease their function.

The reduction in the number of follicles over time, with aging, also correlates with a decrease in the quality of the oocytes they contain. This decline results in gradual changes in hormonal production, menstrual cycle regularity, and fertility.

The measurement of ovarian reserve has gained extraordinary importance in reproductive medicine. It allows, with a certain degree of approximation, the prediction of menopausal age, the transition from fertile to subfertile and eventually infertile periods, thus providing insights into the duration of reproductive life. In the context of assisted reproductive technology (ART), as we will explore, assessing ovarian reserve provides indications not only on the likelihood of treatment success but also on the type of response (normal, poor, or excessive) that the patient may have to drugs administered for ovarian stimulation. This information enables the optimization of clinical management for these patients.

The Ovarian Reserve and Reproductive Aging

Each woman receives her endowment of follicles during fetal life. In the fourth month of intrauterine life, the ovaries contain 6–7 million oocytes surrounded by a single layer of granulosa cells, constituting the pool of primordial follicles. Due to the abrupt loss of primordial follicles through apoptosis in the second

 DOI: 10.1201/9781003460275-6

half of fetal life, only 1–2 million primordial follicles remain at birth within the ovarian cortex (1). After birth, the loss of follicles slows down so that at menarche, there are still between 300,000 to 400,000 primordial follicles. Throughout the reproductive period, there is a continuous and gradual decline in this number, with an acceleration around the age of 37–38. When menopause is reached, the ovarian pool finally amounts to less than 1,000 follicles, unresponsive to FSH stimulation.

It should be emphasized, however, that the age-related decline in the ovarian follicular pool, which certainly affects all women, does not occur in the same way for everyone. For any given age, the estimate of primordial follicles, and therefore, ovarian reserve, falls within an extremely variable range.

The decrease in the number of follicles is not the sole contributor to the decline in reproductive system performance with aging. There is also a simultaneous reduction in the quality of the oocytes contained in the follicles (2). Oocytes of older women are of poorer quality due to the frequent presence of chromosomal abnormalities. It is unclear whether this is due to an increase in meiotic segregation errors in normal disomic oocytes or the presence of trisomic oocytes inherited from fetal life. In any case, the increased frequency of aneuploidy in the mature oocyte and consequently in the embryo are major causes of embryo implantation failure or early miscarriage, conditions that are notably increased in women of advanced reproductive age.

Ovarian aging also results in a reduction in the quality and quantity of granulosa cells. *In vitro*, granulosa cells from older women show reduced steroid and glycoprotein production, decreased mitotic activity, increased apoptosis, and reduced in vivo production of IGF-1. These alterations in granulosa cell function can themselves be a cause of compromised oocyte maturation.

The consequence of profound changes in the number of follicles and the quality of oocytes during the third and fourth decades of life is that female fertility decreases significantly and is clinically detectable. Population studies demonstrate that the loss of natural fertility (represented by maternal age at the last pregnancy) occurs at an average age of 41, with a range from 23 to 51 years.

As age advances, the low number of follicles and the decreased function of granulosa cells lead to irregularities in menstrual cycle regularity. This stage of reproductive aging is called the menopausal transition and lasts until the last menstruation. The onset of the menopausal transition occurs around the age of 46, with a range from 34 to 54 years. The last menstrual flow (menopause) can only be established retrospectively and occurs at an average age of 51, with a range from 40 to 60 years.

Markers of Ovarian Reserve

The compromise of ovarian reserve becomes clinically evident only in advanced stages, typically characterized by signs such as shortened menstrual cycles or irregularities. Nevertheless, various clinical, hormonal, and ultrasound markers enable the estimation of declining follicle numbers even before the onset of perimenopausal symptoms. It's crucial to note that these ovarian reserve markers primarily indicate quantity rather than quality or fertility. For instance, women with low ovarian reserve possess a similar likelihood of live birth rate (LBR) as women of the same age with higher anti-Müllerian hormone (AMH) values.

FSH

The follicle-stimulating hormone (FSH) is the hormonal marker of ovarian reserve that has been known for a long time and has been widely used in the past. It is an indirect marker since the pituitary release of FSH varies based on the feedback from inhibin B and estradiol produced by the cells in the follicles. As FSH levels vary in different phases of the menstrual cycle, measuring baseline values must be done in the early follicular phase for reproducibility. FSH, measured on the 2nd–5th day of the menstrual cycle, physiologically increases with a woman's age. Studies on large datasets have shown that in the population of women with mild infertility factors, spontaneous pregnancy occurs more frequently in women with FSH values <8 IU/L compared to women of similar age but with higher FSH values, and the probability of spontaneous pregnancy within 12 months decreases as the baseline FSH increases.

In assisted reproductive technology (ART), where ovarian reserve correlates with treatment response, a baseline FSH higher than 10 IU/mL may predict a poor response of the ovary to stimulation therapy. Some authors report that a cutoff of 15 IU/L, in addition to predicting ovarian response to hormonal stimulation, also allows for predicting, with a certain statistical approximation, the likelihood of success or failure in reproductive outcomes after ART application. From a practical standpoint, any reasonable cutoff can be adopted in daily clinical use; however, the higher the chosen cutoff, the lower the sensitivity and the higher the specificity.

It should be considered that FSH values >8–10 IU/L are frequently encountered in the female population around the age of 40. In these cases, FSH measurement adds limited information for the clinician compared to what can be deduced based on the woman's age. Detecting high FSH levels in young women is indeed indicative of reduced ovarian reserve compared to expected values for age; however, numerous studies demonstrate that in young patients with diminished ovarian reserve, the probability of pregnancy after ART remains acceptable, albeit reduced compared to the average probability estimated solely based on age.

It is still unclear whether patients over 40 with non-elevated FSH levels can have a better reproductive outcome compared to their peers with physiologically "skewed" FSH. FSH should be considered a more quantitative than a qualitative marker of ovarian reserve. Another issue related to FSH measurement is its wide inter-cycle variability. FSH variations between one follicular phase and another are reported to be greater than 50% of the measured value, inevitably reducing the overall predictive performance of this marker. For all these reasons, FSH alone cannot be used to exclude couples from assisted reproductive programs, and in recent years, studies have led to the use of other, more precise markers when estimating ovarian reserve for the management of patients undergoing ART.

Furthermore, it has been suggested that the measurement of baseline FSH should not be part of routine tests for a subfertile woman if she has regular cycles, as approximately half of women with high baseline FSH values and regular cycles still conceive (3).

Estradiol

The determination of baseline estradiol values had been proposed as a predictor of ovarian response to stimulation *in vitro* fertilization cycles, as one study reported that estradiol values higher than 60 pg/mL are associated with a higher percentage of canceled cycles due to poor ovarian response and cycles with a low oocyte retrieval rate (4). However, subsequent studies have not confirmed the significance of this correlation, much less the ability of estradiol values to predict the likelihood of achieving pregnancy in assisted reproductive technology (ART) (5).

Currently, the role of this marker is limited to facilitating a proper interpretation of the third-day FSH value. Since FSH is inhibited by estradiol produced by ovarian follicles in women with poor ovarian reserve, it may falsely appear regular if associated with a very high serum estradiol level.

Inhibin B

Inhibin B is a dimeric polypeptide predominantly secreted during the follicular phase by granulosa cells of antral follicles and has been studied as a marker of ovarian reserve. However, it has been observed that, due to the site of production, inhibin B reflects ovarian activity at a given moment rather than the ovarian reserve, leading to significant intra-cycle variability. Several studies have reported that inhibin B has limited value in predicting ovarian response or the likelihood of pregnancy after controlled ovarian stimulation (6). Finally, the demonstration that inhibin B levels deviate grossly from the curve defining the age-related decline of primordial follicles discourages its use as a marker of ovarian reserve.

Anti-Müllerian Hormone (AMH)

Anti-Müllerian hormone (AMH) is a dimeric glycoprotein exclusively produced by granulosa cells of preantral (primary and secondary) and small antral follicles. AMH production begins when primordial follicles progress to the primary follicle stage and continue until the follicles reach diameters of 8–10 mm (7). AMH's main actions in the ovary are the inhibition of recruitment from the pool of primordial follicles and the inhibition of follicular growth induced by FSH. Although AMH primarily acts through autocrine and paracrine mechanisms, it can also be measured in the serum. Pathological studies have shown that the number of small antral follicles is directly correlated with the primordial follicle pool and, therefore, ovarian reserve. As ovarian reserve decreases with aging, the number of produced antral follicles and serum AMH levels decrease, becoming nearly undetectable near menopause (8). It is now recognized that serum AMH levels are a direct marker of the quantitative ovarian reserve of patients and can provide an indication of the response to ovarian stimulation in assisted reproductive technology (ART) cycles and the age of menopause. In women with various degrees of hypogonadotropic hypogonadism, AMH appears to be the best indicator that reflects the loss of follicles and is likely the best marker for premature ovarian insufficiency (POI). Conversely, serum AMH is two to four times higher in women with polycystic ovary syndrome (PCOS) than in normal ovulatory women due to the high number of antral follicles in their ovaries. There is ongoing discussion about the possibility of including AMH among the diagnostic criteria for PCOS. Lastly, AMH seems to be an excellent predictor of reproductive potential post-chemotherapy in women with neoplastic diseases. The existence of nomograms representing the decline in serum AMH levels in the general population allows the physician to provide scientifically accurate information to the patient about the normal hormone range for age relative to individual data (8). The clinical use of AMH as a marker of ovarian reserve has been strongly advocated in recent years in the field of ART due to a vast body of scientific evidence uniformly highlighting the high correlation of circulating AMH with ovarian response to stimulation with exogenous gonadotropins, particularly with the number of retrieved oocytes. The literature reports a range of cutoff values varying between 0.7 and 1.3 ng/ml, below which poor response, i.e., a weak ovarian response to stimulation with exogenous FSH, is predicted with more than acceptable performance (9). For lower AMH values (<0.4 ng/ml), an absent ovarian response to FSH with subsequent cycle cancellation is more likely. Conversely, AMH values >3.5 ng/ml allow for predicting hyper-response, i.e., excessive ovarian response to stimulation, with good sensitivity and specificity (9). In the past, several studies, often limited to small casuistries, did not find good predictive capacity of AMH for the ultimate success of ART, i.e., pregnancy and live birth.

Moreover, some authorities have reported a higher percentage of pregnancies and births in patients with high AMH values compared to their peers with low concentrations of the same hormone. The association between AMH and live birth rates after ART may be related to the high correlation between serum hormone levels and the number of oocytes retrieved at pick-up rather than their better quality (10). Certainly, the correlation between AMH and the quality of ovarian reserve will be a relevant research focus in the immediate future. In favor of this marker, it is worth noting its low intra- and inter-cycle variability. The majority of studies confirm that AMH is relatively stable, and therefore, it can be measured at any time during the cycle (11). It should be remembered, however, that AMH levels significantly decrease reversibly during hormonal contraception and pregnancy. Against AMH, we recall problems related to assay kits, which have evolved from old immunoassay-based IOT and DSL kits to the more recent AMH GenII, which continued to generate discrepancies in measured serum concentrations and poor inter-laboratory comparability. These issues should now be resolved with the introduction of fully automated assay systems (Elecsys and Access), which should ensure repeatability of measured values and excellent reliability.

Antral Follicular Count (AFC)

In each menstrual cycle, a small portion of follicles develops beyond 2 mm in diameter and reaches the stage of preantral and then antral follicles. These follicles are referred to as "recruitable" as they are highly sensitive and responsive to FSH, and they can be visualized and measured with transvaginal ultrasound. Antral follicle count (AFC) refers to the total number of antral follicles between 2 and 10 mm in both ovaries. This follicular pool is the same one that produces AMH and, as mentioned earlier, is correlated with the number of primordial follicles and, consequently, ovarian reserve. Therefore, a strong correlation exists between AFC and AMH values, and although cases are reported where the values of the two markers are discordant (which may be due, for example, to the fact that ultrasound may not detect smaller follicles capable of producing AMH, or conversely, may not reveal the possible atresia of granulosa cells in follicles, which affects AMH production), in general, the performance of AFC and AMH in estimating quantitative ovarian reserve appears to be comparable. Like AMH, AFC decreases with increasing age of women due to the reduction in the pool of primordial follicles and, consequently, antral follicles. Nomograms for AFC with age-related reference values expressed in centiles are available in the literature (12).

AFC shows low inter-cycle variability; however, its intra-cycle variability remains significant, and for this reason, it should be measured in the early stages of the menstrual cycle (unlike AMH, which can be measured at any phase of the cycle). The main problem with measuring this marker lies in its considerable intra- and inter-observer variability, as the measurement depends on the ultrasound examination, which is known to be highly operator-dependent. This variability can be partially reduced with proper training of operators involved in the measurement and the use of recent 3D automated ultrasound counting techniques.

AFC is undoubtedly one of the most widely used ovarian reserve markers in clinical practice. This popularity is primarily due to the ease of transvaginal ultrasound use in all assisted reproductive technology (ART) centers and, secondarily, to the recognized strong correlation between AFC and the number of oocytes retrieved after ovarian stimulation. AFC is also capable of predicting extremes of ovarian response (poor response and hyper-response). In particular, the optimal cutoff for predicting poor ovarian response seems to be an AFC <5–7 (13), while to identify women at risk of hyper-response and ovarian hyperstimulation syndrome (OHSS), it seems appropriate to choose cutoff values between >9 and >16 (14).

The association between AFC and live birth rate following ART remains controversial. However, as with AMH, it has been suggested that the higher live birth rate observed in women with high AFC may be attributed more to the increased number of oocytes retrieved during pick-up rather than to superior oocyte quality.

Key Points

- Female fertility diminishes as age advances, primarily due to a gradual decline in ovarian reserve, characterized by a reduction in the number of primordial follicles and oocyte quality.
- Ovarian reserve markers are valuable for quantitatively assessing the decline in female fertility. However, it's important to note that these markers primarily reflect quantity and do not directly indicate oocyte quality or infertility.
- Ovarian reserve can be assessed through various markers, including FSH, estradiol, inhibin B, anti-Müllerian hormone (AMH), and antral follicle count (AFC). Among these, AMH and AFC are the most commonly employed.
- The measurement of ovarian reserve, particularly AMH and AFC, plays a pivotal role in assisted reproductive technology (ART), providing insights into treatment success and optimizing clinical management.

REFERENCES

1. Markström E et al. Survival factors regulating ovarian apoptosis—dependence on follicle differentiation. *Reproduction*. 2002;123(1):23–30.
2. te Velde ER, Pearson PL. The variability of female reproductive aging. *Hum Reprod Update*. 2002;8(2):141–54.
3. van Montfrans JM et al. Predictive value of basal follicle-stimulating hormone concentrations in a general subfertility population. *Fertil Steril*. 2000;74:97–103.
4. Evers JL et al. Elevated levels of basal estradiol-17beta predict poor response in patients with normal basal levels of follicle-stimulating hormone undergoing in vitro fertilization. *Fertil Steril*. 1998;69:1010–14.

5. Scott RT et al. Follicle-stimulating hormone levels on cycle day 3 are predictive of in vitro fertilization outcome. *Fertil Steril*. 1989;51:651–654
6. Broekmans FJ et al. A systematic review of tests predicting ovarian reserve and IVF outcome. *Hum Reprod Update*. 2006;12:685–718.
7. La Marca A, Volpe A. Anti-Mullerian hormone (AMH) in female reproduction: is measurement of circulating AMH a useful tool? *Clin Endocrinol (Oxf)*. 2006;64:603–10.
8. La Marca A et al. Normal serum anti-Mullerian hormone levels in the general female population and the relationship with reproductive history. *Eur J Obstet Gynecol Reprod Biol*. 2012;163(2):180–4.
9. La Marca A, Sunkara SK. Individualization of controlled ovarian stimulation in IVF using ovarian reserve markers: from theory to practice. *Hum Reprod Update*. 2014;20:124–40.
10. Arce JC et al. Antimullerian hormone in gonadotropin releasing-hormone antagonist cycles: prediction of ovarian response and cumulative treatment outcome in good-prognosis patients. *Fertil Steril*. 2013;99:1644–53.
11. La Marca A et al. Anti-Mullerian hormone measurement on any day of the menstrual cycle strongly predicts ovarian response in assisted reproductive technology. *Hum Reprod*. 2007;22:766–71.
12. La Marca A et al. Age specific nomogram for the decline in antral follicle count throughout the reproductive period. *Fertil Steril*. 2011;95:684–8.
13. Ferraretti AP et al. ESHRE consensus on the definition of 'poor response' to ovarian stimulation for in vitro fertilization: the Bologna criteria. *Hum Reprod*. 2011;26:1616–24.
14. Broer SL et al. AMH and AFC as predictors of excessive response in controlled ovarian hyperstimulation: a meta-analysis. *Hum Reprod Update*. 2011;17(1):46–54.

7

Hypothyroidism and Its Role in Infertility and Recurrent Pregnancy Loss

Sara Arian

Hypothyroidism

Causes

Hypothyroidism is a condition marked by insufficient production of thyroid hormones by the thyroid gland. The most prevalent cause of hypothyroidism is autoimmune thyroiditis, specifically Hashimoto's thyroiditis, which is the most common cause of primary hypothyroidism. In Hashimoto's thyroiditis, the immune system produces antibodies against thyroid proteins, such as thyroid peroxidase (TPO) and thyroglobulin, leading to the gradual destruction of thyroid tissue.

In addition to autoimmune causes, hypothyroidism can also result from iatrogenic factors, such as surgical removal of the thyroid gland (thyroidectomy) or radioactive iodine therapy, both of which are common treatments for hyperthyroidism and thyroid cancer.

Medications can also induce hypothyroidism. Drugs such as lithium, commonly used in the treatment of bipolar disorder, can inhibit thyroid hormone release and synthesis. Amiodarone, an antiarrhythmic medication, has a high iodine content, which can disrupt thyroid function, leading to hypothyroidism. Additionally, iodine deficiency or excess can impair thyroid hormone production. Iodine is a critical component of thyroid hormones, and both insufficient and excessive iodine intake can lead to thyroid dysfunction.[1] Congenital hypothyroidism, present from birth, is another important cause. This condition is often due to thyroid dysgenesis (abnormal development of the thyroid gland) or dyshormonogenesis (defects in thyroid hormone synthesis).[2]

Clinical Presentation

The clinical presentation of hypothyroidism is often subtle and nonspecific, making it a challenge to diagnose, especially in its early stages. The symptoms result from the body's metabolic processes slowing down due to the lack of thyroid hormones. Common symptoms of hypothyroidism include fatigue, weight gain, and cold intolerance. Patients often report feeling tired and sluggish, even after adequate rest and may struggle with unexplained weight gain despite no changes in diet or physical activity. Cold intolerance is another hallmark symptom, with patients feeling unusually sensitive to cold temperatures. Dermatologic manifestations include dry, rough skin, brittle nails, and hair loss. These symptoms are the result of decreased circulation and reduced activity of the sebaceous and sweat glands, leading to dry skin. Cardiovascular symptoms are significant in hypothyroidism. Patients may experience bradycardia (a slower-than-normal heart rate), which can lead to fatigue and exercise intolerance. Hypothyroidism is also associated with dyslipidemia, characterized by elevated levels of LDL cholesterol and triglycerides, increasing the risk of atherosclerosis and cardiovascular disease. Neurological symptoms are also

DOI: 10.1201/9781003460275-7

present in hypothyroidism, including cognitive decline, memory impairment, mood swings, and depression. These symptoms, often described as "brain fog," can significantly affect a patient's quality of life and may lead to misdiagnosis as a primary psychiatric disorder.

Reproductive health is notably affected by hypothyroidism, particularly in women. Menstrual irregularities, such as oligomenorrhea (infrequent menstruation) or amenorrhea (absence of menstruation), are common. These irregularities are due to the impact of hypothyroidism on the hypothalamic-pituitary-ovarian axis, leading to disruptions in gonadotropin release and ovarian function. As a result, women with hypothyroidism may experience difficulties with ovulation, contributing to infertility. However, current evidence does not support routine testing for antithyroid antibodies in the evaluation of male or female infertility, and widespread testing is not recommended without specific clinical indications that would justify their assessment.[3] Furthermore, hypothyroidism is associated with an increased risk of recurrent pregnancy loss (RPL). This is thought to be due to the thyroid's role in maintaining a healthy endometrium and supporting early pregnancy through adequate levels of thyroid hormones.

Endometrial Development

For successful implantation and the maintenance of early pregnancy, the endometrium must be receptive. This receptivity is partly regulated by a delicate balance of hormones, including estrogen, progesterone, and thyroid hormones. Thyroid hormones, particularly T3, have direct and indirect effects on the endometrium. They enhance the expression of certain genes and proteins involved in endometrial growth, differentiation, and vascularization.

Progesterone Production

After ovulation, the corpus luteum (the structure that forms from the collapsed follicle that releases the oocyte) produces progesterone. This hormone is crucial for maintaining the endometrium and creating a conducive environment for the embryo to implant and grow. Thyroid hormones indirectly influence progesterone production by supporting the function of the corpus luteum. Hypothyroidism can result in luteal phase defects, where the endometrium is not properly maintained, increasing the risk of implantation failure or early pregnancy loss and recurrent miscarriages.

Immune Modulation

Thyroid hormones also play a role in modulating the immune environment within the uterus.[4] During early pregnancy, the maternal immune system must tolerate the semi-allogeneic fetus (the embryo, which is genetically distinct from the mother). Thyroid hormones contribute to this immune tolerance by regulating the expression of immune-modulatory molecules and cytokines in the endometrium.

Vascularization and Blood Flow

The thyroid hormones are also involved in the regulation of blood flow to the uterus.[5] They promote angiogenesis (the formation of new blood vessels) within the endometrium, ensuring that the developing embryo receives adequate oxygen and nutrients. In hypothyroidism, reduced thyroid hormone levels can impair this process, leading to a poorly vascularized endometrium that is less capable of supporting an implanted embryo.

Placental Function

As pregnancy progresses, the placenta takes over the production of hormones necessary to sustain pregnancy. Adequate thyroid hormone levels are important for the proper development and function of the placenta.[6] They influence placental growth, nutrient transfer, and the secretion of hormones like human chorionic gonadotropin (hCG) and progesterone.

Thyroid disorders, including overt hypothyroidism and hyperthyroidism, may influence sperm production, though they are not definitively linked to male infertility. Some experts still advocate testing for thyroid dysfunction during infertility assessments. In hyperthyroidism, total testosterone levels may be elevated, but free testosterone can be low, often accompanied by high FSH and LH levels and reduced sperm motility. However, mild or subclinical thyroid issues generally do not appear to affect male fertility.

Diagnosis

Diagnosing hypothyroidism involves several laboratory tests, with serum TSH measurement being the most sensitive initial test.[7] In primary hypothyroidism, TSH levels are elevated due to decreased feedback inhibition from low circulating thyroid hormones. The hypothalamus responds to low thyroid hormone levels by increasing the release of thyrotropin-releasing hormone (TRH), which in turn stimulates the pituitary gland to secrete more TSH. However, the thyroid gland's impaired ability to produce thyroid hormones leads to persistently high TSH levels.

Free T4, the active form of thyroxine, is typically low in hypothyroidism. Measuring free T4 provides a direct assessment of thyroid hormone levels in the blood, confirming the diagnosis of hypothyroidism when TSH is elevated.

In cases of suspected autoimmune thyroiditis, measurement of antithyroid antibodies, such as anti-TPO and antithyroglobulin antibodies, can help confirm the diagnosis.[8] These antibodies are often elevated in Hashimoto's thyroiditis, reflecting the underlying autoimmune process.

Some studies suggest that using targeted screening for thyroid dysfunction in women at high risk for thyroid or autoimmune diseases may fail to detect up to one-third of cases with subclinical or overt hypothyroidism (TSH >3.5 to 4.2 mU/L). However, prospective trials comparing universal screening with targeted screening or no screening found no significant improvement in pregnancy outcomes.

Management

The mainstay of hypothyroidism treatment is levothyroxine, a synthetic form of thyroid hormone thyroxine (T4). The dose of levothyroxine is individualized based on the patient's TSH levels, body weight, age, and the presence of comorbid conditions, such as cardiovascular disease.

The goal of treatment is to maintain TSH within the reference range, typically between 0.5 and 2.5 mIU/L for most patients, though individual targets may vary. In pregnant women or those planning to conceive, stricter TSH targets may be necessary to optimize reproductive outcomes and reduce the risk of pregnancy complications. Monitoring is typically done every 6 to 12 weeks after initiating or adjusting therapy until stable TSH levels are achieved. Once stable, annual monitoring is generally sufficient.

Hypothyroidism and Recurrent Pregnancy Loss

Hypothyroidism is a well-established cause of infertility and recurrent pregnancy loss. The hormonal imbalance caused by hypothyroidism can disrupt the normal function of the hypothalamic-pituitary-ovarian axis, leading to anovulation (lack of ovulation) and luteal phase defects. Anovulation occurs because the lack of thyroid hormones affects the release of gonadotropins, particularly luteinizing hormone (LH), which is necessary for the release of an egg during the menstrual cycle.

Untreated hypothyroidism during pregnancy is associated with an increased risk of miscarriage, preterm birth, preeclampsia, and impaired fetal development, including cognitive impairments. Therefore, it is crucial to diagnose and treat hypothyroidism in women of reproductive age, particularly those with a history of infertility or recurrent pregnancy loss (RPL). Levothyroxine therapy can restore normal ovulation and menstrual function, improving the chances of conception and reducing the risk of miscarriage.

In women with subclinical hypothyroidism (elevated TSH with normal free T4), treatment with levothyroxine is also recommended, particularly in those with TSH levels above 4.0 mIU/L or those planning to conceive.

One study found that maternal free T4 levels below the 2.5th percentile, even with normal TSH, were not linked to negative pregnancy outcomes. However, data from the FaSTER consortium (First- and Second-Trimester Evaluation of Risk for aneuploidy) showed that women with hypothyroxinemia and normal TSH had a higher risk of preterm labor, macrosomia, and gestational diabetes. Similarly, the Generation R Study[9] reported an increased risk of preterm delivery in women with hypothyroxinemia compared to euthyroid women.

Hyperthyroidism and Its Role in Infertility and Recurrent Pregnancy Loss

Causes

The most common cause of hyperthyroidism is Graves' disease, an autoimmune disorder where thyroid-stimulating immunoglobulins (TSI) bind to and activate the TSH receptor on the thyroid gland.[10] This leads to uncontrolled thyroid hormone production and thyroid gland enlargement (goiter).

Other causes of hyperthyroidism include toxic multinodular goiter, where multiple autonomously functioning thyroid nodules produce excess thyroid hormones independent of TSH regulation. This condition is more common in older adults and regions with iodine deficiency.

Thyroiditis, an inflammatory condition of the thyroid gland, can also cause hyperthyroidism. In thyroiditis, thyroid hormone stored in the thyroid gland is released into the bloodstream due to glandular damage, leading to transient hyperthyroidism. Subtypes of thyroiditis include subacute thyroiditis (often following a viral infection) and postpartum thyroiditis, which occurs after pregnancy.

Exogenous thyroid hormone intake, either accidentally or intentionally, can cause hyperthyroidism.

Trophoblastic disease, including molar pregnancy and choriocarcinoma, can lead to hyperthyroidism through the production of high levels of human chorionic gonadotropin (hCG). hCG can mimic TSH and stimulate the thyroid gland to produce excess thyroid hormones.

Clinical Presentation

The clinical presentation of hyperthyroidism reflects the hypermetabolic state induced by excess thyroid hormones. General symptoms include unexplained weight loss, despite an increased appetite. Patients may report feeling unusually warm or intolerant to heat, even in cool environments. Hyperthyroidism also leads to excessive sweating and frequent bowel movements.

Cardiovascular manifestations are prominent in hyperthyroidism. Patients may experience palpitations, tachycardia (rapid heart rate), and, in severe cases, atrial fibrillation, which increases the risk of stroke.[11] These symptoms result from the increased adrenergic activity caused by excess thyroid hormones. Neurological symptoms include tremors, anxiety, irritability, and hyperreflexia (exaggerated reflexes). Patients may also report difficulty concentrating and insomnia. These symptoms are due to the stimulatory effects of thyroid hormones on the central nervous system. Dermatologic findings include warm, moist skin and hair thinning. Onycholysis, or separation of the nail from the nail bed, can also occur. In Graves' disease, patients may present with specific eye findings, such as exophthalmos (protrusion of the eyes), which is a result of inflammation and swelling of the tissues behind the eyes.

Hyperthyroidism also significantly impacts reproductive health. Women with hyperthyroidism may experience menstrual irregularities, such as oligomenorrhea (infrequent menstruation) or amenorrhea (absence of menstruation).

In addition to menstrual irregularities, hyperthyroidism is associated with an increased risk of miscarriage. This risk is likely due to the effects of excess thyroid hormones on the endometrium and luteal phase. The endometrium may become inhospitable for implantation, or the luteal phase may be shortened, leading to early pregnancy loss.

Effects on the Endometrium

For successful implantation, the endometrium must be in an optimal state, both structurally and functionally, to support the embryo. This involves appropriate thickness, vascularization, and a receptive cellular environment.[12] Excess thyroid hormones can alter the expression of certain genes and proteins that are crucial for endometrial receptivity. These hormones influence the balance of estrogen and progesterone, which are the primary regulators of endometrial development. The endometrial cells may not undergo the necessary changes (decidualization) required to support the embryo, leading to implantation failure or early pregnancy loss.

Altered Immune Environment

The immune environment within the endometrium is critical for the successful implantation of an embryo. Normally, the immune system is modulated to allow the embryo, which is genetically distinct from the mother, to implant and grow without being attacked. However, hyperthyroidism can disrupt this immune modulation by altering cytokine profiles and immune cell activity within the endometrium. This can create an environment that is either too inflammatory or not supportive enough for the embryo, increasing the risk of miscarriage.

Impaired Vascularization

Adequate blood supply to the endometrium is essential for supporting the growing embryo after implantation. Hyperthyroidism can affect the vascularization of the endometrium by influencing the production of angiogenic factors—proteins that promote the growth of new blood vessels.

Shortened Luteal Phase

In hyperthyroidism, excessive levels of thyroid hormones can disrupt the normal functioning of the corpus luteum. This disruption can lead to a shortened luteal phase, known as luteal phase defect. A shortened luteal phase means that progesterone levels drop sooner than they should, causing the endometrium to shed prematurely. This premature shedding can lead to the loss of an implanted embryo, resulting in an early miscarriage. Thyroid imbalance, hypo- or hyper-, can interfere with reproductive health by shortening the luteal phase, which may impact the ability to sustain a fertilized egg.[13]

Inadequate Progesterone Production

Even if the luteal phase is not shortened, hyperthyroidism can still interfere with progesterone production by the corpus luteum. Additionally, inadequate progesterone can lead to suboptimal conditions for the embryo, increasing the risk of chromosomal abnormalities and other issues that can result in early pregnancy loss. Hyperthyroidism creates a state of overall hormonal imbalance that can disrupt the intricate interplay between the thyroid hormones, estrogen, progesterone, and other reproductive hormones. This imbalance can lead to irregular menstrual cycles, anovulation (failure to ovulate), and inadequate endometrial preparation, all of which contribute to increased risk of miscarriage.

Moreover, the stress that hyperthyroidism places on the body, including increased metabolic demands and cardiovascular strain, can also contribute to a less favorable environment for maintaining a pregnancy. The elevated heart rate, anxiety, and other symptoms associated with hyperthyroidism can exacerbate the physiological stress on the reproductive system, further increasing the risk of miscarriage.[14]

Diagnosis

Serum TSH is typically suppressed in hyperthyroidism due to the negative feedback effect of elevated thyroid hormone levels on the hypothalamus and pituitary gland. Free T4 and free T3 levels are elevated, confirming the diagnosis of hyperthyroidism.

Pregnant women with overt hyperthyroidism in the first trimester often present with very low serum TSH levels (below 0.01 mU/L), alongside elevated free T4 and/or free T3 levels, which are higher than the normal pregnancy range. Transient subclinical hyperthyroidism, characterized by low TSH levels with normal serum total or free T4 and T3 concentrations, is a common physiological occurrence in the first trimester of pregnancy. It does not typically require treatment, as it is not linked to adverse pregnancy outcomes.

Management

The management of hyperthyroidism involves several treatment options, depending on the cause and severity of the condition.

Antithyroid medications are commonly used as the first line of treatment. These medications, such as methimazole and propylthiouracil (PTU), inhibit thyroid hormone synthesis by blocking the enzyme thyroid peroxidase, which is responsible for the iodination of thyroglobulin. Methimazole is generally preferred due to its longer half-life, allowing for once-daily dosing, and its lower side effect profile compared to PTU. However, PTU is preferred during the first trimester of pregnancy due to the potential teratogenic effects of methimazole.

Beta-blockers, such as propranolol, are often used for symptom control in hyperthyroidism. These medications do not reduce thyroid hormone levels but can help manage symptoms such as palpitations, tremors, and anxiety by blocking the effects of thyroid hormones on the cardiovascular and nervous systems.[15] While these medications can effectively manage maternal symptoms, long-term use may lead to adverse fetal effects such as intrauterine growth restriction and fetal bradycardia.

Radioactive iodine ablation is another treatment option, particularly for patients with Graves' disease or toxic multinodular goiter who do not respond to or are intolerant of antithyroid medications. After RAI therapy, some women may experience temporary menstrual irregularities or amenorrhea (absence of menstruation). However, studies generally suggest that these effects are transient, and normal ovarian function usually returns within several months to a year post-treatment. However, the American Thyroid Association suggests women avoid pregnancy for 6–12 months following RAI therapy to allow the body to clear the radioactive iodine and to reduce any potential risk to the developing fetus.

Thyroidectomy, or surgical removal of the thyroid gland, is an option for patients with large goiters, suspicion of malignancy, or those who cannot tolerate other treatments.

Role in Infertility and Recurrent Pregnancy Loss

The excess thyroid hormones can disrupt the normal function of the hypothalamic-pituitary-ovarian axis, leading to anovulation and menstrual cycle irregularities. Anovulation occurs because the excess thyroid hormones affect the release of gonadotropins, particularly luteinizing hormone (LH), which is necessary for the release of an egg during the menstrual cycle.

In addition to anovulation, hyperthyroidism can lead to luteal phase insufficiency and defects, where the corpus luteum fails to produce enough progesterone to maintain the endometrium and support early pregnancy. This can lead to implantation failure or early miscarriage.

Untreated hyperthyroidism during pregnancy increases the risk of miscarriage, preterm labor, preeclampsia, and other adverse pregnancy outcomes. Excess thyroid hormones can also negatively impact fetal development, leading to complications such as intrauterine growth restriction and neurodevelopmental delays.

In women with subclinical hyperthyroidism (suppressed TSH with normal free T4 and free T3 levels), treatment decisions should be individualized based on the underlying cause, the severity of the TSH suppression, and the presence of symptoms. In asymptomatic women with mild TSH suppression, observation may be appropriate. However, in women with more severe TSH suppression or those with symptoms, treatment with antithyroid medications may be necessary to achieve a euthyroid state before conception.

Subclinical Thyroid Disorders and Their Role in Infertility and Recurrent Pregnancy Loss

Subclinical thyroid disorders represent a spectrum of conditions where there is an abnormal TSH level with normal free T4 and free T3 levels. These conditions are often asymptomatic but can have significant implications for reproductive health, particularly in women with infertility or recurrent pregnancy loss.

Subclinical Hypothyroidism

Subclinical hypothyroidism (SCH) is defined by an elevated TSH level with normal free T4 levels. Although subclinical hypothyroidism may not produce overt symptoms, it is associated with an increased risk of infertility, miscarriage, and adverse pregnancy outcomes. The exact mechanisms are not fully understood, but it is thought that even mild thyroid dysfunction can disrupt the hypothalamic-pituitary-ovarian axis, leading to ovulatory dysfunction and luteal phase defects.[16] In women with infertility and subclinical hypothyroidism, between 44% to 84% of those treated with levothyroxine (T4) successfully conceived during the treatment period. Also, in patients with subclinical hypothyroidism undergoing assisted reproductive technologies (ART), treatment with thyroid hormone replacement (T4) compared to placebo has been shown to improve certain pregnancy outcomes, such as live birth rates and reduced miscarriage rates.

Levothyroxine therapy is recommended in symptomatic women, those with a TSH level greater than 4.0 mIU/L, or those planning to conceive. The goal is to normalize TSH levels to optimize reproductive outcomes. Regular monitoring of TSH and free T4 levels is essential during treatment, especially during pregnancy, as thyroid hormone requirements increase.

Subclinical Hyperthyroidism

A suppressed TSH level with normal free T4 and free T3 levels define subclinical hyperthyroidism. Although subclinical hyperthyroidism is often asymptomatic, it can lead to complications such as osteoporosis, atrial fibrillation, and adverse pregnancy outcomes if left untreated. The impact of subclinical hyperthyroidism on fertility and pregnancy is less clear than that of subclinical hypothyroidism, but some studies suggest an increased risk of miscarriage and preterm birth. Poorly controlled subclinical hyperthyroidism can have a controversial association with a higher risk of complications like preterm birth and preeclampsia, and these risks are lower compared to overt hyperthyroidism. Some guidelines suggest treating subclinical hyperthyroidism in women with fertility issues or recurrent pregnancy loss, while others recommend a more conservative approach unless symptoms worsen. Management of subclinical hyperthyroidism depends on the underlying cause, the severity of the TSH suppression, and the patient's clinical status. In symptomatic patients or those at risk for complications, antithyroid drugs may be considered to achieve a euthyroid state.

It is recommended by theASRM that laboratory-specific TSH cutoff levels be used to diagnose subclinical hypothyroidism (SCH) for nonpregnant patients and for pregnant patients by trimester (Figure 7.1).[17] When laboratory cutoffs are not available, defined upper limits of normal TSH levels should be used. Women should be advised that TSH levels between 2.5 and 4 mIU/L are not associated with an increased risk of miscarriage.

As per the ASRM practice committee document guidelines, there is insufficient evidence to counsel women that SCH is associated with infertility. It is recommended to counsel women that SCH is not associated with increased obstetric risk, and that women be counseled that SCH is not associated with adverse neurodevelopmental outcomes in offspring.

It is not recommended to treat women desiring pregnancy or already pregnant who have a diagnosis of SCH with levothyroxine, as treatment has not been proven to reduce pregnancy loss or to improve clinical pregnancy outcomes.

Treatment with levothyroxine for SCH diagnosed in pregnancy is not recommended for the indication of improving developmental outcomes. ASRM also does not recommend screening for thyroid

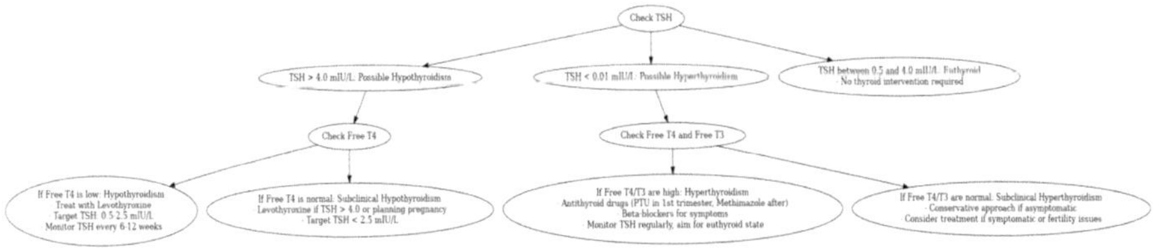

FIGURE 7.1 ASRM Recommendations for Management of Subclinical Hypothyroidism (from ref 17 with permission).

autoimmunity in asymptomatic women with infertility or pregnancy. Targeted screening may be considered in women with a history of RPL. Universal screening of thyroid function during pregnancy is also not recommended. Screening of thyroid function during pregnancy with a serum TSH level is recommended for patients at increased risk. TSH and T4 levels should be tested in patients with signs or symptoms of hypothyroidism (including irregular menstrual cycles) rather than in all patients with infertility.

Indications for Referral to an Endocrinologist

Most cases of thyroid disease in reproductive-aged women including subclinical and clinical hypothyroidism can be managed by a reproductive endocrinology and infertility (REI) specialist. Referral to an endocrinologist for management of thyroid disease may be indicated for a number of reasons, including thyroid nodules, thyroid hormone blood level fluctuations unresponsive to medical treatment and dose adjustments, an enlarged thyroid gland, or goiter, persistence of thyroid symptoms that have not improved with treatment, Graves' disease, women with a new diagnosis of hyperthyroidism, and suspected thyroid malignancy.

Key Points

- In women with subclinical hypothyroidism (TSH above 4.0 mIU/L with normal free T4), treatment with levothyroxine is recommended.
- TSH levels between 2.5 and 4 mIU/L are not associated with an increased risk of miscarriage.
- There is insufficient evidence to counsel women that subclinical hypothyroidism is associated with infertility.
- Hyperthyroidism is associated with menstrual irregularities, and an increased risk of miscarriage and referral to a medical professional qualified to treat the condition is warranted.

REFERENCES

1. Sohn SY. Risks of iodine excess. *Endocr Rev* 2024;45(6):858–79.
2. Hannoush ZC, Weiss RE. Defects of thyroid hormone synthesis and action. *Endocrinol Metab Clin North Am* 2017;46:375–88.
3. Kallen CB, Arici A. Immune testing in fertility practice: truth or deception? *Curr Opinion Obstet Gynecol* 2003;15:225–31.
4. Wenzek C et al. The interplay of thyroid hormones and the immune system - where we stand and why we need to know about it. *Eur J Endocrinol* 2022;186:R65–77.
5. Silva JF et al. Thyroid hormones and female reproduction. *Biol Reprod* 2018;99:907–21.
6. Chan SY et al. The role of the placenta in thyroid hormone delivery to the fetus. *Nat Clin Pract Endocrinol Metab* 2009;5:45–54.
7. Sheehan MT. Biochemical testing of the thyroid: TSH is the best and, oftentimes, only test needed - a review for primary care. *Clin Med Res* 2016;14:83–92.
8. Dwivedi SN et al. Thyroid autoantibodies. *J Clin Pathol* 2023;76:19–28.

9. Korevaar TI et al. Hypothyroxinemia and TPO-antibody positivity are risk factors for premature delivery: the generation R study. *J Clin Endocrinol Metab* 2013;98:4382–90.
10. Barbesino G, Tomer Y. Clinical review: clinical utility of TSH receptor antibodies. *J Clin Endocrinol Metab* 2013;98:2247–55.
11. Biondi B, Kahaly GJ. Cardiovascular involvement in patients with different causes of hyperthyroidism. *Nature Rev Endocrinol* 2010;6:431–43.
12. Teh WT et al. What is the contribution of embryo-endometrial asynchrony to implantation failure? *J Assist Reprod Genet* 2016;33:1419–30.
13. Gude D. Thyroid and its indispensability in fertility. *J Hum Reprod Sci* 2011;4:59–60.
14. Ramya S et al. Role of hormones and the potential impact of multiple stresses on infertility. *Stresses* 2023;3:454–74.
15. Levey GS, Klein I. Catecholamine-thyroid hormone interactions and the cardiovascular manifestations of hyperthyroidism. *Am J Med* 1990;88:642–46.
16. Mikhael S et al. Hypothalamic-pituitary-ovarian axis disorders impacting female fertility. *Biomedicines* 2019;7:5.
17. Practice Committee, ASRM. Subclinical hypothyroidism in the infertile female population: a guideline. *Fertil Steril* 2024;121:765–82.

8

Pituitary Disease in Infertility

Gary Frishman and Kerri Luzzo

Introduction

The pituitary gland is a roughly pea size organ in the brain. This gland plays a critical part in reproduction via its role in the hypothalamic-pituitary-ovarian axis. The pituitary gland is divided into two "halves": the anterior (front lobe) pituitary and posterior (back lobe) pituitary. The different lobes of the pituitary secrete and release a variety of hormones (Table 8.1).

The World Health Organization (WHO) separated women with ovulatory disorders into three groups.

Group I: Low gonadotropins and estradiol

Hypogonadotropic hypogonadism, hypothalamic amenorrhea pituitary insufficiency, hyperprolactinemia

Group II: "Gonadotropin disorder" and normal estradiol

Hypothalamic/pituitary dysfunction (PCOS)

Group III: High gonadotropins and low estradiol

Primary Ovarian Insufficiency (Premature menopause)

Group I includes women with hypothalamic conditions, Group II includes PCOS, and Group III includes diminished ovarian reserve.

Hypopituitarism

A full discourse on hypopituitarism is outside the scope of this chapter and that of most Ob/Gyn practices, and consultation should be made with a provider specializing in this. Briefly, hypopituitarism can be categorized based on the lack of hormone production:

- Isolated pituitary deficiency: Deficit of a single pituitary hormone
- Panhypopituitarism: Deficit of all pituitary hormones

The etiology of hypopituitarism can be further classified as follows:

- Primary hypopituitarism: This results from damage or disorders with the pituitary gland itself.
- Secondary hypopituitarism: This results from direct damage (e.g. trauma, radiation therapy, or surgery) or disorders outside the gland (e.g. hemochromatosis or bacterial meningitis) resulting in damage to the pituitary stalk or hypothalamus.
- Idiopathic hypopituitarism: No cause can be found.

DOI: 10.1201/9781003460275-8

TABLE 8.1

Pituitary Gland Hormones

Pituitary Lobe	Effect
Anterior Pituitary	
Prolactin (PRL)	Milk production
Follicle-stimulating hormone (FSH)	Helps control menstrual cycle and oocyte production
Luteinizing hormone (LH)	Helps control menstrual cycle and triggers ovulation
Thyroid-stimulating hormone (TSH)	Stimulates release of thyroid hormone from thyroid
Adrenocorticotropic hormone (ACTH)	Stimulates release of cortisol by adrenal cortex
Growth hormone (GH)	Helps regulate growth and development including puberty
Posterior Pituitary	
Oxytocin	Stimulates uterine contractions in labor and childbirth and aids in lactation
Antidiuretic hormone (ADH)	Helps regulate water reabsorption by kidneys
Intermediate Pituitary Lobe	
Melanocyte-stimulating hormone (MSH)	Stimulates melanin production and release in melanocytes

Symptoms of hypopituitarism depend on which hormones are impacted. The most common manifestation impacting fertility is thyroid disease, which is covered in Chapter 7.

Hyperprolactinemia

The incident of hyperprolactinemia in women undergoing an evaluation for infertility is close to 20%. Pituitary adenomas are one of the most common central nervous system tumors with a prevalence of 17% in infertile women with hyperprolactinemia, which is at least ten times higher than in the general population.[1]

Both functional and clinically non-functioning tumors are of monoclonal cell origin and are comprised of one of the cell types that exist in the anterior pituitary: lactotrophs, corticotrophs, somatotrophs, gonadotrophs, and thyrotrophs. Of these tumors, the most common is a prolactin secreting tumor (prolactinoma), which will be the main focus of this chapter.

Elevated prolactin levels can lead to disruption of the normal gonadotropin-releasing hormone pathway. Women with hyperprolactinemia as the cause of their infertility typically present with irregular or absent cycles. Fortunately, prolactinomas are rarely malignant, straightforward to diagnose, and typically easy to manage medically, rarely requiring surgery.

Causes of Hyperprolactinemia

Anything that interferes with dopamine secretion or delivery can lead to hyperprolactinemia. Etiologies include conditions such as tumors and infiltrative diseases (including non-lactotroph adenomas), trauma, or surgery. Physical lesions are often treated surgically with dopamine agonists also being used (Table 8.2). In addition, there may be no identifiable etiology for a patient's hyperprolactinemia.

Clinical Presentation

Hyperprolactinemia interferes with GnRH release and, possibly, even gene expression in the GnRH neurons via prolactin receptors on these cells. As noted earlier, the most common presentation of an infertile woman with hyperprolactinemia is irregular or absent cycles. Symptoms typically correlate with serum prolactin levels and significantly elevated levels are more likely to be associated with more severe disruptions of the menstrual cycle.

TABLE 8.2

Causes of Hyperprolactinemia

Physiological Causes:			
	Pregnancy-related		
	Stress		
Pathological Causes:			
	Hypothalamic disorders		
		Tumors	
			Non-secreting pituitary adenomas
			Craniopharyngiomas, meningiomas, dysgerminomas
		Cranial radiation exposure	
		Trauma	
		Invasive processes	
			Sarcoidosis, Langerhans Cell Histiocytosis (Histiocytosis X)
	Pituitary disorders		
		Prolactinoma	
		Thyroid disorders	
		Cushing disease, acromegaly	
		Empty Sella Syndrome	
		Lymphocytic hypophysitis	
	Drugs (Dopamine antagonists)		
		Antipsychotics	
			Thioxanthenes, Butyrophenones, Phenothiazines
		Tricyclic antidepressants	
			SSRIs, Monoamine oxidase inhibitors
		Antihypertensive agents	
			Alpha-methyldopa, verapamil
		Opioids	
			Methadone, morphine
		Antiemetics	
			Domperidone, metoclopramide, prochlorperazine
Idiopathic hyperprolactinemia			

In addition to irregular or absent cycles, the other major presenting symptom in patients with a prolactinoma is galactorrhea. Importantly, galactorrhea can be present even with regular menstrual cycles, and hyperprolactinemia may be present without galactorrhea. Furthermore, menstrual cycle dysfunction is not linked to the presence or absence of galactorrhea.

When taking a history about galactorrhea, one should determine the typical presentation: Galactorrhea is more likely to be contributing to infertility if frequent, spontaneous, and bilateral when compared to occurring only during sexual activity and/or breast stimulation. A helpful technique during the physical examination assessing galactorrhea is to ask the patient to express their milk themselves. In addition to the patient being more likely to be forceful during this examination (compared to the clinician), it is helpful to see if the milk production is seen with gentle manipulation or only when the patient is strongly manipulating their breast. Importantly, if there are any worrisome signs (i.e. evidence of a breast tumor, bloody or otherwise atypical breast discharge, etc.), the clinician should complete a thorough examination and follow up accordingly.

Tables 8.3 and 8.4 summarize the most common signs and symptoms resulting from hyperprolactinemia and those associated with the mass effect of macroadenomas, respectively.

Diagnosis

Hyperprolactinemia can impact the menstrual cycle ranging from slightly irregular periods to complete amenorrhea and may or may not be associated with a pituitary adenoma (also known as a prolactinoma). Assessing a serum prolactin is essential for all women presenting with infertility with irregular or absent cycles. Prolactin levels should ideally be obtained as a fasting morning specimen free from recent breast stimulation and, ideally, free from medications that may increase its release (three days of a drug-free period is typically adequate[2]).

A patient with menstrual abnormalities should also have their thyroid assessed with a TSH to rule out primary hypothyroidism. In addition to hypothyroidism, renal insufficiency and liver failure are accepted causes of hyperprolactinemia.

If there is persistent hyperprolactinemia with a normal TSH, an MRI of the pituitary should be obtained. Although levels great than 500 ng/mL are virtually always a macroadenoma, one should consider obtaining an MRI with *any* elevation of prolactin, as even minimal increases may be resulting from a prolactinoma[2]. Patients with an elevated serum prolactin without a visible tumor on MRI, including those with a prolactin less than 100 ng/mL, should be treated the same as those with a microadenoma.

Prolactinomas are divided into microadenomas and macroadenomas based on size (<1 cm and ≥ 1 cm, respectively). Microadenomas are typically quite stable and 95% do not enlarge when observed over 4–6 years. Furthermore, although observation alone without follow up is not recommended, approximately one-third of women may have improvement of their symptoms without treatment[3]. If a microadenoma does grow, this indicates treatment based on that alone.

TABLE 8.3

Most Common Signs and Symptoms of Hyperprolactinemia

Irregular or absent cycles
Infertility
Galactorrhea
Decreased libido

TABLE 8.4

Signs and Symptoms Associated with Mass Effect from Macroadenomas

<u>More common findings</u>
Headaches
Vision changes
Visual field defects (reduced bilateral peripheral vision, bitemporal hemianopsia)
Decreased visual acuity
Blurred or double vision
<u>Uncommon findings</u>
Cranial nerve palsies
Seizures

Although serum prolactin levels typically correlate with the size of the adenoma, this is not always the case. Having said that, as a rule of thumb, microadenomas will usually have serum prolactin values of less 200 ng/mL, macroadenomas 1 to 2 cm in size typically have values between 200 and 1000 ng/mL, and those greater than 2 cm are typically associated with serum prolactin values greater than 1000 ng/mL. Extremely high serum prolactin concentrations may be seen with lactotroph macroadenomas, whereas prolactin levels due to non-adenoma causes rarely exceed 200 ng/mL.

Both ASRM and ACOG (adopting ASRM's guidelines) recommend against obtaining serum prolactin levels in asymptomatic infertile women but do recommend checking prolactin in infertile patients with recurrent pregnancy loss, oligomenorrhea, amenorrhea, or galactorrhea.[4,5]

This advice is consistent with the National Institute for Health and Care Excellence (NICE) in the UK which states:

> Women who are concerned about their fertility should not be offered a blood test to measure prolactin. This test should only be offered to women who have an ovulatory disorder, galactorrhoea or a pituitary tumour.

In contrast, prolactin is recommended to be checked in patients with recurrent pregnancy loss based on its association with ovulatory dysfunction and potential alternation in the hypothalamic-pituitary-ovarian axis. These changes may negatively impact oocyte growth and maturation and/or the luteal phase[6]. Furthermore, treatment of hyperprolactinemia has been shown to achieve successful outcomes in patients with recurrent pregnancy loss.

Uncommon Scenarios

Macroprolactinemia

There is a "big" form of prolactin (40–60 kDa compared to the typical 23 kDa). In 10–25% of patients with hyperprolactinemia, this larger form may be present and detected with the assay. As these forms are biologically inactive, these impacted patients typically have disproportionately minor symptoms for their serum levels. Special assay preparations (prolactin recovery after polyethylene glycol precipitation) can usually differentiate true hyperpro-lactinemia and macroprolactinemia.

Hook Effect

In cases with the hook effect, extremely high concentrations of prolactin can interfere with the assay (saturating both antibodies and preventing sandwich formation), resulting in only moderately elevated levels of prolactin. Although this is less common with modern assays, if a patient's symptoms are concerning (e.g. suspicion for a macroadenoma) with only mild elevations in serum prolactin, the hook effect should be considered.

Management

Lifestyle Interventions

In contrast to menstrual cycle irregularities due to conditions such as hypothalamic amenorrhea or PCOS, there are no lifestyle interventions that may be effective for patients with prolactinomas.

Medical Therapies

Dopamine agonist medications are usually the first-line treatment for all patients with hyperprolactinemia of any cause. Dopamine agonists work by binding to the dopamine cell-surface receptors resulting in reduced synthesis and secretion of prolactin as well as a reduction in the size of the adenoma cells.

Two medications, both ergot derivatives and available in generic formulations, are front line for treatment of hyperprolactinemia in the United States: cabergoline and bromocriptine. Cabergoline is typically considered first-line based on superior efficacy in decreasing prolactin levels and tumor shrinkage, ease of administration, and lesser side effects. Furthermore, cabergoline needs to be taken only once or twice a week compared to bromocriptine at twice a day. Cabergoline's superiority has been well demonstrated in multiple studies, being effective in approximately 95% of patients compared to 80–90% of patients using bromocriptine[7]. In a study of 85 patients with hyperprolactinemia (of which 29 had a macroprolactinoma), all had their hyperprolactinemia normalized with resumption of regular cycles and 94% conceived. Of note, approximately 74% of these women were either bromocriptine intolerant or resistant[8]. Bromocriptine's major advantage is a slight price advantage, and some insurance companies may require it to be first-line.

If the patient does not conceive despite regular cycles achieved with an ergot derivative, additional therapy with a medication like clomiphene citrate can be used.

Common side effects that may occur with either medication include "brain fog" and postural hypotension. Importantly, side effects are dose-related and can often be avoided or minimized by starting on a low dose and taking the medication with food or at bedtime minimizes nausea and sleepiness[7].

Use in Pregnancy

Bromocriptine was the historical gold standard with decades of use prior to the establishment of cabergoline's superiority. This includes more data available on its safety in pregnancy[9].

However, given meaningful data suggesting the safety of cabergoline in pregnancy, alongside its more tolerable side effect profile (e.g. lesser nausea) and less frequent dosing, it is often considered first-line even in women attempting conception.

Dosing

For cabergoline, start patients on a half of a 0.5 mg pill (i.e. 0.25 mg) twice a week and one-half tablet of a 2.5 mg (i.e. 1.25 mg) bromocriptine pill once a day after dinner or at bedtime.

While on treatment, repeat the serum prolactin, alongside assessing side effects of treatment, one month after the starting dose. If there is no drop in prolactin levels, the dose should be gradually increased, repeating the prolactin level in one month. The upper limit of dosing for cabergoline is 1 to 1.5 mg two to three times a week and for bromocriptine is 5 mg twice a day, increasing the dosing to twice a day (adding a dose after breakfast) after one week.

Consideration should be given to co-management of patients on more than 2 mg of cabergoline a week, as cardiac ultrasonography should be entertained based on the risk of valvular heart disease. However, this recommendation is based on long-term exposure in patients with Parkinson disease and has not been seen with shorter exposure with lower doses as in treatment of prolactinomas.

The dosing for macroadenomas is the same as for microadenomas; however, an MRI should be repeated in 6 to 12 months to assess treatment impact on size[2].

If normal menstrual cycles resume despite a slightly elevated prolactin level, it is reasonable to consider the endpoint of normalization of menstrual cycle function rather than "chasing" the prolactin level. However, in the patient who is tolerating increased medication dosing, striving for a normal prolactin is also acceptable.

Medication-Induced Hyperprolactinemia

A common subset of patients whose adenomas are resistant to dopamine agonists includes those taking a medication (typically an antipsychotic drug). Although stopping all psychiatric medications temporally to confirm their impact on symptoms makes sense in theory, this is not typically an option clinically. If there are persistently elevated levels or prolactin on these medications, one should still order an MRI to confirm the absence of a concomitant pituitary tumor[2].

Treatment of these patients should be in close consultation with their prescribing provider, including investigating the safety in pregnancy of all medications the patient is taking as well as considering alternative therapies which may be less likely to cause symptoms. Aripiprazole has been shown to decrease prolactin levels when used alongside antipsychotic medications.

If the patient is advised against stopping their psychiatric medication, consideration can be given to starting a dopamine agonist alongside their psychiatric medication, again, in close consultation with their psychiatrist.

Some antihypertensives, such as verapamil and methyldopa, may also induce hyperpro-lactinemia. In these cases, alternative medications can be entertained.

Management of Side Effects

For the rare woman with persistent nausea despite low oral doses, efficacy can still be achieved via a vaginal route bypassing the gut. Of note, vaginal administration is less likely to alleviate side effects other than nausea.

For patients unable to tolerate bromocriptine or in whom a response is not seen, switch to cabergoline.

Impulse Control Disorders

The onset or worsening of impulse control disorders, such as hypersexuality, compulsive gambling, eating, or shopping is an uncommon but accepted adverse side effect. In one study of over 300 patients with lactotroph adenomas being treated with a dopamine agonist for three months or more, 17% developed some impulse control disorder of which compulsive eating was the most common manifestation in female patients. Of note, these patients were being followed in a tertiary referral center which may reflect a more challenging or atypical patient profile.

Ongoing Management of Patients on Medical Treatment with a Dopamine Agonist

Monitoring serum prolactin is the mainstay technique for assessing treatment efficacy as, although variations exist, decrease in adenoma size typically correlates with the reduction in prolactin levels.

Prolactin levels typically decrease within two to three weeks of treatment, although the ability to document a decrease in tumor size via imaging takes longer. For those women whose menses return, this typically occurs within the first eight weeks of therapy[7]. Because of the potential increased risk of miscarriage with oligo-ovulation, consideration should be given to recommending barrier birth control in couples actively trying to conceive until normal menstrual cycles resume.

In patients in whom normalization of menstruation is not able to be achieved and/or medication cannot be tolerated, attempts at ovulation induction can be entertained. In rare circumstances transsphenoidal surgery to treat the adenoma can be considered, although this is almost always only pursued in the presence of a macroadenoma.

In patients stable on longer term treatment, medication dosing can often be decreased over time and should be considered with normal levels after one year of treatment. After two years of normal serum prolactin levels, if an MRI shows resolution of the adenoma, treatment can be stopped. In this case, prolactin levels should be checked after three months and then yearly to ensure continued resolution[2]. In patients who no longer desire fertility (e.g. completed childbearing), the hypoestrogenic impact of amenorrhea can be corrected with exogenous estrogen with periodic progestin exposure if a uterus is present, if preferred by the patient. Oral contraceptives are a reasonable option.

Management in Pregnancy

Bromocriptine is known to cross the placenta and *dopamine agonist therapy should be stopped in women who become pregnant*. This should be individualized for patients with a macroadenoma[2].

Fortunately, as noted earlier, the literature is very reassuring, with thousands of babies having been exposed to bromocriptine in utero in the early gestation having comparable outcomes. This includes similar paths in postnatal development to those without exposure. These studies also reported no increased risk of miscarriage or ectopic pregnancy. With few exceptions, the data on cabergoline is equally reassuring[7].

Given normal marked elevations of prolactin during pregnancy, following serum levels is not indicated. Although microadenomas may enlarge either asymptomatically (2.6% risk) or as noted by imaging (4.5% chance) during pregnancy, the risk is low enough such that routine monitoring in asymptomatic patients is not mandated[10].

Although breast feeding stimulates prolactin release, it is not associated with tumor growth, and breast feeding is typically not contraindicated in patients with hyperprolactinemia.

Visual fields should be examined and documented prior to pregnancy in women with prolactinomas to serve as a baseline, and patients should be alerted to the risk of a microadenoma growing during pregnancy. Fortunately, this is unlikely with symptomatic growth occurring in approximately 2.5% of patients with a microadenoma. A macroadenoma has a higher chance with an untreated one having approximately 23% clinically significant growth. Patients should also be asked about headaches as another symptom of adenoma growth.

Surgical Interventions

There is a body of evidence showing that surgery and radiotherapy are able to provide benefit in patients who are either resistant to, or intolerant to, dopamine agonists.

Summary

The pituitary gland can impact fertility in a number of ways both intrinsically, such as with hyperprolactinemia, and by playing a role in other conditions such as PCOS and thyroid disease.

A serum prolactin and TSH should be ordered in all infertile women with irregular or absent menses or galactorrhea. An MRI should be obtained in those with a persistently elevated prolactin. Cabergoline is considered the first-line therapy for hyperprolactinemia based on ease of use, side effect profile, and efficacy. Regardless of choice of ergot derivative, the medication should be stopped with a pregnancy. Macroadenomas may be best co-managed but typically do not negate the ability to conceive.

Key Points

1. ASRM and ACOG recommend obtaining a serum prolactin level in patients with recurrent pregnancy loss, and as part of the infertility evaluation in the setting of galactorrhea, oligomenorrhea, or amenorrhea.
2. Important factors to consider in the setting of hyperprolactinemia include pituitary tumors, medications, hypothyroidism, and renal failure. Obtain a pituitary MRI in patients with persistent hyperprolactinemia and a normal TSH.
3. Initial treatment for hyperprolactinemia includes a dopamine agonist. Cabergoline is typically first-line based on superior efficacy and lesser side effects.
4. For women attempting conception, the pregnancy safety data in the literature is reassuring for both cabergoline and bromocriptine. Dopamine agonist therapy should be discontinued in pregnancy.

REFERENCES

1. Souter I et al. Prevalence of hyperprolactinemia and abnormal magnetic resonance imaging findings in a population with infertility. *Fertil Steril*. 2010,94(3):1159–1162.
2. Melmed S et al. Diagnosis and treatment of hyperprolactinemia: an Endocrine Society clinical practice guideline. *J Clin Endocrinol Metab*. 2011;96(2):273–288.
3. Schlechte J et al. The natural history of untreated hyperprolactinemia: a prospective analysis. *J Clin Endocrinol Metab*. 1989;68(2):412–418.
4. Practice Committee, ASRM. Fertility evaluation of infertile women: a committee opinion. *Fertil Steril*. 2021;116(5):1255–1265.
5. Infertility Workup for the Women's Health Specialist: ACOG Committee Opinion 781. *Obstet Gynecol*. 2019;133(6):e377–e384.
6. Practice Committee, ASRM. Evaluation and treatment of recurrent pregnancy loss: a committee opinion. *Fertil Steril* 2012;98(5):1103–1111.
7. Webster J et al. A comparison of cabergoline and bromocriptine in the treatment of hyperprolactinemic amenorrhea. Cabergoline Comparative Study Group. *N Engl J Med*. 1994;331(14):904–909.
8. Ono M et al. Individualized high-dose cabergoline therapy for hyperprolactinemic infertility in women with micro- and macroprolactinomas. *J Clin Endocrinol Metab*. 2010;95(6):2672–2679.
9. Turkalj I et al. Surveillance of bromocriptine in pregnancy. *JAMA*. 1982;247(11):1589–1591.
10. Molitch ME. Pregnancy and the hyperprolactinemic woman. *N Engl J Med*. 1985;312(21):1364–1370.

On-line resources for patients include:

https://pituitary.org/disorders/prolactinomas

www.pituitary.org.uk/information/prolactinoma/

9

Evaluation and Management of Male Infertility

Stephen Lazarou and Quetrell D. Heyward

Introduction

Approximately 15% of couples are unable to conceive after one year of unprotected intercourse. A male factor is responsible in about 20% of infertile couples and contributory in up to 40%.[1] Male infertility is generally determined by the finding of an abnormal semen analysis, although other factors may play a role in the setting of a normal semen analysis.

Male infertility can be due to a variety of conditions. Some of these conditions are potentially reversible, such as obstruction of the vas deferens and hormonal imbalances. Other conditions are not reversible, such as bilateral testicular atrophy secondary to a viral infection.

Treatment of various conditions may improve male infertility and allow for conception through intercourse. Even men who have absent sperm on their semen analyses (azoospermia) may have sperm production by their testicles. Detection of conditions for which there are no treatments spares couples the distress of attempting therapies that are not effective. Identifying certain genetic causes of male infertility allows couples to be informed about the potential to transmit genetic conditions that may affect the health of offspring. Therefore, a comprehensive evaluation of the male partner allows the couple to better understand the basis of their infertility and to obtain genetic counseling where necessary. Male infertility may be the presenting manifestation of an underlying life-threatening condition, such as testicular or pituitary tumors.[2]

If corrective treatment is not available, assisted reproductive techniques such as testicular or epididymal sperm retrieval in combination with *in vitro* fertilization (IVF)/intracytoplasmic sperm injection (ICSI) may be utilized. Other options for couples include donor insemination or adoption.

When to Evaluate the Male

A couple attempting to conceive should have an evaluation for infertility if pregnancy does not occur within one year of regular unprotected intercourse. An evaluation should be done before one year if male infertility risk factors exist, such as a history of bilateral cryptorchidism (undescended testes) or chemotherapy. Other reasons may include female infertility risk factors, including advancing female age (over the age of 35) or a couple that questions the male partner's fertility potential. While a man may have a history of previous involvement in a pregnancy, this does not exclude the possibility of a newly acquired factor preventing normal fertility (secondary infertility). Men with secondary infertility should be evaluated in the same comprehensive way as men who have never initiated a pregnancy.

DOI: 10.1201/9781003460275-9

Evaluation of the Infertile Male

The evaluation of the infertile male should be performed by a urologist and include a complete reproductive and medical history, physical examination, and at least two semen analyses. The reproductive and medical history should include coital frequency and timing, duration of infertility and prior fertility, childhood illnesses and developmental history, medications, systemic medical illnesses (e.g., diabetes mellitus and upper respiratory diseases) and prior surgeries (e.g., hernia repair), sexual history including sexually transmitted infections, and exposure to toxins from heat, chemicals, and radiation, including smoking and family reproductive history, review of systems, and allergies.

Physical Examination

A general physical examination is an essential part of the evaluation. In addition to the general physical examination, particular attention is made to the genitalia including 1) examination of the penis including the location of the urethral meatus or presence of plaque/lesion; 2) palpation of the testes and measurement of their size; 3) presence and consistency of both the vasa and epididymides; 4) presence of a varicocele; 5) secondary sex characteristics including body habitus, hair distribution, and breast development; and 6) digital rectal exam.

Based on the results of the full evaluation, the urologist may recommend other procedures and tests to determine the cause of a patient's infertility. These tests may include additional semen analyses, hormone evaluation, post-ejaculatory urinalysis, ultrasonography, specialized tests of semen, and genetic screening.

Semen Analysis

A semen analysis is the principal laboratory evaluation of the infertile male and helps to define the severity of the male factor. An abstinence period of two to seven days is necessary before semen should be collected by masturbation or by intercourse using special semen collection condoms that do not contain substances detrimental to sperm (i.e. lubricants/spermicide). The specimen may be collected at home or at the laboratory. The specimen should be kept at room, or ideally body temperature, during transport and examined within one hour of collection.[3]

The semen analysis provides information on semen volume as well as sperm concentration, motility, and morphology (Table 9.1). Values that fall outside these ranges indicate the need for consideration of additional clinical/laboratory evaluation of the patient. It is important to note that reference values for semen parameters are not the same as the minimum values needed for conception, and men with semen variables outside the reference ranges may be fertile. In fact, patients with values within the reference range may still be subfertile.[4]

Absent sperm in the ejaculate, or azoospermia, is not diagnosed unless the specimen is centrifuged and the pellet is examined. The evaluation of sperm morphology (shape) has changed considerably over time.

TABLE 9.1

World Health Organization Reference Limits for Human Semen Characteristics 2021 (ref. 3)

Semen Parameter	Lower Reference Threshold
Semen Volume	1.4 ml
pH	7.2
Sperm Concentration	16 million/ml
Total Sperm Number	39 million/ejaculate
% Motile	42%
Progressive Motility	30%
Normal Morphology	4% Strict Kruger morphology

It remains controversial and many clinics do not perform the evaluation. Sperm morphology assessment by strict (Kruger) criteria has been used to identify couples who have a poor chance of fertilization with standard *in vitro* fertilization (IVF)[3,5,6] or a better chance of fertilization with ICSI[7] (see Figure 5.13).

Endocrine Evaluation

Hormonal abnormalities of the hypothalamic-pituitary-testicular axis are well known causes of male infertility. Endocrine laboratory work should be obtained if there is an abnormal semen analysis, impaired sexual function, or other clinical signs or symptoms suggestive of a specific endocrinopathy. The initial hormonal evaluation should consist of measurements of serum follicle-stimulating-hormone (FSH), luteinizing hormone (LH), testosterone, and prolactin. The relationship of free and bound testosterone, LH, FSH, and prolactin helps to identify various clinical conditions, such as primary steroidogenic/spermatogenic dysfunction or pituitary dysfunction. A normal serum FSH level does not guarantee the presence of intact spermatogenesis. However, an elevated FSH level even in the upper end of normal reference may be indicative of an abnormality in spermato-genesis.

Post-Ejaculatory Urinalysis

Low-volume or absent ejaculate suggests retrograde ejaculation (semen going back into the bladder instead of out the urethra), lack of emission, ejaculatory duct obstruction, hypogonadism (low testosterone), or congenital bilateral absence of the vas deferens (CBAVD). Other explanations of low-volume ejaculate are incomplete collection and short periods (<2 days) of abstinence. Retrograde ejaculation can occur in men who have diabetes and those with testicular cancer who have undergone a lymph node dissection that can disrupt the sympathetic nerves. In order to diagnose possible retrograde ejaculation, a post-ejaculatory urinalysis (analysis of urine sample after ejaculation) should be performed for any man whose ejaculatory volume is low and who has not been diagnosed with hypogonadism or CBAVD.

The post-ejaculatory urinalysis is performed by centrifuging the specimen and microscopically inspecting the pellet. The presence of any sperm in a post-ejaculatory urinalysis of a patient with azoospermia is suggestive of retrograde ejaculation. Significant numbers of sperm must be found in the urine of patients with low ejaculate volume oligospermia in order to suggest the diagnosis of retrograde ejaculation.

Ultrasonography

Scrotal Ultrasonography

Most scrotal abnormalities are visible and palpable on physical examination. This includes varicoceles (dilated veins in the scrotum; see Figure 9.1), spermatoceles (epididymal cysts; see Figure 9.2), absence of the vas deferens, epididymal induration, and testicular masses. Scrotal ultrasonography may identify nonpalpable varicoceles. Scrotal ultrasonography may be useful to clarify ambiguous findings on examination, such as may occur in patients with testes that are in the upper scrotum, small scrotal sacs, or other anatomy that makes physical examination difficult.

Transrectal Ultrasonography

The finding of dilated seminal vesicles, dilated ejaculatory ducts, and/or midline prostatic cystic structures on transrectal ultrasonography (TRUS) is suggestive of complete or partial ejaculatory duct obstruction.[8] Normal seminal vesicles are less than 2.0 cm in anteroposterior diameter.[9] Patients with complete ejaculatory duct obstruction produce low-volume, fructose-negative, acidic, azoospermic ejaculates and may have dilated seminal vesicles identified by ultrasound (Figure 9.3). Patients with CBAVD may also have these findings because they often have absent or atrophic seminal vesicles. Patients with partial ejaculatory duct obstruction often present with low-volume, diminished sperm concentration and/or poor motility. Cysts at the ejaculatory ducts may be identified by ultrasonography and are occasionally

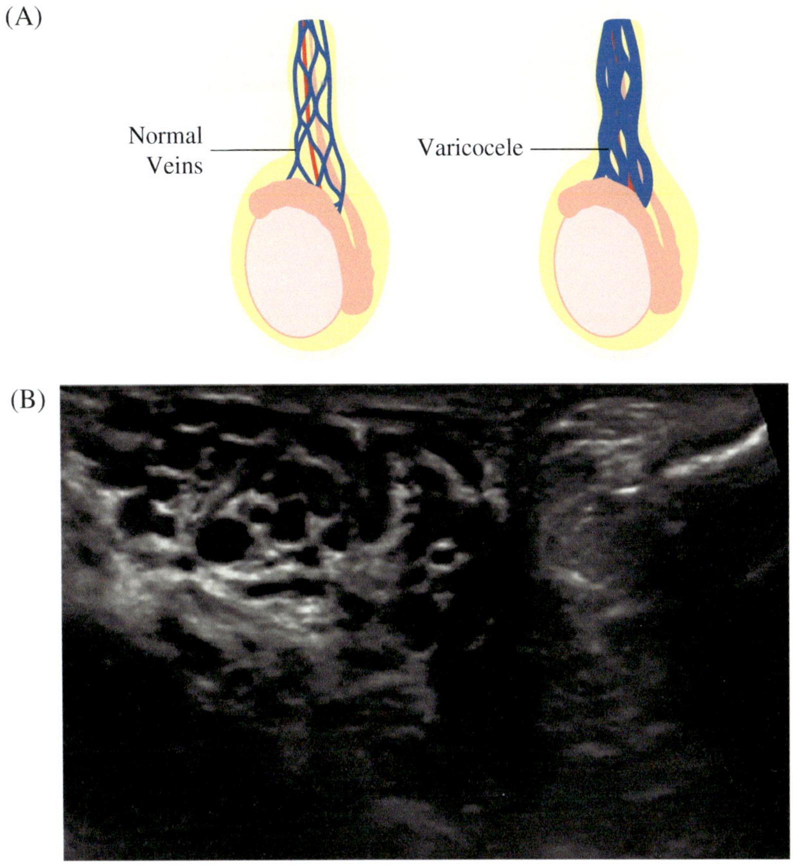

FIGURE 9.1 (A) Normal appearance and varicocele with dilated veins (from Shutterstock.com, under license); (B) varicocele identified by scrotal ultrasonography (from Raheem AA, Ultrasound imaging of the infertile male, in Rizk B et al., eds, Male Infertility in Reproductive Medicine, CRC Press 2019, with permission).

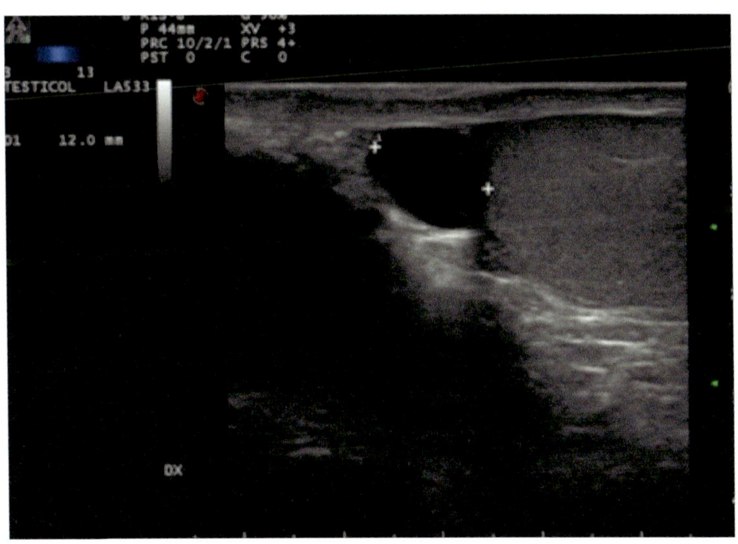

FIGURE 9.2 Ultrasonographic images of epididymal cysts (spermatocele)(from Boscarelli A, Bellini T. Epididymal cyst in children. Eur J Pediatr 2021;180(9):2723-2729 with permission).

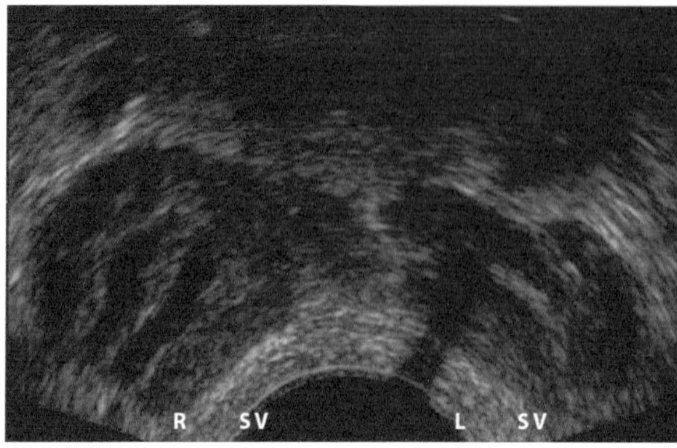

FIGURE 9.3 Transurethral ultrasound examination confirming a dilated seminal vesicle as a result of obstruction (from Raheem AA et al., Ultrasound imaging of the infertile male, in Rizk B et al., eds, Male Infertility in Reproductive Medicine, CRC Press 2019, with permission).

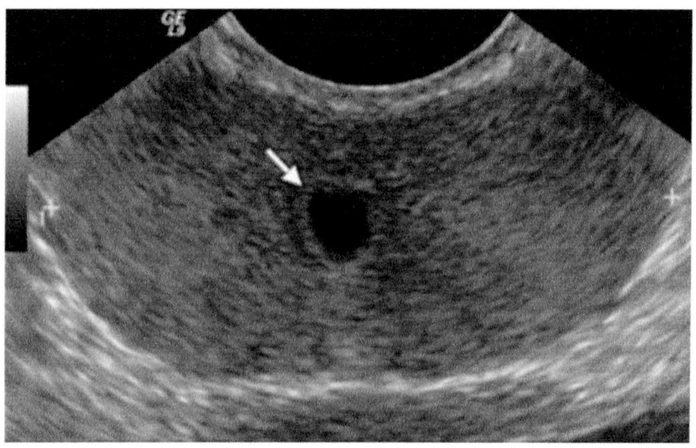

FIGURE 9.4 Ejaculatory duct cyst associated with an obstruction (from Arafa M et al., A new algorithm for management of ejaculatory duct obstruction due to prostatic cyst in infertile males, *Internet J Radiol* 2013;16/1: https://ispub.com/IJRA/16/1/2941, with permission).

amenable to transurethral resection ("unroofing"), which may allow sperm to present in the ejaculate (Figure 9.4).

Specialized Clinical Tests on Semen and Sperm

In some cases, semen analyses fail to accurately predict a man's fertility. Specialized clinical tests should be reserved only for those cases in which identification of the cause of male infertility will direct treatment.

Strict Sperm Morphology

The clinical implications of poor morphology are controversial. Initial studies evaluating the utility of strict sperm morphology in predicting fertilization rates during IVF used a score of greater than 14% for normal. However, subsequent studies report fertilization rates being lowest for patients with morphology scores of less than 4%. Pregnancy rates have also been reported to be suboptimal with lower scores, but some recent studies have reported no relationship of morphology to IVF results.[10, 11] The relationship between morphology scores and pregnancy rates with intrauterine insemination (IUI) and intercourse have been examined.[12–15] However, there is no consensus on the implications of poor morphology scores.

Furthermore, the interpretation of sperm morphology varies between labs. Certain rare morphological abnormalities, such as sperm without acrosomes, are highly predictive of failure to fertilize eggs. Yet, in a number of cases, fertilization and pregnancy are possible even with very low morphology scores. Many physicians utilize strict morphology in practice, although most studies have not addressed the significance of isolated low morphology in patients with otherwise normal semen parameters.[16]

DNA Integrity

DNA integrity testing refers to a variety of assays utilized to evaluate the degree of sperm DNA fragmentation. Assessment of sperm DNA integrity has been evaluated for correlation with the ability to conceive by intercourse, IUI, IVF, and IVF using ICSI. Studies demonstrate a statistically significant lower pregnancy rate in those patients with impaired sperm DNA integrity. Nonetheless, these studies also show that many couples with impaired sperm DNA integrity can conceive by intercourse.[17–20] The tests are inadequate as screening tests for pregnancy by intercourse. One large study has suggested that abnormal DNA integrity in the sample used for IUI was predictive of pregnancy rates.[19] Most studies have examined the predictive value of sperm DNA integrity testing in routine IVF and IVF using ICSI. Meta-analysis of published studies has found a small statistically significant predictive effect of DNA integrity results upon pregnancy rates for IVF with or without ICSI.[21, 22] Data also suggest DNA integrity testing may be of value in identifying those at risk for recurrent pregnancy loss.[23–25] Given the evidence, sperm DNA testing is recommended for couples with recurrent pregnancy loss and failed ART cycles.[26]

Reactive Oxygen Species (ROS)

Elevated reactive oxygen species (ROS) have been implicated as a cause of male infertility. Both sperm and white blood cells in the semen can produce ROS. ROS may interfere with sperm function by peroxidation of sperm lipid membranes and creation of toxic fatty acid peroxides. Controversy exists regarding the best method of testing for ROS and whether therapies are effective at reducing seminal ROS and improving fecundity. Routine clinical testing and treatment of ROS are not indicated. Treatment of oxidative stress with which types and doses of antioxidants is controversial and is the focus of multiple research studies. Commonly used antioxidants include zinc, vitamins C and E, l-carnitine, co-enzyme Q10, and several others. It is unclear as to whether or not these antioxidants improve fertility outcomes, but the cost and side effect risk is low enough that many physicians routinely recommend them to infertile men.[27]

Quantitation of Leukocytes in Semen

An elevated number of leukocytes (white blood cells) in the semen has been associated with decreased sperm function and motility. Under microscopy, both leukocytes and immature germ cells appear similar and are properly termed "round cells." The lab must make sure that the two types of cells are evaluated to differentiate between a possible infection and immature sperm. Men with true pyospermia (greater than 1 million leukocytes per ml) should be evaluated for a genital tract infection or inflammation. A semen culture may also be of value to determine the presence of microorganisms. Antibiotics, anti-oxidants, and frequent ejaculation are all potential options recommended by various guidelines.[28, 29]

Sperm Viability Tests

Sperm viability can be assessed by mixing fresh semen with a dye such as eosin or trypan blue or by the use of the hypoosmotic swelling (HOS) test. These assays determine whether nonmotile sperm are viable by identifying which sperm have intact cell membranes. Though outcomes may be inferior to those of motile sperm, nonmotile but viable sperm may be successful in cases utilizing ICSI.[30–32]

Computer-Aided Sperm Analysis

Computer-aided sperm analysis (CASA) requires sophisticated instruments for quantitative assessment of sperm from a microscopic image or from videotape. CASA is used to measure sperm numbers, motility, and morphology. CASA is useful for assessing sperm motility and motion, such as velocity or speed and head movement, which are important factors in determining sperm fertility potential.

Genetic Screening

Genetic abnormalities may cause infertility by affecting sperm production and/or transport. The three most common genetic factors known to be related to male infertility are cystic fibrosis gene mutations associated with congenital absence of the vas deferens (CBAVD), chromosomal abnormalities resulting in impaired testicular function, and Y-chromosome microdeletions (YCMD) associated with impaired spermatogenesis. Azoospermia and severe oligospermia (sperm concentration <5 million/ml) are more often associated with genetic abnormalities. Men with nonobstructive azoospermia (NOA) and severe oligospermia should be informed that they might have chromosomal abnormalities or YCMD. Genetic counseling should be offered whenever a genetic abnormality is found.

Cystic Fibrosis Gene Mutations

The most common cause of CBAVD is a mutation of the CFTR gene. Almost all males with clinical cystic fibrosis have CBAVD. Approximately 70% of men with CBAVD and no clinical evidence of cystic fibrosis have an identifiable abnormality of the CFTR gene.[33,34] Since normal vasa are palpable within the scrotum, the diagnosis of vasal absence (agenesis), either bilateral or unilateral, is established by physical examination. Imaging studies and surgery are not necessary to confirm the diagnosis but may be useful for diagnosing abnormalities associated with vasal agenesis. Most patients with vasal agenesis also have malformed or absent seminal vesicles. Since the majority of semen is derived from the seminal vesicles, almost all patients with CBAVD have low semen volume.

It is recommended that both partners undergo genetic counseling and testing of the CFTR gene (including assessment of the 5T allele) to rule out abnormalities. Failure to identify a CFTR abnormality in a man with CBAVD, however, does not absolutely rule out the presence of a mutation, since several are undetectable by routine testing methods. It is important to test the partner for CFTR gene abnormalities prior to performing a treatment that utilizes the male's sperm because of the risk that the female may be a carrier.

Karyotype

A karyotype analyzes all chromosomes for the gain or loss of entire chromosomes as well as structural defects, including chromosome rearrangements (translocations), duplications, deletions, and inversions. Chromosomal abnormalities account for about 6% of all male infertility, and the prevalence increases with poorer semen parameters. Paternal transmission of chromosome defects can result in pregnancy loss, birth defects, male infertility, and other syndromes. Karyotypes should be ordered in men with severe oligospermia (sperm concentrations less than 5 million/mL) and azoospermia, as well as for couples with recurrent pregnancy loss and failed ART cycles.

Y-Chromosome Microdeletions

Approximately 13% of men with nonobstructive azoospermia or severe oligospermia have an underlying Y-chromosome microdeletion (YCMD).[35] YCMD responsible for infertility (azoospermic factor regions a, b, c) are detected using sequence tagged sites (STS) and polymerase chain reaction (PCR) analysis. Successful testicular sperm extraction for ICSI approaches 70% of men with AZFc deletions. The couple must be counseled on the transmission of the gene to all male offspring.[36–38]

Treatments for Male Infertility

There are several causes of infertility for which there is no treatment. For instance, there are no current treatments to stimulate sperm production when the seminiferous tubules have been severely damaged; examples include Klinefelter syndrome and YCMD.

In contrast, some azoospermic conditions, such as those with obstruction, may have sperm that can be extracted from the epididymis and/or testis. If mature sperm are obtained, they can be cryopreserved or used immediately to fertilize oocytes through *in vitro* fertilization. Even in cases with primary testicular failure, such as Klinefelter syndrome, sperm retrieval techniques can be employed along with intracytoplasmic sperm injection.[39] There are important genetic ramifications for these procedures.

Specific endocrine treatment is available for men whose infertility results from hypogonadotropic hypogonadism, i.e. from a pituitary/hypothalamic abnormality in which the pituitary gland does not properly release gonadotropic hormones that stimulate the testes. If hypogonadotropic hypogonadism results from hyperprolactinemia, the hypogonadism can often be corrected and fertility restored by lowering the serum prolactin concentration. If the hyperprolactinemia results from a medication, that medication should be discontinued. If the hyperprolactinemia results from a pituitary tumor identified by an MRI, the adenoma can be treated with a dopamine agonist, such as cabergoline or bromocriptine. Resumption of normal spermatogenesis usually does not occur for at least 3 to 6 months.

Removal of Gonadotoxic Agents

A wide range of chemical substances can affect sperm quality and/or quantity, including medications. The medications listed here are not exhaustive, but are commonly associated with male infertility and should be avoided where possible:

- Anabolic steroids/exogenous testosterone
- Antihypertensives (e.g., spironolactone)
- Chemotherapeutic agents (e.g., cyclophosphamide)
- Colchicine
- Finasteride
- Antibiotics (e.g., gentamycin, erythromycin, tetracycline)
- Opiates
- Antipsychotics

Radiation

Testes directly exposed to ionizing radiation suffer germ cell loss and Leydig cell dysfunction. The chances of having future offspring are lessened by radiation doses to the testes of 7.5 Gy and above.[40] Injury to the testis may occur even if not directly irradiated.

Treatment of Low Testosterone

It is estimated that up to 40% of infertile men may have hypogonadism. Clinicians may use aromatase inhibitors, hCG, selective estrogen receptor modulators such as clomiphene citrate, or a combination thereof for infertile men with low testosterone.

Men who have hypogonadotropic hypogonadism due to hypothalamic disease can be treated with gonadotropin-releasing hormone (GnRH). Human chorionic gonadotropin has the biologic activity of luteinizing hormone. The hCG dose is adjusted upward according to symptoms of hypogonadism, serum testosterone concentrations, and semen parameters. Some patients with acquired hypogonadotropic states can be stimulated with hCG alone to produce sufficient sperm. Utilization of human menopausal gonadotropin (hMG) or recombinant FSH is common as well. Pulsatile subcutaneous or intravenous treatment with gonadotropin releasing hormone (GnRH) has also been successfully used to treat gonadotropin deficient patients.[41]

Treatment of Genital Infections

Infertile men rarely present with symptoms or signs of acute genital infections or prostatitis, but they are sometimes diagnosed as having infections of the urogenital tract by the presence of increased leukocytes in the semen. It is unclear if leukocytospermia plays a pathogenic role in infertility. The presence of leukocytes may decrease sperm functional capacity by the release of reactive oxygen species. Semen cultures should be obtained when there are over one million leukocytes in the semen; however, the yield is usually poor and nondiagnostic[42].

Despite the absence of symptoms, patients who have leukocytospermia even if the culture is negative are treated with at least a 10-day course of antibiotics such as doxycycline or quinolone. A second course of therapy may be given if leukocytes persist in the semen after antibiotics. However, poor results make it difficult to demonstrate a cause-and-effect relationship between genital infections and male infertility. Exceptions are patients with a past history of gonorrhea, tuberculosis, and other specific sexually-transmitted diseases which lead to genital tract obstruction at the epididymis and/or vas deferens.[43]

Retrograde Ejaculation

Retrograde ejaculation (sperm backing up into the bladder) occurs in neurological conditions such as urogenital tract surgery, sympathetic denervation, and diabetes. Intrauterine insemination (IUI) can be performed using semen collected after alkalinization of the urine and extensive washing of the sperm. The washed sperm can also be used for *in vitro* fertilization or ICSI procedures. Concurrent use of alpha agonists, such as pseudoephedrine (Sudafed) prior to producing a sample, may be helpful in closing the bladder neck and converting retrograde ejaculation to antegrade ejaculation.

Varicocele

Varicoceles are dilated veins of the scrotum that are commonly associated with diminished semen parameters. They are thought to have deleterious effects by increasing the temperature of the scrotum and potentially creating back pressure and toxins.[44–46] Although the presence of varicoceles can be associated with normal semen parameters and normal fertility, many men with varicoceles have abnormal semen parameters including low-sperm concentration, motility, and abnormal morphology. When patients are carefully screened, and the goals as well as the time frame to achieve pregnancy are clearly determined, varicocele repair may significantly improve semen parameters and thereby improve the success of conceiving naturally and/or with assisted reproduction.

Atrophic testes, elevated serum FSH levels, and/or severe oligospermia or azoospermia indicate severe damage and are associated with a diminished likelihood of fertility after varicocele repair. A subinguinal approach has been shown to be effective treatment with low chance of adverse events. In some centers, laparoscopic varicocelectomy or vascular catheter embolization of spermatic veins are utilized.[47] An alternative to varicocele ligation or embolization is an assisted reproductive technique. Subfertile men with varicoceles should be offered repair with the understanding it may take anywhere from three to 12 months before there may be an improvement in semen parameters. Furthermore, couples may still require IUI or IVF in future depending on a variety of cofactors.

Obstructive Azoospermia

Obstructive azoospermia is determined by finding testes of normal size, normal serum FSH concentration, and absent sperm in the ejaculate. Both surgery and ART may be beneficial in such patients. As an example, obstruction of the epididymis or ejaculatory duct can be treated surgically. These procedures may lead to the presence of ejaculated sperm, but the results are variable and depend on the site of connection (reanastomosis), the skill of the surgeon, and the duration of obstruction. Patients should have the opportunity for sperm extraction and cryopreservation at the time of the reversal in the event they wish to proceed immediately with assisted reproduction or in the event of reversal failure and obstruction.

The results are best when obstructive azoospermia is due to a vasectomy.[48] The appearance of sperm after a vasectomy reversal can be over 90% with pregnancy in over 50% in selected patients.[49]

Ejaculatory duct obstruction presents with decreased semen volume and azoospermia or severe oligo/asthenozoospermia. Transrectal ultrasonography (TRUS) demonstrates dilated seminal vesicles, and aspiration of the seminal vesicles show spermatozoa suggesting obstruction. This condition may be treated by transurethral resection (opening via the urethra) of the ejaculatory ducts with resulting improved semen quality and pregnancy in the partner.[50, 51]

Assisted reproductive techniques can be combined to use sperm from men who have obstructive azoospermia to fertilize ova of their partners and achieve pregnancy. Sperm obtained by microsurgical aspiration from the epididymis (MESA) or from the testes by biopsy (TESE) or fine needle aspiration (TESA) can be used with eggs aspirated from the female partner for *in vitro* fertilization or ICSI.[52] The fertilization rate of microsurgical sperm aspiration along with ICSI, despite epididymal or testicular sperm of low quality, is approximately 50%, and the pregnancy rate is about 40% per cycle and 20% per microsurgical aspiration[53]. Given the continuous improvements in sperm retrieval and ICSI techniques, surgical reversal versus ART must be discussed before an informed decision can be made.[54]

Testicular Microdissection (microTESE)

Extraction of sperm from patients with NOA can be performed with microdissection of the testis to extract sperm (microTESE) from the seminiferous tubules. This has been successful in obtaining sperm in over 50% of patients with nonobstructive azoospermia, including patients with Klinefelter syndrome.[55–57]

ART

Assisted reproductive techniques (ART) are commonly used for the treatment of the female partner of men with oligospermia or azoospermia. Intrauterine insemination (IUI) consists of washing an ejaculated semen specimen to remove prostaglandins, concentrating the sperm in a small volume of culture media, and injecting the sperm suspension directly into the upper uterine cavity using a small catheter through the cervix. The insemination is timed to take place just prior to ovulation. In couples with mild male-factor infertility, IUI improves pregnancy rates compared to intracervical insemination or timed natural cycles. However, in cases of moderate to severe male-factor infertility where total motile sperm counts are significantly affected, IUI treatments have a lower chance of success.[58, 59]

In Vitro Fertilization with Intracytoplasmic Sperm Injection (ICSI)

ICSI has revolutionized treatment and improved the prognosis for infertile men with severe oligospermia, asthenospermia (low-sperm motility), teratospermia (a higher rate of abnormal sperm morphology), and even azoospermia. This technique involves the direct injection of a single sperm into the cytoplasm of a human oocyte, usually obtained from follicles produced under controlled ovarian hyperstimulation. This technique has also been successful in some men with Klinefelter syndrome where sperm are obtained from testicular biopsies.[60, 61] The overall fertilization rate is about 60%, and the clinical pregnancy rate per cycle is about 20% while the multiple pregnancy rate is about 29% to 38%. The ICSI results are not influenced by either the cause of the azoospermia or the origin of the spermatozoa.

When there are no sperm in the ejaculate but there are sperm producing cells (Sertoli cells) in the testes, ICSI can be performed with sperm isolated from testicular extraction.[62,63] Success is dependent on retrieving adequate numbers of sperm. Successful pregnancy can occur using injection of fresh or cryopreserved (frozen) sperm, but not with spermatocytes (immature sperm). Extracted testicular sperm may fertilize oocytes even in azoospermic men with maturation arrest, defective spermatogenesis, Klinefelter syndrome, and in men with long-standing azoospermia after chemotherapy.[64–68]

Artificial Insemination with Donor Semen

The alternative to ART for many couples is artificial insemination with donor sperm. This method has a very high success rate in otherwise normal females with close to 50% pregnancy rate within six cycles of insemination.

Conclusion

It is important to realize that infertility is often secondary to a male factor. In the past, men with infertility had relatively few options for treatment. In this era, however, it is often possible to determine the etiology of male subfertility and provide treatment options which offer help to many couples. Men with abnormal semen parameters or other known infertility risks factors should have a urological evaluation.

Key Points

1. Obstetricians and gynecologists, and in particular REIs, are historically the gatekeepers and first-line providers for couples initially seeking an infertility evaluation. It is important to recognize that 40% of these couples will have a male factor contributing to their infertility, with a male factor as the singular reason in approximately 20% of infertile couples.
2. Timely referral to a reproductive urologist may improve pregnancy outcomes in certain clinical scenarios and represents an opportunity for male health evaluation.
3. Circumstances which should prompt referral to a reproductive urologist include abnormal semen analysis, IUI and IVF failures, a clinically significant varicocele, idiopathic recurrent pregnancy loss, erectile and/or ejaculatory disorders.
4. Men with infertility are also at higher risk for other comorbid conditions such as hormonal and metabolic disorders and, therefore, evaluation is an opportunity to improve men's health.
5. Male infertility may be the presenting manifestation of an underlying life-threatening condition, such as testicular or pituitary tumors.

REFERENCES

1. Thonneau Pet al. Incidence and main causes of infertility in a resident population (1,850,000) of three French regions (1988–1989). *Hum Reprod* 1991; 6:811–816.
2. Honig SC et al. Significant medical pathology uncovered by a comprehensive male infertility evaluation. *Fertil Steril* 1994;62:1028–1034.
3. WHO. *WHO Laboratory Manual for the Examination and Processing of Human Semen*; 6th edition Geneva: World Health Organization, 2021.
4. Guzick DS et al. Sperm morphology, motiity, and concentration in fertile and infertile men. *N Engl J Med* 2001;345:1388–1393.
5. Kruger TF et al. Predictive value of abnormal sperm morphology in in vitro fertilization. *Fertil Steril* 1988;49:112–117.
6. Menkveld R et al. The evaluation of morphological characteristics of human spermatozoa according to stricter criteria. *Hum Reprod* 1990;5:586–592.
7. Pisarska MD et al. Fertilization after standard in vitro fertilization versus intracytoplasmic sperm injection in subfertile males using sibling oocytes. *Fertil Steril* 1999;71:627–632.
8. Carter SS et al. Transrectal ultrasonography in disorders of the seminal vesicles and ejaculatory ducts. *Urol Clin North Am* 1989; 16:773–790.
9. Jarow JP: Transrectal ultrasonography of infertile men. *Fertil Steril* 1993;60:1035–1039.
10. Coetzee K et al. Predictive value of normal sperm morphology: a structured literature review. *Hum Reprod Update* 1998;4:73–82.

11. Keegan BR et al: Isolated teratozoospermia does not affect in vitro fertilization outcome and is not an indication for intracytoplasmic sperm injection. *Fertil Steril* 2007; 88:1583–1588.
12. Van Waart J et al. Predictive value of normal sperm morphology in intrauterine insemination (IUI): a structured literature review. *Hum Reprod Update* 2001;7:495–500.
13. Spiessens C et al. Isolated teratozoospermia and intrauterine insemination. *Fertil Steril* 2003;80:1185–1189.
14. Shibahara H et al. Prediction of pregnancy by intrauterine insemination using CASA estimates and strict criteria in patients with male factor infertility. *Int J Androl* 2004;27:63–68.
15. Gunalp S et al. A study of semen parameters with emphasis on sperm morphology in a fertile population: an attempt to develop clinical thresholds. *HumReprod* 2001;16:110–114.
16. Kohn TP et al. Role of sperm morphology in deciding between various assisted reproduction technologies. *Eur Urol Focus* 2018;4(3):311–313.
17. Evenson DP et al. Utility of the sperm chromatin structure assay as a diagnostic and prognostic tool in the human fertility clinic. *Hum Reprod* 1999;14:1039–1049.
18. Evenson DP ,Wixon R: Data analysis of two in vivo fertility studies using Sperm Chromatin Structure Assay-derived DNA fragmentation index vs. pregnancy outcome. *Fertil Steril* 2008;90:1229–1231.
19. Bungum M et al. Sperm DNA integrity assessment in prediction of assisted reproduction technology outcome. *Hum Reprod* 2007; 22: 174–179.
20. Spano M et al. Sperm chromatin damage impairs human fertility. The Danish first pregnancy planner study team. *Fertil Steril* 2000;73:43–50.
21. Collins JA et al. Do sperm DNA integrity tests predict pregnancy with in vitro fertilization? *Fertil Steril* 2008;89:823–831.
22. Zini A, Sigman M. Are tests of sperm DNA damage clinically useful? Pros and cons. *J Androl* 2009;30:219–229.
23. Zini A et al. Sperm DNA damage is associated with an increased risk of pregnancy loss after IVF and ICSI: systematic review and meta-analysis. *Hum Reprod* 2008; 23:2663–2668.
24. Tan J et al. Association between sperm DNA fragmentation and idiopathic recurrent pregnancy loss: a systematic review and meta-analysis. *Reprod Biomed Online* 2019;38(6):951–960.
25. Sakkas D, Alvarez JG. Sperm DNA fragmentation: mechanisms of origin, impact on reproductive outcome, and analysis. *Fertil Steril* 2010;93(4):1027–1036.
26. ESHRE Guideline Group on RPL. ESHRE guideline: recurrent pregnancy loss: an update in 2022. *Hum Reprod Open* 2023;2023(1):hoad002.
27. de Ligny W et al. Antioxidants for male subfertility. *Cochrane Database Syst Rev* 2022;5(5):CD007411.
28. Brunner RJ et al. Review of guidelines for the evaluation and treatment of leukocytospermia in male infertility. *World J Mens Health* 2019;37(2):128–137.
29. Jung JH et al. Treatment of leukocytospermia in male infertility: a systematic review. *World J Mens Health* 2016;34(3):165–172.
30. Nagy ZP et al. Special applications of intracytoplasmic sperm injection: the influence of sperm count, motility, morphology, source and sperm antibody on the outcome of ICSI. *Hum Reprod* 1998;(13 Suppl 1):143–54.
31. Park YS et al. Influence of motility on the outcome of in vitro fertilization/intracytoplasmic sperm injection with fresh vs. frozen testicular sperm from men with obstructive azoospermia. *Fertil Steril* 2003;80(3):526–30.
32. Aboukhshaba A et al. Testicular sperm characteristics in men with nonobstructive azoospermia and their impact on intracytoplasmic sperm injection outcome. *Fertil Steril* 2022;117(3):522–527.
33. Anguiano A et al. Congenital bilateral absence of the vas deferens. A primarily genital form of cystic fibrosis. *JAMA* 1992;267:1794–1797.
34. Chillon M et al. Mutations in the cystic fibrosis gene in patients with congenital absence of the vas deferens. *New Engl J Med* 1995;332:1475–1480.
35. Reijo R et al. Severe oligozoospermia resulting from deletions of azoospermia factor gene on Y chromosome. *Lancet* 1996;347:1290–1293.
36. Silber SJ, Repping S. Transmission of male infertility to future generations: lessons from the Y chromosome. *Hum Reprod Update* 2002;8:217–229.
37. Foresta C et al. Y chromosome microdeletions and alterations of spermatogenesis. *Endocr Rev* 2001;22:226–239.

38. Schiff JD et al. Success of testicular sperm extraction and intracytoplasmic sperm injection in men with Klinefelter syndrome. *J Clin Endocrinol Metab* 2005;90:6263–6267.
39. Lanfranco F et al. Klinefelter's syndrome. *Lancet* 2004;364:273–283.
40. Green DM et al. Fertility of male survivors of childhood cancer: a report from the Childhood Cancer Survivor Study. *J Clin Oncol* 2010;28(2):332–9.
41. Crowley WF et al. The physiology of gonadotropin-releasing hormone (GnRH) secretion in men and women. *Recent Prog Horm Res* 1985;41:473–531.
42. Hua VN, Schaeffer AJ. Acute and chronic prostatitis. *Med Clin North Am* 2004; 88:483–494.
43. Bar-Chama N et al. Infection and pyospermia in male infertility. Is it really a problem? *Urol Clin North Am* 1994;21:469–475.
44. WHO. The influence of varicocele on parameters of fertility in a large group of men presenting to infertility clinics. *Fertil Steril* 1992;57:1289–1293.
45. Saypol, DC et al. Influence of surgically induced varicocele on testicular blood flow, temperature, and histology in adult rats and dogs. *J Clin Invest* 1981;68:39–45.
46. Mieusset R et al. Association of scrotal hyperthermia with impaired spermatogenesis in infertile men. *Fertil Steril* 1987;48:1006–1011.
47. White, RI. Radiologic management of varicoceles using embolotherapy. In: Whitehead ED, Nagler HM (eds), *Management of Impotence and Infertility*, JB Lippincott, Philadelphia 1994: 228.
48. Southwick, GJ, Temple-Smith, PD. Epididymal microsurgery: current techniques and new horizons. *Microsurgery* 1988; 9:266–277.
49. Belker AM et al. Results of 1,469 microsurgical vasectomy reversals by the Vasovasostomy Study Group. *J Urol* 1991;145:505–511.
50. Meacham RB et al. Evaluation and treatment of ejaculatory duct obstruction in the infertile male. *Fertil Steril* 1993;59:393–397.
51. Jarow JP. Transrectal ultrasonography in the diagnosis and management of ejaculatory duct obstruction. *J Androl* 1996; 17:467–472.
52. Silber SJ et al. Congenital absence of the vas deferens. The fertilizing capacity of human epididymal sperm. *N Engl J Med* 1990;323(26):1788–1792.
53. Silber SJ et al. Fertilizing capacity of epididymal and testicular sperm using intracytoplasmic sperm injection (ICSI). *Reprod Fertil Dev* 1995;7:281–292.
54. Robb P, Sandlow JI. Cost-effectiveness of vasectomy reversal. *Urol Clin North Am* 2009;36:391–396.
55. Donoso P et al. Which is the best sperm retrieval technique for non-obstructive azoospermia? A systematic review. *Hum Reprod Update* 2007;13:539–549.
56. Ramasamy R et al. Successful fertility treatment for Klinefelter's syndrome. *J Urol* 2009;182:1108–1113.
57. Schlegel, PN. Nonobstructive azoospermia: a revolutionary surgical approach and results. *Semin Reprod Med* 2009;27:165–170.
58. Merviel P et al. Predictive factors for pregnancy after intrauterine insemination (IUI): an analysis of 1038 cycles and a review of the literature. *Fertil Steril* 2010;93(1):79–88.
59. Muthigi A et al. Clarifying the relationship between total motile sperm counts and intrauterine insemination pregnancy rates. *Fertil Steril* 2021;115(6):1454–1460.
60. Palermo GD et al. Births after intracytoplasmic injection of sperm obtained by testicular extraction from men with nonmosaic Klinefelter's syndrome. *N Engl J Med* 1998;338:588–590.
61. Reubinoff,BE et al. A birth in non-mosaic Klinefelter's syndrome after testicular fine needle aspiration, intracytoplasmic sperm injection and preimplantation genetic diagnosis. *Hum Reprod* 1998;13:1887–1892.
62. Tournaye H et al. Recent concepts in the management of infertility because of non-obstructive azoospermia. *Hum Reprod* 1995;10 Suppl 1:115–119.
63. Schlegel PN et al. Testicular sperm extraction with intracytoplasmic sperm injection for nonobstructive azoospermia. *Urology* 1997;49:435–440.
64. Silber SJ et al. Normal pregnancies resulting from testicular sperm extraction and intracytoplasmic sperm injection for azoospermia due to maturation arrest. *Fertil Steril* 1996; 66:110–117.
65. Chen SU et al. Fertilization and embryo cleavage after intracytoplasmic spermatid injection in an obstructive azoospermic patient with defective spermiogenesis. *Fertil Steril* 1996;66:157–160.

66. Mulhall JP et al. Azoospermic men with deletion of the DAZ gene cluster are capable of completing spermatogenesis: fertilization, normal embryonic development and pregnancy occur when retrieved testicular spermatozoa are used for intracytoplasmic sperm injection. *Hum Reprod* 1997;12:503–508.
67. Tournaye H et al. Testicular sperm recovery in nine 47,XXY Klinefelter patients. *Hum Reprod* 1996;11:1644–1649.
68. Chan PT et al. Testicular sperm extraction combined with intracytoplasmic sperm injection in the treatment of men with persistent azoospermia postchemotherapy. *Cancer* 2001;92:1632–1637.

10

Clinical Algorithms

Naveena Daram, Denis Vaughan, and Nina Resetkova

Clinical algorithms aid the physician in the day-to-day management of the infertile couple. Each infertile individual or couple presents with a different set of circumstances, and the scope of the testing and recommended treatment will vary accordingly. These clinical algorithms are meant to serve as guides to diagnosis and treatment.

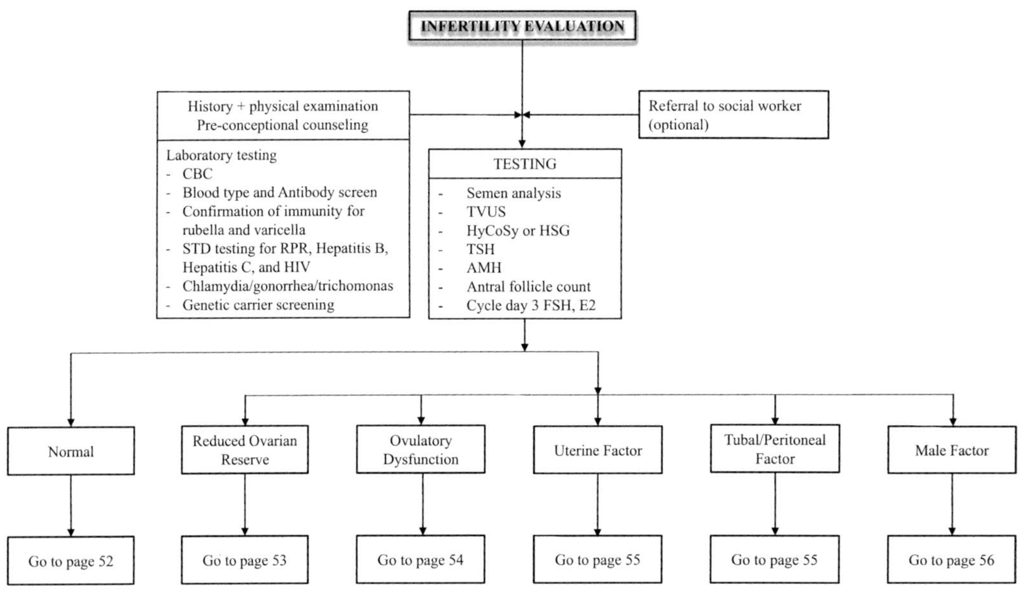

FIGURE 10.1 Infertility Evaluation. *Abbreviations:* CBC, complete blood count; TSH, thyroid stimulating factor; RPR, rapid plasma regain; HIV, human immunodeficiency virus; FSH, follicle stimulating hormone; HSG, hysterosalpingogram; AMH, anti-Müllerian hormone.

BIBLIOGRAPHY

Carson SA, Kallen AN. Diagnosis and management of infertility: a review. *JAMA* 2021;326(1):65–76.
Danforth DN. *Danforth's Obstetrics and Gynecology*. Lippincott Williams & Wilkins, 2008.
Penzias A et al. Fertility evaluation of infertile women: a committee opinion. *Fertil Steril* 2021;116(5):1255–1265.

DOI: 10.1201/9781003460275-10

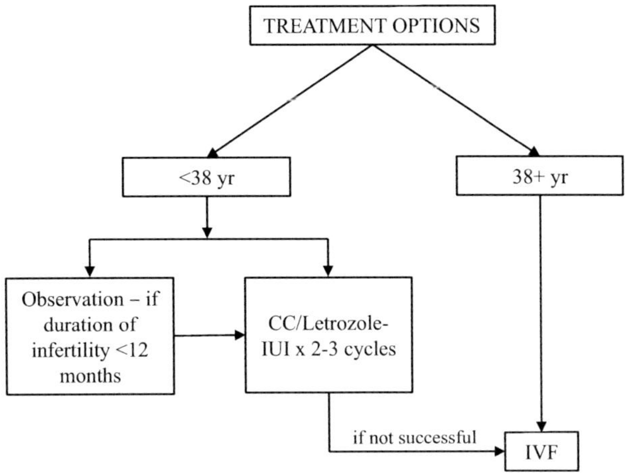

FIGURE 10.2 Unexplained infertility.

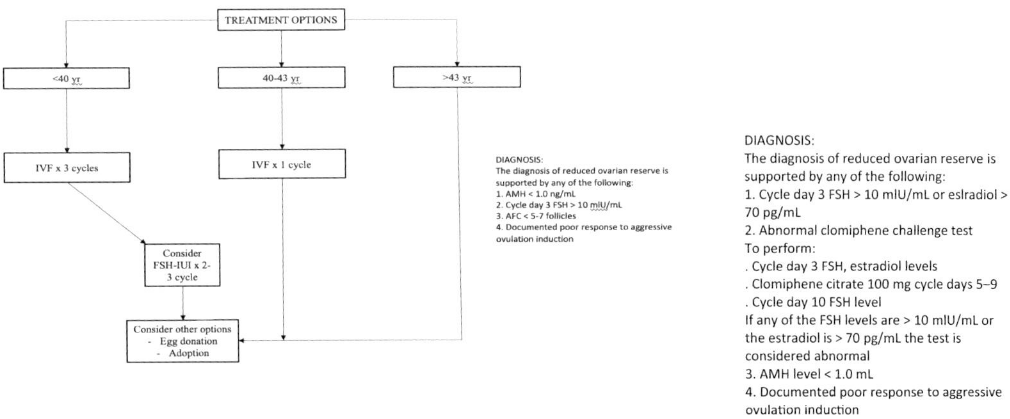

FIGURE 10.3 Reduced ovarian reserve.

DIAGNOSIS:

The diagnosis of reduced ovarian reserve is supported by any of the following:

1. **Cycle day 3:** FSH >10 mIU/mL or estradiol >70 pg/mL
2. Abnormal clomiphene challenge test
   To perform:
   - **Cycle day 3:** FSH, estradiol levels
   - **Cycle days 5–9:** Clomiphene citrate 100 mg
   - **Cycle day 10:** FSH level

   If any of the FSH levels are >10 mIU/mL or the estradiol is >70 pg/mL, the test is considered abnormal.
3. AMH level <1.0 mL
4. Documented poor response to aggressive ovulation induction

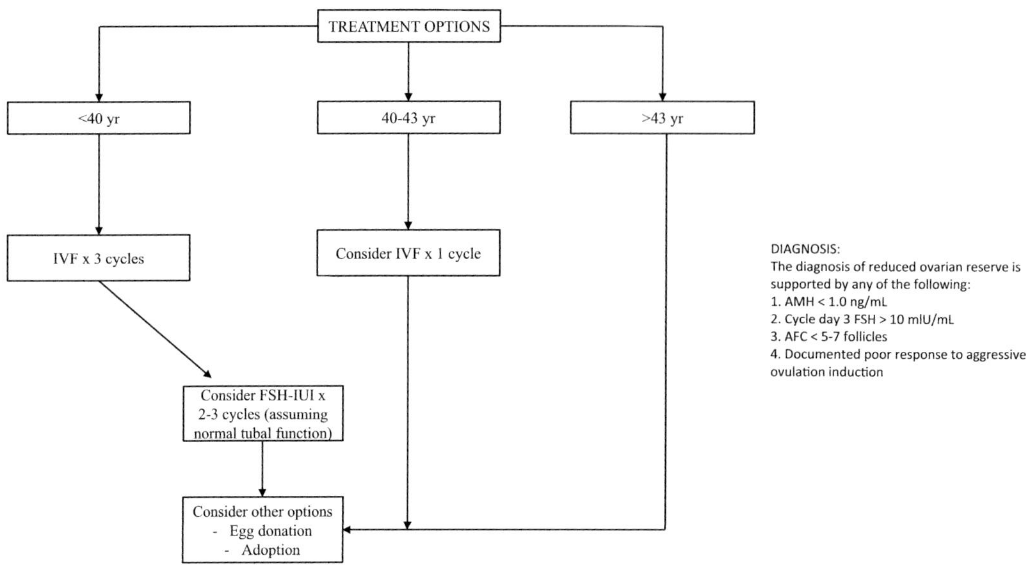

FIGURE 10.4 Diminished ovarian reserve.

DIAGNOSIS:

The diagnosis of reduced ovarian reserve is supported by any of the following:

1. AMH <1.0 ng/mL
2. Cycle day 3: FSH >10 mIU/mL
3. AFC <5-7 follicles
4. Documented poor response to aggressive ovulation induction

BIBLIOGRAPHY

Cohen J et al. Diminished ovarian reserve, premature ovarian failure, poor ovarian responder—a plea for universal definitions. *J Assisted Reproduct Genet* 2015;32):1709-1712.

Infertility Workup for the Women's Health Specialist: ACOG Committee Opinion 781. *Obstet Gynecol* 2019;133:e377–e384.

Testing and interpreting measures of ovarian reserve: a committee opinion. *Fertil Steril* 2020;114:1151–1157.

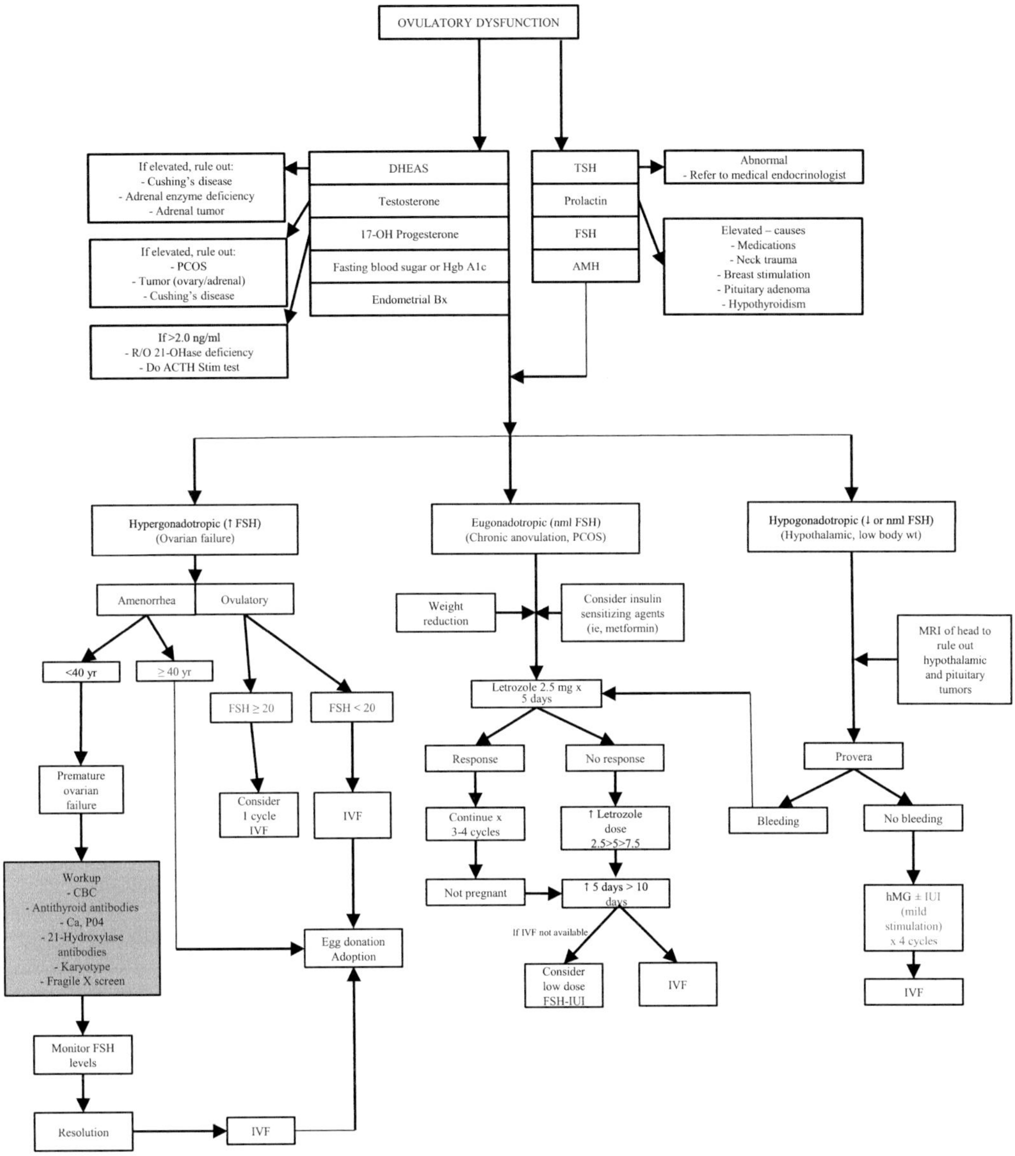

FIGURE 10.5 Ovulatory dysfunction.

BIBLIOGRAPHY

Casper R, Mitwally M. Ovulation induction with letrozole [internet], UpToDate, 2020 (updated 2024).

Madani T et al. Double mild stimulation and egg collection in the same cycle for management of poor ovarian responders. *J Gynecol Obstet Hum Reprod* 2019;48:329–333.

Mandelbaum RS et al. A comparison of letrozole regimens for ovulation induction in women with polycystic ovary syndrome. *F&S Reports* 2024;5(2):170-175.

Rahmani E et al. Dosage optimization for letrozole treatment in clomiphene-resistant patients with polycystic ovary syndrome: a prospective interventional study. *Obstet Gynecol Int* 2012;1:758508.

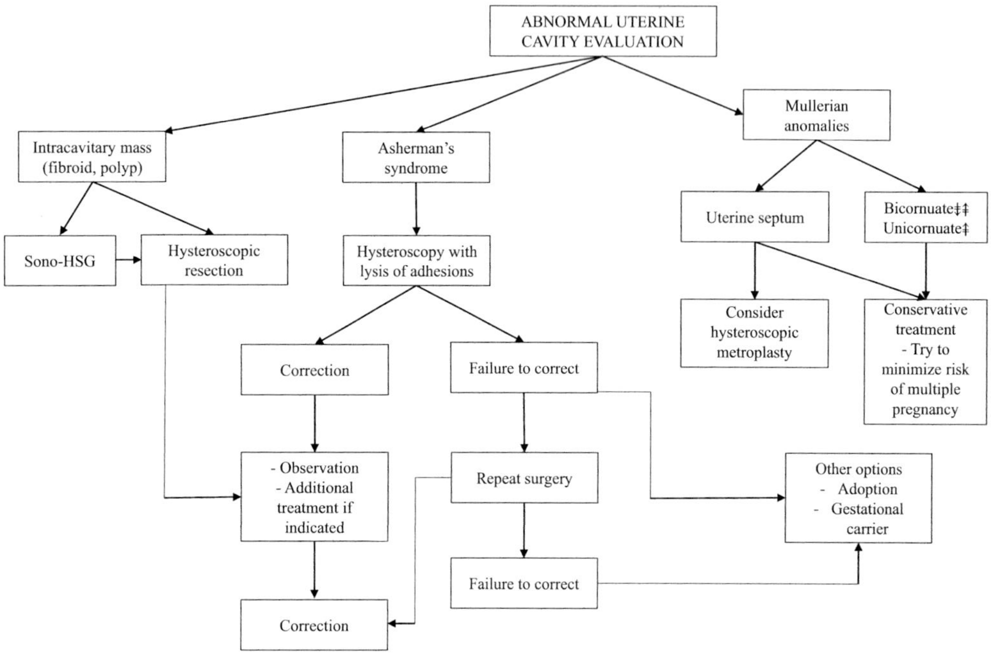

‡ 3D vaginal ultrasound and/or MRI will help to differentiate a uterine septum and a bicornuate uterus.
‡ Renal ultrasound to rule out anomalies in cases of unicornuate or bicornuate.

FIGURE 10.6 Uterine factor infertility.

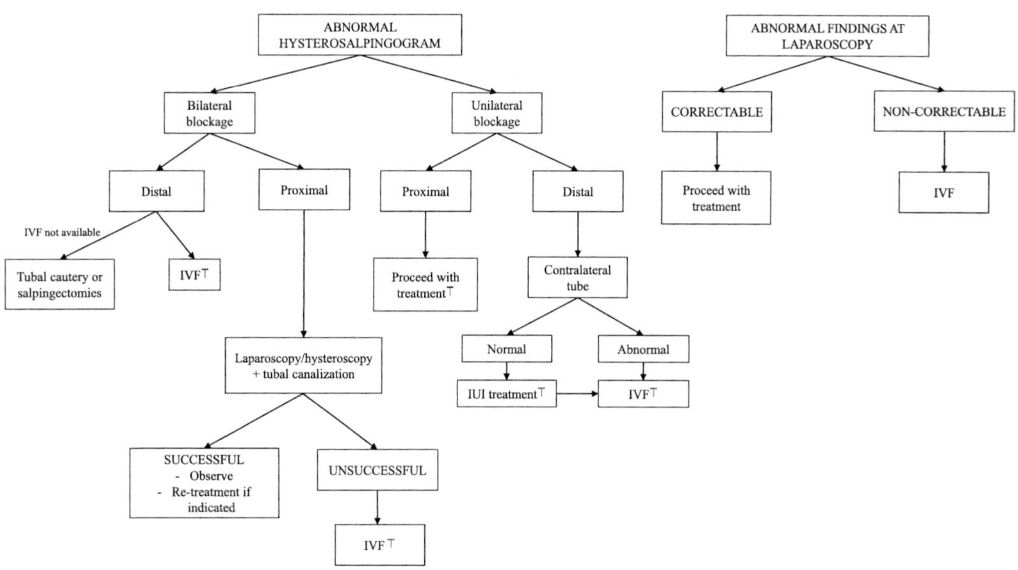

⊤ If hydrosalpinx present, salpingectomy prior to treatment is advised to optimize treatment outcomes.

FIGURE 10.7 Tubal/peritoneal factor.

BIBLIOGRAPHY

Roberts A. Fallopian tube recanalization for the management of infertility. *CVIR Endovasc*. 2023;6(1):13.

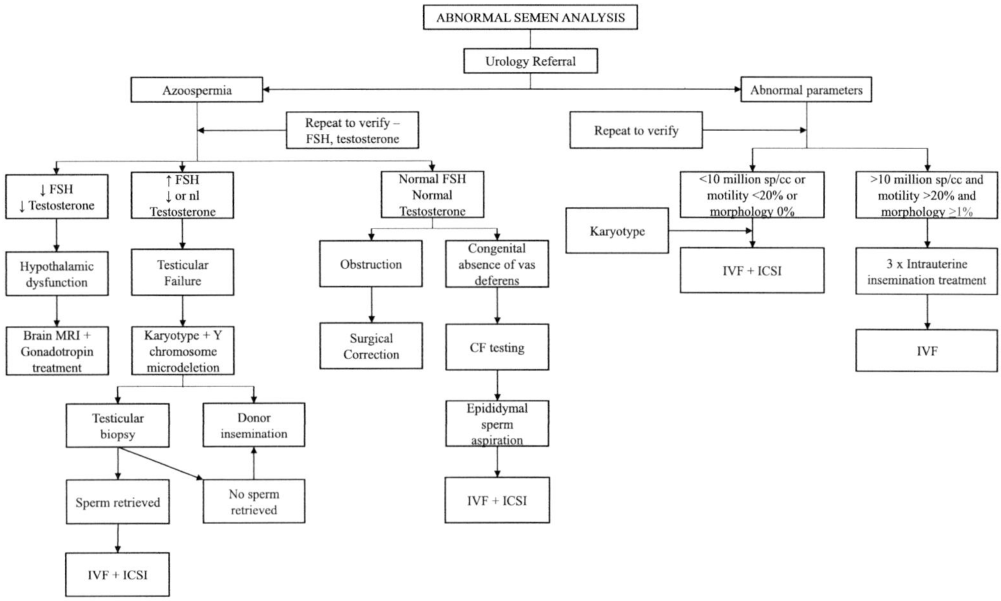

FIGURE 10.8 Male factor.

BIBLIOGRAPHY

Andrade DL et al. Differential diagnosis of azoospermia in men with infertility. *J Clin Med* 2021;10/14: 3144. (For abnormal sperm parameters)

Mulhall JP et al. Abnormal semen analysis. In: *Clinical Care Pathways in Andrology*. Springer, New York, 2014:1-10.

11

Treatment Options: I. Ovulation Induction

George Kovalevsky

Approximately 20% of infertile patients present with underlying ovulatory dysfunction as a major contributing factor to their infertility. Compared to other etiologies, ovulatory problems are often the easiest to overcome. However, before any treatment is started, it is important to delineate the underlying cause of the ovulatory dysfunction. The causes of ovulatory dysfunction are varied and can be categorized into *hypergonadotropic* (ovarian insufficiency), *eugonadotropic* (chronic anovulation), and *hypogonadotropic* (hypothalamic and pituitary dysfunction) states. When possible, the underlying etiology of ovarian dysfunction should be treated and corrected or improved. Women who have ovarian insufficiency or are perimenopausal generally do not respond favorably to medical treatment. Other causes of ovulatory dysfunction, such as thyroid disorders and hyperprolactinemia, can be easily identified and usually successfully treated to restore normal ovulation. However, the large majority of ovulatory dysfunction (>80%) is due to Polycystic Ovarian Syndrome (PCOS). In the majority of these cases, the underlying etiology cannot be fixed, making induction of ovulation necessary. There are several treatment options that can be used to induce ovulation, including medical treatment, lifestyle changes, and surgery (Box 11.1).

When ovarian stimulation is utilized, the choice of medication depends on the clinical presentation and the goal of the specified treatment. Ovarian stimulation can be conceptually separated into two types, ovulation induction and superovulation. Ovulation induction describes the stimulation of ovulation in the anovulatory patient. The goal is to achieve the growth of a single follicle with subsequent release of its egg. Superovulation refers to stimulation of growth of multiple follicles with the goal of releasing more than one egg. This chapter will focus primarily on the current approach to ovulation induction.

Lifestyle Changes

Body weight outside of the normal range is associated with ovulatory dysfunction. Change of weight towards normal range has been shown to result in resumption of ovulatory cycles.

Obesity, with or without diagnosis of Polycystic Ovarian Syndrome (PCOS), is associated with ovulatory dysfunction. Weight loss utilizing a healthy diet with exercise should be recommended. These

BOX 11.1 OVULATION INDUCTION

1. Identify and correct any underlying etiology when possible.
2. For eugonadotropic patients with conditions such as PCOS, institute lifestyle changes focusing on diet, exercise, and weight management.
3. If medical therapy is required, start with letrozole 2.5 mg daily for 5 days.
4. Monitor for an ovulatory response with urinary LH kits or serum progesterone.

DOI: 10.1201/9781003460275-11

lifestyle changes can restore ovulation through several mechanisms. Weight reduction lowers circulating insulin levels and reduces insulin resistance. Increased physical activity improves insulin sensitivity.

Weight loss is difficult to accomplish for many and assistance may be beneficial. Referral to weight loss programs is helpful for many. In recent years, glucagon-like peptide-1 receptor (GLP-1) agonists have been shown to be highly effective in accomplishing rapid weight loss. However, safety data for use in pregnancy is limited, and the current recommendation is to discontinue these medications two months prior to pregnancy. Lastly, when weight loss with conservative methods is unsuccessful, bariatric surgery may be considered.

Conversely, body weight below normal is also associated with ovulatory dysfunction. However, the mechanism is different, with these patients usually exhibiting hypogonadotropic hypogonadism and hypothalamic amenorrhea. Further investigation may uncover an eating disorder or excessive exercise. These should be appropriately addressed, and healthy weight gain should be recommended.

Inositol

Inositol is a sugar alcohol with two notable stereoisomers, Myo-inositol and D-chiro-inositol. Both have a role in insulin signaling and have been associated with increased chance of ovulation in patients with PCOS with minimal adverse effects. Evidence demonstrating efficacy is very limited. The optimal ratio of Myo to D-chiro has been demonstrated to be 40:1. A standard suggested dose is 2000 mg of Myo-inositol and 50 mg of D-chiro-inositol twice per day. Maximum efficacy is expected in three to six months. In the United States, inositol is considered a supplement and is available over the counter (1).

Letrozole

Letrozole is an aromatase inhibitor, FDA approved for the treatment of hormonally responsive breast cancer in post-menopausal women. It is now commonly used for ovarian stimulation, but it is not FDA approved for this indication. By inhibiting the aromatase enzyme, letrozole blocks the conversion of androgens to estrogens, thereby causing a drop in estrogen levels. This removes the negative feedback to the hypothalamus. The hypothalamus responds to the pseudo-hypoestrogenic state by increasing GnRH pulse frequency which, in turn, increases the secretion of FSH and LH from the anterior pituitary.

Letrozole is available in 2.5 mg tablets and is taken once a day for five days, beginning in the early follicular phase (cycle days 3–5). The standard starting dose is 2.5 mg per day, increasing up to 7.5 mg a day following either a spontaneous or progesterone-induced menstrual period. Many practitioners begin letrozole in anovulatory women following confirmation of a negative pregnancy test without inducing menses. Variable cycle monitoring can be utilized to determine timing for sexual intercourse or intra-uterine inseminations. Over-the-counter urine tests are available that can detect elevations of luteinizing hormone (LH) to predict imminent ovulation. Elevations of serum progesterone approximately 10–14 days after treatment has completed provide evidence that ovulation has occurred. After the treatment is started, if ovulation is confirmed but no pregnancy occurs, then the current dose should be continued for more attempts. If there is no indication of ovulation, the dosage of the letrozole should be increased to 5 mg for 5 days. If this dose is inadequate, then the dose should be increased to 7.5 mg. If the patient with chronic anovulation does not respond to a dose of 7.5 mg daily, then other treatment strategies should be considered. These include adding adjunct medications such as metformin or dexamethasone or proceeding with injectable gonadotropins.

If pregnancy is not achieved after three ovulatory cycles or sooner, then other factors should be ruled out, if a complete evaluation has not yet been performed. If no other factors are identified, then intrauterine inseminations can be added. IVF can also be considered.

The side effects of letrozole are usually mild and include hot flashes, nausea, dizziness, and headaches. The risk of a multiple pregnancy is from 5–10%, most of which are twins. High order multiple pregnancies are rare. Ovarian hyperstimulation syndrome is theoretically possible but exceedingly rare.

Historically, there was a concern regarding the use of letrozole for fertility after an initial report concluding that there was an increased rate of fetal anomalies with letrozole (2). However, larger studies have *not* shown any increased risk to the offspring (3, 4). The half-life of letrozole is only 2 days. It is completely eliminated within 10 days, which is before any significant embryo development if letrozole is used for ovulation induction. Care should be taken to avoid administering it to anyone who could already be pregnant.

Since the publication of a large multicenter randomized clinical trial in 2014, letrozole has become the first choice for ovulation induction in women with PCOS (5). This trial demonstrated that when compared to clomiphene citrate, letrozole resulted in higher rates of ovulation, conception, and live birth in this population. Letrozole also showed a trend toward a lower twin pregnancy rate, but this finding did not reach statistical significance as the study appeared to be underpowered to appropriately evaluate this outcome.

Clomiphene Citrate

Clomiphene citrate (CC) was first introduced in 1961 and was, for many years, the most common agent for ovulation induction, including patients with PCOS. Those patients with hypothalamic dysfunction who fail to have withdrawal bleeding following a progesterone challenge will in most cases not respond well to CC.

CC is a triphenylethylene derivative that is a selective estrogen receptor modulator (SERM) but functions primarily as an estrogen antagonist. It binds for an extended period of time to intranuclear estrogen receptors, which decreases the replenishment of these receptors. This results in decreased negative feedback to the hypothalamus, which subsequently leads to increased FSH release, similar to the effect of letrozole.

CC has a half-life of 5 days and can be detected in the blood and stool up to 6–8 weeks after administration. Despite the long half-life of CC, there are no reported increases in congenital anomalies that can be attributed to the use of this medication.

CC is usually well-tolerated. However, since CC is a synthetic hormonal agent, side effects are common and are not dose-related. Many of the side effects that result relate to the pseudo-hypoestrogenic state that is created. The more common side effects and their incidence are shown in Table 11.1.

The use of ovulation inductions agents, especially CC, may result in more pain associated with ovulation. Prolonged administration of CC through its anti-estrogenic action can diminish cervical mucus production and thin the endometrial lining, which could lower the chance of pregnancy.

CC is available in 50 mg tablets. The recommended initial dose of CC for treatment of anovulatory infertility is 50 mg daily for 5 days following either a spontaneous or progesterone-induced menstrual period. Many practitioners begin CC in anovulatory women following confirmation of a negative pregnancy test without inducing menses. Variable cycle monitoring can be utilized to determine timing for sexual intercourse or intrauterine inseminations. Over-the-counter urine tests are available that can detect elevations of luteinizing hormone (LH) to predict imminent ovulation. Elevations of serum progesterone approximately 10–14 days after treatment has completed provide evidence that ovulation occurred. After

TABLE 11.1

Side Effects of Clomiphene Citrate

Irritability, mood changes	20%
Vasomotor symptoms	10%
Abdominal discomfort	6%
Breast discomfort	2%
Nausea/Vomiting	2%
Visual symptoms	1%
Headaches	1%

the treatment is started, if ovulation is confirmed but no pregnancy occurs, then the current dose should be continued for more attempts. If there is no indication of ovulation, the dosage of the CC should be increased to 100 mg for 5 days. If this dose is inadequate, then the dose should be increased to 150 mg. Although higher doses up to 250 mg per day may be attempted, the majority of pregnancies occur at dosages of 150 mg daily or less. If the patient with chronic anovulation does not respond to a dose of 150 mg daily, then other treatment strategies should be considered. These include switching to letrozole, adding adjunct medications such as metformin or dexamethasone, or proceeding with injectable gonadotropins.

If pregnancy is not achieved after three ovulatory cycles or sooner, then other factors should be ruled out if a complete evaluation has not yet been performed. If no other factors are identified, then intrauterine inseminations can be added to the CC treatment since CC may have an adverse effect on cervical mucus in 15% of cases. IVF can also be considered.

Proceeding in the stepwise fashion as described previously, the ovulatory rates on the 50 mg, 100 mg, and 150 mg dosage regimens are 50%, 22%, and 12%, respectively (6). However, despite 80% of anovulatory patients ovulating with CC treatment, only 40–50% of women will achieve pregnancy (7). The multiple pregnancy rate is 10% with the large majority being twins and the risk of triplets less than 1%.

Medications That Can Be Used as an Adjunct to Letrozole and Clomiphene Citrate

In cases of resistance to letrozole or CC, other medications may be considered, which can be administered in addition to the primary ovulation induction agent (Box 11.2).

Metformin (Oral Hypoglycemic Agent)

It is believed that insulin resistance plays a central role in the pathogenesis of PCOS. Insulin resistance is a condition in which insulin action is hampered either by a defective insulin receptor or a post-receptor defect. With insulin resistance, higher circulating insulin levels are necessary to maintain normal glucose homeostasis. Hyperinsulinism can explain many of the associated findings of PCOS. Insulin increases ovarian and adrenal androgen production, decreases the production of sex hormone binding globulin, and stimulates the pituitary secretion of LH. All of this leads to an androgenic *milieu* that

BOX 11.2 MANAGEMENT OF LETROZOLE AND CLOMIPHENE CITRATE FAILURES

Lack of ovulation:

- Serial increases in dose.
- If using CC, switch to letrozole.
- Metformin pretreatment with 1500–2000 mg qd for 4–6 weeks prior to another course of treatment (8).
- Dexamethasone 0.5 mg PO qd starting same day as main treatment and continuing for 10 days or until LH surge—particularly for cases where the DHEAS is elevated (>430 mg/dL) but may be helpful even without DHEAS elevation.
- Switch to gonadotropin use or proceed to IVF.

Ovulation but no pregnancy:

- In order to optimize timing of sexual intercourse, add a surrogate LH surge with an injection of hCG 10,000 units or recombinant hCG 250 mcg subcutaneously when the lead follicle is 18–25 mm in diameter.
- Add a progesterone supplement starting three days after the LH surge detected by an ovulation predictor kit or after the hCG injection (9).
- Add intrauterine inseminations.

interferes with normal follicular development and ovulation. Insulin resistance is a metabolic disorder, and ovulatory dysfunction is only one of its manifestations. Other medical issues associated with insulin resistance include Type II diabetes, hypertension, dyslipidemia, centripetal obesity, and an increased risk of cardiovascular disease.

Those with adult-onset diabetes mellitus have been treated effectively with oral hypoglycemic agents, such as metformin which improves the actions of insulin in several ways. It increases the uptake of glucose into fat and muscle cells. In addition, it decreases intestinal absorption of glucose and reduces hepatic gluconeogenesis. There is published data that has confirmed that metformin improves the insulin resistance in patients with PCOS, which results in a correction of the ovulatory dysfunction (8, 10, 11). This was a significant breakthrough in the treatment of PCOS. Many women with PCOS respond poorly to CC and have to be treated with injectable gonadotropins to induce ovulation, which is associated with a higher multiple pregnancy rate and greater chance of OHSS. In a previous meta-analysis, it was concluded that metformin alone improved the rate of ovulation (12, 13). The ovulation rates were different between the metformin and placebo groups, 46% vs. 26%. Also, the rate of ovulation in those who took metformin plus CC or CC alone was 76% vs. 42%, respectively. While metformin may be effective by itself, it may take up to six months to appreciate ovulatory cycles (11, 13). After these studies were published, metformin treatment became a common initial treatment for PCOS patients. However, many of the initial studies included a small number of patients. A well-designed study published by Legros et al. provided the data that helped to define the role of metformin treatment in PCOS (14). This multicenter, blinded study involved 626 infertile women with PCOS who were randomly assigned to one of three arms: clomiphene citrate plus placebo (CC), metformin plus placebo (MET), and metformin plus clomiphene citrate (MET/CC). Patients were then followed for six months after the treatment began. The live birth rate was 22.5% in the CC group, 7.2% in the MET group, and 26.8% in the MET/CC group. The difference in pregnancy rates was statistically significant between CC vs. MET and MET/CC vs. MET groups but not for CC vs. MET/CC. The conclusion from this study is that CC is significantly more effective than metformin for the PCOS patient. However, metformin does have a role in the treatment of the PCOS patient, primarily as an adjunct.

Evaluation

Renal studies (creatinine, BUN) and liver function tests (SGOT, SGPT) should be considered. One potential risk of metformin treatment is lactic acidosis. The incidence of this side effect is increased in those patients with renal or hepatic dysfunction.

Recommended Dosage

Metformin is available in standard and extended release (XR) formulations. Initiation of metformin should be done in a gradual fashion to decrease the incidence of side-effects. One tablet (500 mg) should be taken daily for 1 week, then twice a day for 1 week, and then 3–4 times a day (1500–2000 mg per day). The medication should be taken with meals. There are benefits in the XR formulation—for some it is better tolerated, and the total dose can be taken at once on a daily basis.

Side Effects

Gastrointestinal symptoms, including nausea, vomiting, diarrhea, bloating, and flatulence, occur in 30% of patients who take metformin. These side effects are usually temporary, but in some patients the side effects do not abate. In these cases, decreasing the dose may reduce the side effects, and at some time in the future a higher dose may be tried again. Lactic acidosis is a serious metabolic disorder that may be increased in those with renal and/or hepatic dysfunction. There have been reports of metformin-induced lactic acidosis following the administration of intravenous iodine contrast agents, which can result in transient nephrotoxicity. Therefore, metformin should be withheld 24 hours before and 48 hours after the performance of the x-ray procedure. PCOS patients are at increased risk of miscarriage, and there has been some controversy as to whether metformin decreases the chance of a first trimester loss if taken throughout the early part of pregnancy. A meta-analysis concluded that metformin does not decrease the chance of a first trimester loss (15).

Long-Term Treatment

In some cases, long-term treatment with metformin can be considered for up to 6–12 months. This is an especially attractive treatment for those women with obesity and possibly other associated consequences of insulin resistance (i.e., hypertension, glucose intolerance) who may not be in the best health for a pregnancy. Metformin should also be considered in those women who want to avoid a multiple pregnancy that is associated with ovarian stimulation medications. For the patient with obesity, good nutrition and an exercise program should be stressed. A referral to a nutritionist should strongly be considered. Weight loss will increase the effectiveness of metformin. The patient should follow-up with the physician periodically every 6–8 weeks to monitor for treatment efficacy.

Short-Term Treatment

For those patients who have failed to respond to moderate doses of CC or letrozole, pretreatment with metformin (4–8 weeks) before moving on to another cycle may prove efficacious.

Dexamethasone

Dexamethasone can be considered for the anovulatory woman who fails to respond to increasing doses of CC and letrozole, particularly if she is noted to have an elevated dehydroepiandrosterone sulfate (DHEAS) level. An elevated DHEAS level may suggest an attenuated adrenal enzyme deficiency, but in most cases a mild increase is associated with PCOS. Other causes include an adrenal tumor and Cushing's syndrome, which must be considered but are, nonetheless, rare. If associated with an elevated 17-OH-progesterone level, a 21-hydroxylase deficiency must be ruled out. The administration of dexamethasone will decrease the adrenal androgen contribution to the pool of androgens. In some cases, this will be enough to improve the response to CC. Dexamethasone can be administered at night at a dose of 0.5 mg. One month after starting the dexamethasone, a morning cortisol level should be checked. A cortisol level less than 2 mcg/dL suggests significant depression of cortisol synthesis by the adrenal gland, which could interfere with a stress response by the adrenal gland. In this circumstance, the dose or frequency of administration should be decreased. The use of dexamethasone should be avoided during pregnancy.

Dexamethasone can also be considered in CC and letrozole failures in the absence of elevated androgen levels. In a previous RCT, 223 CC resistant patients were randomized to receive CC 200 mg days 5–9 + dexamethasone (DEX) 2.0 mg days 5–14, and the other group was given CC 200 mg days 5–9 + a placebo (16). In the CC+Dex group 88% ovulated compared to only 20% in the CC+placebo group.

Dexamethasone treatment options:

- 0.5 mg qd. Check morning serum cortisol plasma level 3–4 weeks after treatment started and if <2.0 mcg/dL, reduce the dose.
- 0.5–2.0 mg cycle days 5–14 during CC cycle.

Gonadotropins

Gonadotropins (FSH and LH) are injectable medications that are effective in correcting ovulatory dysfunction. For the majority of patients, only FSH is needed since most anovulatory patients produce adequate LH. Gonadotropin use is rarely the first choice for ovulation induction due to the high cost, need for daily injections, and associated risks. In particular, one must exercise caution when administering these agents to correct ovulatory dysfunction (as compared to their use in the context of superovulation) to minimize the risk of a multiple pregnancy. It is important that low doses of FSH (50–75 IU daily) be administered initially, the patient's response is monitored, and the dose is increased slowly in small increments. The patient should be counseled that the process can be lengthy and labor-intensive.

Gonadotropin use for ovulation induction is primarily reserved for patients with hypothalamic/pituitary dysfunction and those who were resistant to therapy with oral agents.

Hypothalamic and Pituitary Dysfunction

Since these patients are deficient in both FSH and LH, both hormones need to be replaced. Letrozole and CC may be tried but have a low chance of achieving ovulation. Previously, human menopausal gonadotropins was the drug of choice. Currently, treatment usually consists of using FSH with LH activity added in the form of HCG, injected as a combined product or individually.

1. Begin with FSH 50–75 IU daily (with HCG added in or 10 IU given separately) x 5–7 days, then check estradiol level and pelvic ultrasound to assess response.
2. If no follicular development and no rise in E2 is seen, increase FSH by 25–37.5 IU x 3 days, then repeat the monitoring. Increase FSH by no more than 37.5 IU every 3–4 days.
3. When a response is detected (follicle >12 mm and/or rise in E2), continue the same dose and repeat monitoring 2–3 days.
4. Administer hCG (trigger shot) when lead follicle is ≥16mm.

Caution

These patients are at significant risk of a multiple pregnancy—the goal of the stimulation is 1–2 follicles. If more than 2 follicles ≥ 16 mm or if several secondary follicles are present >12 mm, consideration should be given to canceling the cycle or converting to IVF.

Ovarian hyperstimulation syndrome (OHSS) can be a risk related to gonadotropin use. In addition to the aforementioned mature follicles, careful study of the ultrasound is needed to assess the number of small follicles 10–14 mm.

Polycystic Ovarian Disease

These patients are deficient in FSH and may have elevated circulating levels of LH. Therefore, only FSH containing medications are needed to correct the ovulatory dysfunction.

1. FSH 37.5 to 75 IU x 5 days, then check E2 and ultrasound
   a. If E2 <50, increase by 37.5 IU x 3 days, then repeat the E2/US. Increase hMG by no more than 1/2 amp every 3–4 days
   b. If E2 >50, continue the same dose and repeat monitoring 2–3 days
2. Administer hCG when lead follicle is ≥16mm

Caution

These patients are at risk of a multiple pregnancy and OHSS—the goal of the stimulation is 1–2 follicles. However, the success rate in the PCO population is lower than those patients with hypothalamic dysfunction. If more than 3–4 follicles ≥ 16m develop on ultrasound examination or if several secondary follicles >12 mm are present, then consideration should be given to canceling the cycle or converting to IVF.

Ovarian Drilling

Ovarian drilling is a surgical technique for patients with PCOS that consists of limited destruction of ovarian tissue containing hormone producing follicles and thereby restoring a normal hormonal balance and resumption of ovulation. Currently, it is not frequently performed in the United States for multiple reasons:

- Requires surgery with associated risk of complications.
- Effects are temporary and hormonal dysfunction eventually returns.
- Damaging the ovaries may cause subsequent adhesions and damage to the ovarian reserve, in turn leading to additional causes of infertility.

The main advantages of ovarian drilling are:

- High efficacy rate.
- Allows for unassisted pregnancies to occur without the need for cycle monitoring.
- Elimination of the risks and side effects associated with medical ovulation induction, in particular multiple gestation and OHSS.

Given the noted benefit-to-risk ratio, for most individuals, ovarian drilling is reserved for cases where medical therapy has failed and IVF is not feasible.

Unexplained Infertility

In clinical practice, CC or letrozole are commonly prescribed for the woman with unexplained infertility. Theoretically, it seems that this would improve fecundity by increasing the number of eggs that are released at the time of ovulation and may also correct subtle ovulatory dysfunction. However, previous studies, including a Cochrane review of seven trials, fail to show that CC improves fertility over doing nothing at all (17–19). Nevertheless, some couples and clinicians feel that this is a reasonable initial treatment to pursue. As with any therapy, most pregnancies are achieved within the first few months of treatment. Therefore, the duration of treatment should be limited to 3–4 cycles, at which time the treatment plan should be reassessed. Adding IUI may help improve the low pregnancy rates. Main risk is multiple gestations. Gonadotropins may also be used for treatment of unexplained infertility. However, the extra cost, risk, and effort usually outweigh any small improvement in pregnancy rates.

Recommended Dosage

CC 50–100 mg or letrozole 5 mg administered cycle days 3 through 7. Limit duration of treatment to three to four months. Instruct couples to use an ovulation predictor kit or have intercourse every other day between cycle days 10 and 18.

REFERENCES

1. Fitz V et al. Inositol for polycystic ovary syndrome: a systematic review and meta-analysis to inform the 2023 Update of the International Evidence-based PCOS Guidelines. *J Clin Endocrinol Metab* 2024; 109(6):1630–55.
2. Biljan MM et al. The outcome of 150 babies following the treatment with letrozole or letrozole and gonadotropins. *Fertil Steril* 2005;84(suppl 1);S95.
3. Tulandi T et al. Congenital malformations among 9111 newborns conceived after infertility treatment with letrozole or clomiphene citrate. *Fertil Steril* 2006;85(6):1761–5.

4. Forman S et al. Fetal safety of letrozole and clomiphene citrate for ovulation induction. *J Obstet Gynaecol Can* 2007;29,668–71.
5. Legro RS et al. Letrozole versus clomiphene for infertility in the polycystic ovary syndrome. *N Engl J Med* 2014;371:119–29.
6. Gysler M et al. A decade's experience with an individualized clomiphene treatment regimen including its effect on the post-coital test. *Fertil Steril* 1982; 37:161.
7. Garcia J et al. The use of clomiphene citrate. *Fertil Steril* 2006;86:S187–93.
8. Nestler JE et al. Effects of metformin on spontaneous and clomiphene-induced ovulation in the polycystic ovary syndrome. *N Engl J Med* 1998;338:1876–80.
9. Elkind-Hirsch KE et al. Sequential hormonal supplementation with vaginal estradiol and progesterone gel corrects the effect of clomiphene on the endometrium of oligo-ovulatory women. *Hum Reprod* 2002;17:295–8.
10. Velazquez EM et al. Menstrual cyclicity after metformin therapy in polycystic ovary syndrome. *Obstet Gynecol* 1997;90:392–5.
11. Velazquez EM et al. Metformin therapy in polycystic ovary syndrome reduces hyperinsulinemia, insulin resistance, hyperandrogenemia, and systolic blood pressure, while facilitating normal menses and pregnancy. *Metabolism* 1994;43:647–54.
12. Lord JM et al. Metformin in polycystic ovary syndrome: systematic review and meta-analysis. *BMJ* 2003;327:951–7.
13. Ibanez L et al. Sensitization to insulin induces ovulation in nonobese adolescents with anovulatory hyperandrogenism. *J Clin Endocrinol Metab* 2001;863:595–8.
14. Legros RS et al. Clomiphene, metformin, or both for infertility in polycystic ovary syndrome. *N Engl J Med* 2007;356:551–66.
15. Paolmba S et al. Effect of preconceptional metformin on abortion risk in polycystic ovary syndrome: a systematic review and meta-analysis of randomized controlled trials. *Fertil Steril* 2009;92:1646–58.
16. Parsanezhad ME et al. Use of dexamethasone and clomiphene citrate in the treatment of clomiphene-resistant patients with polycystic ovary syndrome and normal dehydroepiandrosterone sulfate levels: a prospective, double-blind, place-controlled trial. *Fertil Steril* 2002;78:1001–4.
17. Hughes E et al. Clomiphene citrate for unexplained subfertility in women. *Cochrane Database of Syst Rev* 2010;1:CD00005.
18. Hughes EG. The effectiveness of ovulation induction and intrauterine insemination in the treatment of persistent infertility: a meta-analysis. *Hum Reprod* 1997;12:1865–72.
19. Fujii S et al. The effects of clomiphene citrate on normally ovulatory women. *Fertil Steril* 1997;68:997–9.

12

Treatment Options: II. Intrauterine Inseminations

Sonia Elguero and Marsha Forman

Intrauterine insemination (IUI) is a common fertility treatment that involves concentrating motile sperm and placing it high within the uterine cavity. It is utilized in a variety of clinical infertility situations including cervical factor, mild male factor, severe vaginismus, and ejaculatory dysfunction. However, the most common indication for IUI is unexplained infertility. It is also the best approach to therapeutic donor sperm insemination (TDI). Prerequisites for performing IUI include ovulation, patency of at least one fallopian tube, and an adequate number of motile sperm for insemination. While a natural cycle approach may be considered in some instances, in most cases of unexplained or male factor infertility, the use of fertility medications (such as clomiphene citrate or letrozole) to increase the development of multiple follicles has been shown to increase the chance of success. The mechanism by which IUI improves fertility is not totally clear but may be the result of several factors. The sperm washing procedure may eliminate toxins or bacteria in the seminal plasma and has been shown to induce the acrosome reaction causing activation of the sperm. The IUI may also bypass an impediment in the cervical mucus. A likely mechanism by which IUI works is simply a sperm number issue; in contrast to intercourse, the IUI results in a higher number of motile sperm that enter the fallopian tube where fertilization occurs. Finally, the IUI may overcome faulty coital technique on the part of the couple. Despite all these theoretical benefits of IUI, the overall success of IUI treatment is low in comparison to IVF. Nevertheless, for many infertility patients IUI is their first introduction to treatment. This chapter will provide an overview of the treatment.

Approaches to IUI Treatment

Natural Cycle

A natural or non-medicated approach is most often used with TDI. A natural cycle IUI may be suitable in a couple with coital factor infertility such as ejaculatory dysfunction or vaginismus. It may be the desire for the couple who want to completely avoid medications or a multiple pregnancy (which is more likely with adjuvant medications). When considering this treatment approach, it is essential that the patient is ovulatory.

Monitoring

The patient is instructed to start testing her urine with an ovulation predictor kit 3–4 days before the anticipated time of ovulation. For the woman who has cycles that are 28–30 days in length, she is instructed to start testing her urine on day 11. When the ovulation predictor test turns positive, she is instructed to come in the following day for the insemination.

DOI: 10.1201/9781003460275-12

Clomiphene Citrate (CC)

CC can be offered with IUI to help improve success rates. CC is the most widely prescribed fertility medication and has been available for decades. CC is administered at a dose of 100 mg for 5 days between cycle days 3 and 7. Alternatively, it can be administered between cycle days 5 and 9.

Femara (Letrozole)

Letrozole is another option instead of CC to add to the IUI treatment. In women with PCOS and an elevated body mass index greater than 30, letrozole has been shown to be more effective in inducing ovulation with higher live birth rates as compared to CC (1). In the setting of unexplained infertility, letrozole and CC have been shown to have similar live birth rates (2). The starting dose is typically 2.5 mg/day for 5 days (starting on either day 3 or 5 of the cycle) and can be increased up to 7.5 mg/day.

At higher doses, it can be associated with a thin endometrium, similar to CC. For women with unexplained infertility, letrozole may result in lower rates of multiple gestation compared to CC. It is currently used off label as it is not approved by the U.S. Food and Drug Administration for ovulation induction. It can be potentially teratogenic if inadvertently used during early pregnancy, and patients should be counselled about off label use before prescribing.

Monitoring

The patient is instructed to use an ovulation predictor kit beginning on cycle day 11. When the test turns positive, a single insemination treatment is done the following day. In our experience, approximately 90% of patients will detect the LH surge between cycle days 11 and 15. An alternative to the ovulation predictor kit is to perform vaginal ultrasound examinations beginning cycle day 12 and to administer human chorionic gonadotropin (hCG) (10 000 IU or 250 ug of Ovidrel®) when the follicle reaches 18 mm, and the insemination is scheduled 36 hours after hCG. There is no difference in the success rate with CC IUI when ultrasound monitoring and hCG trigger versus monitoring the LH surge with urine testing (3). However, the advantage of doing ultrasound exams is that it provides valuable information about the ovarian response and often ameliorated patient anxiety. The average success rate following CC IUI treatment is 8–10% per cycle and the multiple pregnancy rate is 10% (9% twins; 1% triplets). An important factor that impacts treatment success is maternal age. The Boston IVF experience with IUI was published in 2025 (4); see Table 12.1. Of note, IUI success rates decline dramatically beyond 3–4 IUI cycles, therefore, the recommendation is to strongly consider moving to IVF in that setting.

Gonadotropins

The addition of FSH injections (gonadotropin) as part of IUI treatment increases the success rate compared to clomiphene or letrozole. However, twins and higher-order multiples risk is also higher. The injections of FSH are started on day 3 and continued until mature follicles have developed on ultrasound. The initial dose will be dependent on many factors including previous response and age. In general, the first cycle of treatment requires more caution with the starting dose (75–150 U) since it is unknown how the patient will respond to the medication. This is of less concern for the older patient over the age of 40 who most likely has some reduced ovarian reserve, and the starting dose may be increased to (150–225 U). The goal of the treatment may vary as well. For a younger woman, the goal is to obtain 2–3 mature follicles that are 16 mm or larger. If more than 5 mature follicles are present and/or there are multiple follicles between 12–16 mm, then there is an increased risk of a multiple pregnancy. These cycles should be either cancelled or converted to an IVF treatment cycle.

Monitoring

A serum estradiol level and vaginal ultrasound exam is recommended 4–5 days after starting injections. If the estradiol level is >400 pg/mL, then the dose is reduced by 75 U. The goal is to have the estradiol

TABLE 12.1

Cycle Specific and Cumulative Incidence of Clinical Pregnancy by Group among All Patients (from ref 4 with permission)

	Heterosexual couples n=4014 couples			Same-sex female couples n=795 couples			Unpartnered female patients n=355 patients		
Cycle	Started cycle	Cycle-specific clinical pregnancy	Cumulative clinical pregnancy	Started cycle	Cycle-specific clinical pregnancy	Cumulative clinical pregnancy	Started cycle	Cycle-specific clinical pregnancy	Cumulative clinical pregnancy
1	4014	376 (9.4, 8.4–10.3)	376 (9.4, 8.4–10.3)	795	81 (10.2, 8.3–12.5)	81 (10.2, 8.3–12.5)	355	34 (9.0, 6.9–13.1)	34 (9.0, 6.9–13.1)
2	2779	222 (8.0, 7.0–9.1)	598 (14.9, 13.8–16.0)	606	55 (9.1, 7.0–11.6)	136 (17.1, 14.7–19.9)	267	21 (7.9, 5.2–11.7)	55 (15.5, 12.1–19.6)
3	1414	82 (5.8, 4.7–7.1)	680 (16.9, 15.8–18.1)	447	41 (9.2, 6.8–12.2)	177 (22.3, 19.5–25.3)	193	8 (4.1, 2.1–8.0)	63 (17.7, 14.1–22.1)
4	394	26 (6.6, 4.5–9.5)	706 (17.6, 16.4–18.8)	275	28 (10.2, 7.1–14.3)	205 (25.8, 22.9–28.9)	126	9 (7.1, 3.8–13.0)	72 (20.3, 16.4–24.8)
5	157	10 (6.4, 3.5–11.3)	716 (17.8, 16.7–19.1)	188	16 (8.5, 5.3–13.4)	221 (27.8, 24.8–31.0)	85	0 (0.0, 0.0–4.3)	72 (20.3, 16.4–24.8)
6	77	4 (5.2, 2.0–12.6)	720 (17.9, 16.7–19.2)	137	13 (9.5, 5.6–15.6)	234 (29.4, 26.4–32.7)	60	7 (11.7, 5.8–22.2)	79 (22.3, 18.2–26.9)
7	16	0 (0.0, 0.0–19.4)	720 (17.9, 16.7–19.2)	35	4 (11.4, 4.5–26.0)	238 (29.9, 26.9–33.2)	9	1 (11.1, 2.0–43.5)	80 (22.5, 18.5–27.2)
8	4	0 (0.0, 0.0–49.0)	720 (17.9, 16.7–19.2)	16	0 (0.0, 0.0–19.4)	238 (29.9, 26.9–33.2)	5	0 (0.0, 0.0–43.5)	80 (22.5, 18.5–27.2)
9	2	0 (0.0, 0.0–65.8)	720 (17.9, 16.7–19.2)	9	1 (11.1, 2.0–43.5)	239 (30.1, 27.0–33.3)	2	0 (0.0, 0.0–65.8)	80 (22.5, 18.5–27.2)
10	0	N/A	N/A	7	0 (0.0, 0.0–35.4)	239 (30.1, 27.0–33.3)	0	--	--

Note: Data are shown as numbers (percentages and 95% confidence intervals).

TABLE 12.2

FSH-IUI Success Rates (data from ref 7 with permission)

Age	Number of Cycles	Live Birth Rate, % (95% CI)
<25	15	26.7 (4.3, 49.4)
25–29	219	14.2 (9.6, 18.8)
30–35	556	12.5 (9.8, 15.2)
36–39	221	9.5 (5.6, 13.4)
≥40	106	8.5 (3.2, 13.8)

level increase by 50–100% every 2–3 days. The vaginal ultrasound will determine the number and size of the follicles. A mature follicle is between 16–20 mm in diameter. The final goal of the treatment is to have a peak estradiol level between 500–2000 pg/mL at the time of the hCG administration. A single insemination is performed 36 hours after hCG administration.

Success Rate

As with any fertility treatment, several factors impact success. One important factor is the semen quality. Pregnancy rates are higher when the total motile sperm count is >2 million, post-wash motility is >40%, and/or normal sperm morphology is >4%. (5). However, interpretation of sperm morphology can vary from lab to lab. Age is an important determinant of treatment success (6, 7). Duran et al. reported on over 1000 cycles and reported the live birth rate in the different age groups (see Table 12.2).

Multiple pregnancy is a significant issue with gonadotropin IUI cycles and has led to it being essentially replaced by IVF in many centers. The exception is hypogonadotropic hypogonadal patients who often will not respond to oral medications. In these cases, judicious gonadotropin dosing is prudent.

Preparation of the Semen Sample

A semen sample is produced on the day of the IUI. It is best to collect the sample in a sterile specimen container supplied by the laboratory since it has been tested for sperm survivability. Several plastics are harmful to sperm and may reduce the vitality of the sample. It is preferred that semen is collected via masturbation. However, collection condoms can be purchased online from fertility specialty stores. Contraceptive condoms should never be used since they are developed to kill sperm with or without spermicide. Lubricants should also not be used to produce the sample as they can be spermicidal. Semen samples can be produced on site or at home and then transported to the laboratory. It is best if the sample collected outside of the office can be delivered within 60 minutes after production. The sample should be kept at body temperature from the time of collection until it is received by the laboratory staff. Exposure to temperatures other than body temperature for an extended time between collection and processing may be responsible for poor motility of the specimen. For security reasons, we recommend only accepting semen samples from the person who produced the semen sample and not another party. Identification is confirmed by examination of a government-issued picture ID.

Our sperm washing procedure is as follows:

Once the sample is received by the laboratory staff, it is assessed for its raw characteristics including volume, concentration, and motility. The semen sample is then washed and prepared for insemination. Washing can be performed in a complex or simple fashion. Washing of the sample removes prostaglandins and bacteria found in the seminal plasma. A simple wash will concentrate the sperm, both motile and immotile, into the pellet for insemination. A more complex wash uses a density gradient to filter the seminal fluid resulting in a pellet with elevated motility. Washing also concentrates the sperm into a reduced volume for insemination. If the clinic treats patients with Hepatitis or HIV viral infections, there are altered semen washing processes aimed to remove the infective fraction of the ejaculate while still capturing sperm.

Specimens are processed using sterile techniques and practicing universal precautions. Examination gloves should be always worn, and facial protection should be used if the sample is not processed under a hood. Check the laboratory requisition for any special instructions.

1. The semen sample is produced by masturbation into the provided sterile specimen cup.
2. Allow semen sample to liquefy for 20–60 minutes.
3. Measure volume with a 10 ml serological pipet.
4. Divide sample into two test tubes labeled "pellet" with patient's name.
   a. Simple method: Add an equal volume of sperm wash to each of the tubes and mix well.
   b. Complex method: Layer semen in a 2:1 ratio over 80% gradient.
5. Remove any coagulates that may pellet to bottom of tubes.
6. Centrifuge for 10 minutes at 1200 rpm (300 x g).
7. Remove supernatant and place in labeled "super" tube.
8. Resuspend the pellets in a total of 2 ml fresh sperm wash; the two pellet tubes should be combined at this step. The wash medium should not exceed 2 mls.
9. Centrifuge (second time) for 5 minutes at 1200 rpm (300 x g).
10. Remove supernatant.
11. Resuspend the pellet in a total of 0.5 ml sperm wash.
12. Mix thoroughly and count the sample.
13. Place washed sample on the 37^{0}C warmer until ready to use.

Performing the IUI

Depending on local regulations, nurses or physicians may perform the IUIs. Before the insemination, the patient's name and the name of the person who produced the sperm are verified. The names are once again verified on the test tube containing the washed sperm. To perform the IUI treatment, a speculum examination is performed and the cervix is visualized. The cervix is wiped with a large cotton tip applicator. The washed sperm sample is loaded into a catheter by affixing one end of the catheter to a 1 ml syringe and then placing the distal end of the catheter into the semen sample. The syringe plunger is carefully pulled back until the entire sample is loaded into the syringe. The catheter is then inserted through the cervical canal and into the uterine cavity and the plunger is pressed to expel the washed sample into the uterine cavity. Immediately following the IUI, the patient is discharged, and normal activity can be resumed. A pregnancy test is scheduled 14 days later. Patients should be reassured that mild cramping or discomfort can occur along with increased wetness. Luteal phase support can be considered with IUI cycles particularly in patients utilizing gonadotrophins.

Single Versus Double Inseminations

The decision to do one versus two successive daily inseminations has been the subject of ongoing debate. In a meta-analysis, Polyzos et al. reported on 68 randomized controlled studies including 829 women (8). The pregnancy rate in double versus single insemination groups was 13.6% versus 14.4%, respectively. These findings have been supported by other investigators (9, 10). The odds ratio was 1.33 (95% CI 0.99, 1.73). From a theoretical standpoint, a second insemination may not be necessary if one considers that sperm generally maintain their viability for 48–72 hours and the oocyte has a 12–24-hour window to be fertilized.

Cost Analysis

The financial aspect of treatment may play an important part of the decision-making process. It is clear that IVF is the most successful option, but for many couples the treatment may be too costly. Some states and countries have mandated coverage for infertility treatment and the degree of coverage can vary quite a bit. As an example, in U.S.A., the State of Massachusetts has one of the best insurance coverage mandates and allows the couple to choose IVF versus IUI. Many patients choose to go directly to IVF while others will try a few insemination cycles first. Other states have coverage for IVF treatments, and they include New York, Rhode Island, New Hampshire, California, and several others. The vast majority of infertile couples in the U.S.A. do not have insurance coverage for treatment. Boston IVF participated in a study that helped to put this into better perspective. The fast track and standard treatment trial (FASTT) involved over 500 couples with unexplained infertility (11). The couples were randomized to one of two arms: The first arm included 3 cycles of CC IUI followed by 3 cycles of FSH IUI, and then up to 6 cycles of IVF; the second "accelerated" arm involved 3 cycles of CC IUI and then directly moving to IVF. The conclusions from the study were as follows:

- An increased pregnancy rate was noted in the accelerated group.
- Median time to pregnancy was quicker in accelerated group 8 versus 11 months.
- Per pregnancy rates for CC IUI, FSH IUI, and IVF were 7.6%, 9.8%, and 30.7%, respectively.
- Average charges per delivery were $9800 lower for the accelerated arm.
- FSH IUI treatment had no added value.

The most cost-effective approach for the couple with unexplained infertility is CC IUI x 3 cycles, then move on to IVF.

IUI Versus IVF

Intrauterine insemination is one of the oldest infertility treatments and still has a place in the treatment paradigm, but its utility may be fading. Over the years, IVF success rates have continued to increase, and this has resulted in the transfer of fewer embryos, thus decreasing the chance of a multiple pregnancy. The complications and risks associated with a multiple pregnancy are well-documented. Preimplantation genetic testing for aneuploidy (PGT-A) has led to the mostly uniform transfer of a single euploid blastocyst. IUI with medications (especially gonadotropins) has a higher multiple pregnancy rate compared to IVF with the transfer of a single embryo.

Key Points

- Use of injectable gonadotropins as part of IUI treatment increases the risk of twins and higher higher-order multiples compared to clomiphene or letrozole.
- Studies of 1 vs. 2 IUIs in the same cycle show no difference in outcome.
- IUI success rates decline dramatically beyond 3–4 IUI cycles; therefore, the recommendation is to strongly consider moving to IVF thereafter.

REFERENCES

1. Legro RS et al. Letrozole versus clomiphene for infertility in the polycystic ovarian syndrome. NICHD Reproductive Medicine Network. *N Engl J Med* 2014; 371:119–29.
2. Diamond MP et al. Letrozole, gonadotrophin or clomiphene for unexplained infertility. NICHD Reproductive Medicine Network. *N Engl J Med* 2015; 373:1230–40.

3. Lewis V et al. Clomiphene citrate monitoring for intrauterine insemination timing: a randomized trial. *Fertil Steril* 2006;85:401–6.
4. Heyward QD et al. Reproductive outcomes following insemination in same-sex female couples, unpartnered female patients, and heterosexual couples. *Fertil Steril* 2025;123(1):173–5.
5. Haebe J et al. Success of intrauterine insemination in women aged 40–42 years. *Fertil Steril* 2002;78:29–33.
6. Harris ID et al. Poor success of gonadotropin-induced controlled ovarian hyperstimulation and intrauterine insemination for older women. *Fertil Steril* 2010;94:144–8.
7. Duran HE et al. Intrauterine insemination: a systematic review on determinants of success. *Hum Reprod Update* 2002;8:373–84.
8. Polyzos NP et al. Double versus single intrauterine insemination for unexplained infertility: a meta-analysis of randomized trials. *Fertil Steril* 2010; 94:1261–6.
9. Osuna C et al. One versus two inseminations per cycle in intrauterine insemination with sperm from patients' husbands: a systematic review of the literature. *Fertil Steril* 2004;82:17–24.
10. Bagin T et al. Singe versus double intrauterine insemination in multi-follicular ovarian hyperstimulation cycles: a randomized trial. *Hum Reprod* 2010;25:1684–90.
11. Reindollar RH et al. A randomized clinical trial to evaluate optimal treatment for unexplained infertility: the fast track and standard treatment (FASTT) trial. *Fertil Steril* 2010; 94:888–910.

13

Treatment Options: III. In Vitro *Fertilization-Stimulation Protocols*

Ann Korkidakis, Michael M. Alper, and Thomas L. Toth

In vitro fertilization (IVF) is one of the most significant advances in the field of reproductive medicine. The first IVF baby, Louise Brown, was born in England in 1978. This was the result of a decade of research by Dr. Robert Edwards, who was ultimately awarded the Nobel Prize in Medicine in 2010 for his work (1, 2). Now, over 91,000 babies each year are being born as a result of this technology nationally, representing 2.5% of all babies born in the US (3). Initially IVF was developed for women with tubal disease; however, it has become the treatment of choice for many other reproductive cases (Figure 13.1). Since its introduction, there have been advances in every step of IVF treatment, which has resulted in a continued rise of success rates over the last 20 years. IVF offers the highest chance of live birth of all autologous treatment options, meaning the use of a patient's own eggs. This modality has also provided a platform for the development of other treatments including fertility preservation, egg donation, gestational surrogacy, and preimplantation genetic testing. This chapter will provide a basic overview of the IVF treatment.

The four steps of IVF will be reviewed:

I. Ovarian stimulation
II. Oocyte retrieval
III. Oocyte insemination
IV. Embryo transfer

I. Ovarian Stimulation

IVF treatment initially consisted of non-medicated, or natural, cycles. These cycles were extremely inefficient since few follicles developed and they required very frequent monitoring for the endogenous LH surge. One of the first developments that significantly increased IVF success rates was the use of gonadotropins to stimulate the growth of multiple ovarian follicles. The term "gonadotropins" refers to medications that contain follicle stimulating hormone (FSH) and luteinizing hormone (LH) activity. While this change represented a marked improvement, premature ovulation still complicated approximately 30% of cycles, making timing of the egg retrieval a challenge and leading to a very high cancellation rate. The next breakthrough occurred in the late 1980s when the GnRH agonist was introduced. The addition of the GnRH agonist virtually eliminated any chance of a premature LH surge and resulted in more control of the cycle. Later in the 1990s, the GnRH antagonists were developed and provided another approach to suppressing a premature LH surge. The ovarian hyperstimulation step is extremely important since the success rate is directly related to the number of oocytes that are retrieved, which, in turn, impacts the number of embryos that are available for transfer. Over the years, there has been a change using gonadotropins obtained from the urine of postmenopausal women to those preparations created by recombinant

DOI: 10.1201/9781003460275-13

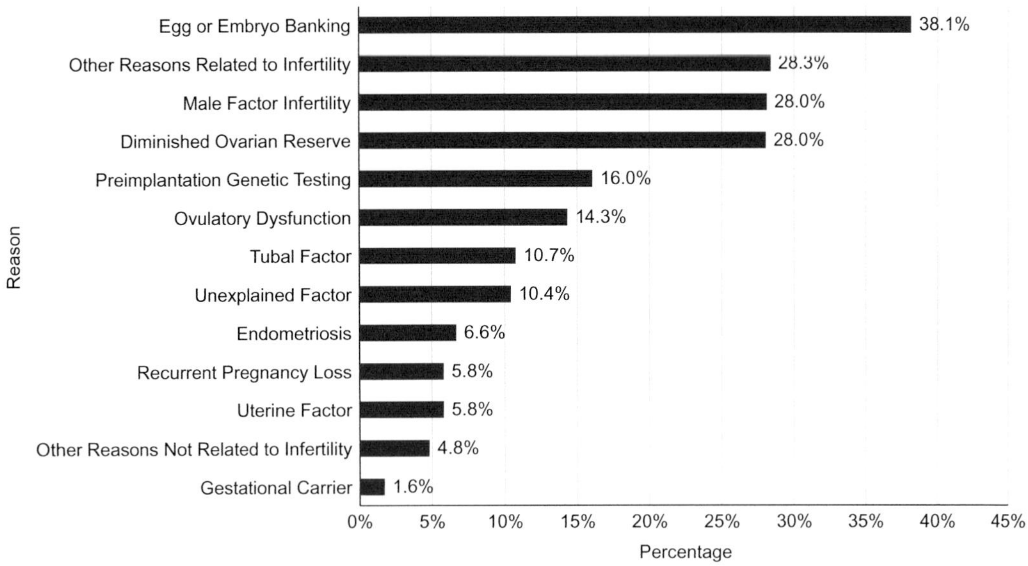

FIGURE 13.1 Percentage of ART cycles by reason for using ART in the United States 2020 (from ref 11 with permission).

DNA technology. The newer gonadotropins are more purified, allowing subcutaneous injection. The ovulation induction protocols that are currently used are described below.

Pituitary Suppression with a GnRH Antagonist

GnRH antagonists are the most commonly used protocols in current ART cycles. They result in the immediate suppression of FSH and LH release from the pituitary gland by competitively binding and blocking the GnRH receptor. Given their binding is reversible, a GnRH agonist trigger can be used in these cycles as it displaces the antagonist from the receptors and induces ovulation. The advantages include fewer injections, avoidance of the profound ovarian suppression that can occur after administration of a GnRH agonist, and a lower chance of ovarian hyperstimulation syndrome (OHSS). These associated effects render GnRH antagonists safer, cost effective, and more patient-friendly than traditional protocols. There are both flexible and fixed GnRH antagonist-start cycles. For both, gonadotropins are started early in the follicular phase. Programs with a fixed start generally routinely initiate the GnRH antagonist after 5–6 days of gonadotropins. In the flexible start, the GnRH antagonist is added once the lead follicle reaches a diameter of 14 mm and/or the serum estradiol level is >500 pg/mL.

Pituitary Down-Regulation with a GnRH Agonist

Prior to the development of GnRH antagonists, pituitary down-regulation with a GnRH agonist was commonly employed. While GnRH agonists initially result in a flare of gonadotropin release, extended use results in "down-regulation" of pituitary GnRH receptors, which reduces pituitary FSH and LH release and prevents an LH surge. However, the GnRH agonist must be administered for a period of 10–15 days before down-regulation occurs. Generally, the GnRH agonist is administered in the mid-luteal phase (cycle day 21) of the preceding cycle. It can also be started in the early follicular phase with the onset of menses. After down-regulation has occurred, the dose of the GnRH agonist is reduced and the ovarian stimulation is initiated with gonadotropin injections. Importantly, as the GnRH receptors are desensitized with this protocol, a GnRH agonist cannot be used as a trigger and a hCG-based trigger is required in these cycles.

Alternative Protocols

There are alternative protocols and protocol modifications that are used for women who have a poor response in a prior cycle or who have evidence of reduced ovarian reserve. These may include a Microdose Lupron Flare protocol, Luteal Phase Estrogen Priming protocol, and Minimal Stimulation protocol. At this time, there is no conclusive evidence of the benefit of one protocol over another, and a personalized approach should be undertaken based on a discussion with the provider.

Monitoring

During the ovarian stimulation, the patient's response is monitored with serum hormone levels and vaginal ultrasound examinations. The estradiol level is used to determine the dose of gonadotropins and whether under- or over-stimulation is occurring. The LH and progesterone levels can be ordered as well to assist in identifying premature ovulation. The goal of the ovarian stimulation is to develop a cohort of mature follicles, often defined as 17 mm in diameter or larger. Once this is achieved, gonadotropins and other medications are discontinued, and a trigger using either hCG or GnRH agonist is given to mature the eggs, improve yield at oocyte retrieval, and optimize subsequent fertilization rates. It is standard that the trigger injection is administered approximately 36 hours before the scheduled egg retrieval, as this will allow adequate maturation of the eggs with little risk of ovulation.

II. Oocyte Retrieval

The egg retrieval is performed under vaginal ultrasound guidance. First the vagina is cleansed with normal saline followed by culture media. Betadine is not used since it may be toxic to the eggs. The vaginal ultrasound probe is then placed in the vagina and the ovarian follicles are identified. A 17-gauge needle is directed through the back wall of the vagina and into the ovarian follicles. The fluid is then aspirated and examined by an embryologist who identifies the egg under microscopy. In general, all follicles within both ovaries are aspirated. Notably, not all follicles are expected to yield an oocyte. Once the eggs are retrieved, they are pipetted into plates with culture media and then placed in the incubator. The procedure is performed under light anesthesia and generally takes less than 10–15 minutes to complete. Prophylactic antibiotics are routinely administered. The overall complication rate is <1%.

III. Oocyte Insemination

Conventional Insemination

On the day of egg retrieval, the sperm concentration and motility are assessed. If the sperm sample is adequate, then a sperm prep is done to isolate the most motile sperm. A total of 50,000 motile sperm are placed with the eggs in a culture dish, which is then placed in the incubator. In the absence of male factor or a history of poor fertilization, conventional insemination is the preferred modality for oocyte fertilization.

Intracytoplasmic Sperm Injection (ICSI)

ICSI is used in cases of male factor or in cases when a prior conventional IVF resulted in poor fertilization (4). It was first introduced in 1992 and revolutionized the field of IVF for cases of male factor infertility (5). ICSI involves the injection of a single sperm directly into the oocyte. Fertilization rates following this procedure are between 60–70%, which are comparable to the rates achieved with a standard insemination with normal semen parameters. Importantly, males with severe oligospermia (counts <5 million sperm/cc) should have further evaluation with a reproductive urologist.

The morning after insemination, the eggs are examined to determine whether fertilization has occurred. Fertilization is determined by the presence of two pronuclei within the egg (one from the sperm and the other from the egg). Subsequently, the nuclei unite and the embryo will start to divide.

IV. Embryo Transfer

The embryo transfer can be performed either day 3 (cleavage stage embryo) or day 5 (blastocyst stage) after the egg retrieval. With the improvement of culture conditions, there has been a shift from day 3 to day 5 embryo transfers in the United States. A good quality embryo on day 3 generally contains between 6–8 cells, whereas a blastocyst on day 5 often contains over 100 cells that have started to organize into embryonic components. The advantage of waiting until day 5 is that it provides the opportunity to select the higher quality embryos, since only 50–60% of embryos have the ability to develop into blastocysts. Published evidence supports a higher implantation potential for a blastocyst embryo compared to a cleavage stage embryo. However, if there are fewer embryos available, there may be a benefit to an earlier transfer, such as lower cycle cancellation rates.

As embryo culture methods and embryo selection have improved over time, the standard has evolved into elective single embryo transfer (Figure 13.2). This practice dramatically reduces the chance of multifetal gestations, which are associated with significant obstetrical risks.

We perform the embryo transfer under transabdominal ultrasound guidance. A full bladder allows the uterus to be easily visualized on ultrasound, which permits the catheter to be clearly seen as it courses through the cervical canal into the uterine cavity. The catheter is positioned 1–2 cm from the top of the cavity where the embryo is placed. Research has demonstrated that both the use of ultrasound guidance and of soft embryo transfer catheters improve implantation and clinical pregnancy rates (6). There is good evidence not to recommend bed rest after an embryo transfer. Any supernumerary high-quality blastocysts can be frozen and stored for future use.

Frozen Embryo Transfer

With the refinement of cryopreservation methodology, the implantation rates of frozen embryo transfers have become equivalent, and in some cases have even surpassed, those associated of fresh embryo transfers. Cryopreserved embryos can be transferred in either a natural/modified natural or medicated/

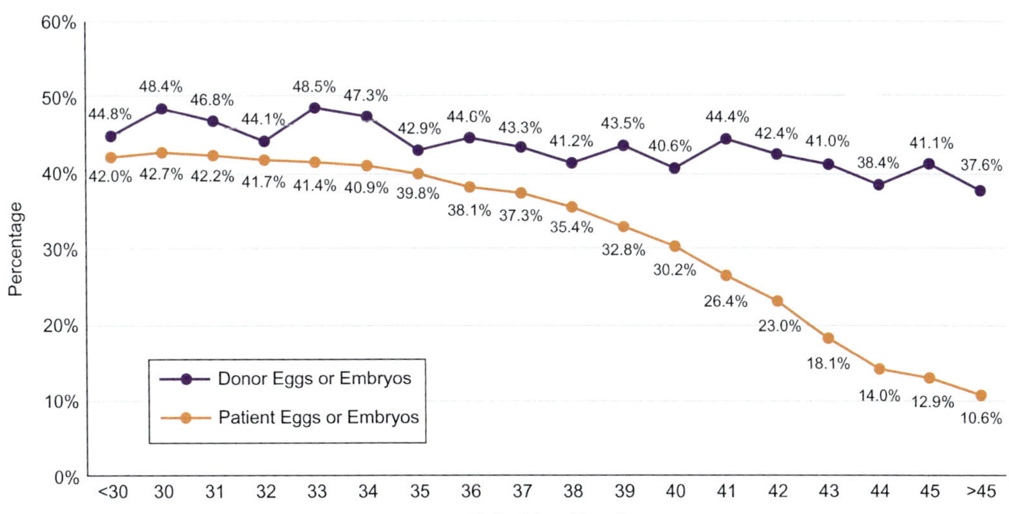

FIGURE 13.2 Percentage of embryo transfers that resulted in a live birth by patient age and egg or embryo source, United States, 2020 (courtesy of CDC.gov).

programmed cycle. While the chance of live birth is similar for both of these cycles, there are possible advantages and disadvantages to each approach that should be considered in creating a personalized treatment plan. Notably, embryos that are frozen with current vitrification technology have a >95% chance of surviving the freeze/thaw process. Additionally, there is no increased risk of congenital anomalies in infants born following the transfer of cryopreserved embryos.

Luteal Phase Support

Progesterone, a hormone produced by the ovary following ovulation, prepares the lining of the uterus for implantation. Studies have shown that women who are undergoing embryo transfers benefit from supplemental progesterone. For this reason, it is standard to administer progesterone following the egg retrieval or in preparation for a frozen embryo transfer. Natural progesterone is available and can be administered vaginally (Crinone®, Endometrin®, Prometrium®) or by intramuscular injection. If pregnancy occurs, the progesterone is continued generally until 8–10 weeks gestation, at which point the placenta has developed and is the organ responsible for producing progesterone for the remainder of the pregnancy. Studies have demonstrated that while vaginal progesterone is sufficient for luteal support in natural or modified natural frozen embryo transfers, there is a clear benefit of intramuscular progesterone administered at least every 3 days in medicated/programmed cycles (7). Studies have supported that there is no increased risk of birth defects or health risks to women who take natural progesterone supplements during pregnancy.

Egg Donation

Egg donation can be considered for patients with a severely diminished ovarian reserve, with poor outcomes from prior IVF cycles, or who are carriers of a genetic condition. There has been a marked increase in the use of donor eggs over time, with 4,471 donor egg recipients cycles reported to SART in 2021. Success rates with donor eggs remain high. The mean live birth rate for patients using donor eggs is higher across all age groups using their own oocytes (Figure 13.3).

Egg donors can be either known (non-anonymous), or unknown (anonymous), to the recipient. While generally non-anonymous donors contribute fresh eggs, anonymous donor eggs can either be obtained directly from a fresh cycle or from frozen egg lots shipped from a donor egg bank. There are additional

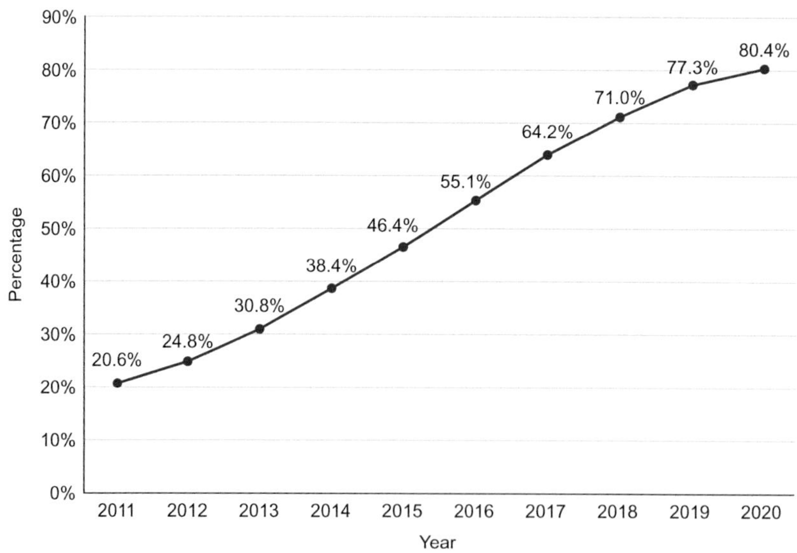

FIGURE 13.3 Percentage of embryo transfer cycles in which a single embryo was transferred, United States, 2011–2020 (from ref 11 with permission).

requirements for known donors, including medical, psychological, and legal counseling. Furthermore, all egg donors need to meet requirements set out by the FDA.

Gestational Surrogacy

A gestational carrier, or a surrogate, carries and delivers a child for another individual or couple. A medical indication is required to proceed with these cycles. For example, gestational surrogacy can be considered if there is absence of a uterus, a medical contraindication to pregnancy, or a biologic inability to conceive. In these cycles, all the steps of IVF treatment are performed except the embryos are transferred into a gestational carrier. An extensive evaluation and counseling involving all parties is required. Similar to egg donors, gestational carriers must meet FDA requirements.

Embryo Donation

There are multiple options that can be considered when an individual or couple's family is complete and they no longer require their embryos. Embryo donation can be considered in certain cases. There are agencies around the country that can assist in matching recipients to donated embryos. Medical, psychological, and legal counseling are important components of the treatment.

Laboratory Procedures

Preimplantation Genetic Testing

Preimplantation genetic testing (PGT) is a popular adjunct to IVF treatment. This technology has several indications, including screening for aneuploidy (PGT-A), chromosomal translocations (PGT-SR), and carrier status for monogenic conditions (PGT-M). At the current time, this screening is generally performed through trophectoderm biopsies, which consist of removing a few cells from a group destined to develop into placental tissue. Processing of this genetic information requires several weeks; therefore embryo cryopreservation is performed after the biopsy. Recent studies show that this procedure does not impair the implantation potential of high-quality embryos.

Many embryos have an extra or missing chromosome (called aneuploidy), which prevents them from implanting or causes a miscarriage. Embryos with the normal chromosome complement (called euploidy) have a higher chance of implanting and lower risk of miscarriage as compared to untested embryos. This technology is most beneficial in cases of more advanced maternal and paternal age due to higher rates of embryonic aneuploidy.

Epididymal/Testicular Sperm Aspiration

Azoospermia is defined as the absence of sperm in a semen specimen. This may be the result of an obstruction (e.g. previous vasectomy, congenital bilateral absence of vas deferens) or of severely impaired sperm production. In certain cases, aspiration of epididymal sperm or testicular sperm by a urologist may be considered. There are several microsurgical and percutaneous options to consider under the guidance of a reproductive urologist. The concentration and motility of sperm is often limited in sperm aspiration samples; therefore the ICSI procedure is anticipated to optimize fertilization. These procedures require close coordination between the reproductive urology and IVF teams.

Other Laboratory Techniques

There are several other laboratory procedures that can be performed but are not standard of care for all patients undergoing IVF. For example, assisted hatching is a procedure in which the zona pellucida, the outer membrane surrounding the embryo, is thinned by either the application of a dilute acidic solution or microscopic laser disruption. This technique may be considered in patients who have undergone several IVF cycles that have been unsuccessful. Artificial oocyte activation involves using calcium ionophores to assist in activating oocytes, which may assist in situations of poor fertilization despite ICSI. Finally, there is ongoing research on sperm selection techniques, such as physiological intracytoplasmic sperm injection (PICSI) and microfluidic sperm selection. These procedures may assist in cases of poor fertilization and/or embryo development.

Success Rates

IVF success rates continue to improve, and the reasons are manyfold, including optimized medical therapies for ovarian stimulation, refined laboratory techniques, and improved embryo transfer techniques. The success rate for any individual patient following IVF is influenced by countless factors, of which age is one of the most important contributors.

Maternal Age

One of the most important factors that influence patients' fertility is the age of the individual providing the eggs. Generally, younger women have a greater quantity and quality of eggs, that once fertilized are more likely to implant in the uterus and result in a pregnancy. Furthermore, the chance of a miscarriage is lower in younger women. The decreased fertility associated with advancing age is a gradual process that begins around age 35 and then accelerates after the age of 40. One reason for the decreased fertility associated with aging is that there is a higher rate of aneuploidy. Women over the age of 40 should be counseled about the decreased chances of pregnancy even with aggressive treatment, such as IVF. IVF using one's own eggs should be discouraged in women who are 44 years and older because of the limited chance of a successful outcome. Alternate options remain, including egg donation and adoption (Figure 13.3).

Fertility Clinic Success Rate and Certification Act of 1992

Since the passage of the Fertility Clinic Success Rate and Certification Act of 1992, it is mandatory that all IVF centers in the United States submit their annual success rates to a federal registry (8). In the past, this was a joint venture of the United States Centers for Disease Control (CDC) and the Society of the Assisted Reproductive Technologies (SART), a subsidiary of the American Society for Reproductive Medicine (ASRM). After the annual data has been compiled, a finalized report is published and made available to the public for review. The published document includes a summary of national and clinic-specific success rates. As patient demographics vary widely among programs, center-to-center comparisons may not be valid.

Complications of Treatment

Ovarian Hyperstimulation Syndrome (OHSS)

OHSS results from an excessive response to ovarian stimulation agents, most commonly to injectable gonadotropins. It can lead to abdominal distension, nausea, and vomiting. These mild symptoms are fairly common and generally resolve within a week. More serious symptoms include shortness of breath, decreased urinary output, abdominal pain, and blood clots. These are caused by the accumulation of fluid in the abdominal, and sometimes pleural, spaces which leads to a contraction of intravascular volume and hemoconcentration. Fortunately, the incidence of severe OHSS is rare (<1%, Figure 13.4). Risk factors include a diagnosis of polycystic ovarian syndrome, high estradiol levels, and those with many smaller follicles (<12 mm) at the time of trigger. However, most patients who develop OHSS do not have any risk factors and are difficult to predict. Generally, symptoms develop within a week of an hCG trigger. If a patient becomes pregnant during a cycle, the hCG produced by the pregnancy can worsen the severity and length of illness.

All patients should be educated on the symptoms of OHSS. Any patient who develops persistent or worsening symptoms of OHSS must be evaluated. Vitals are obtained and a physical examination is

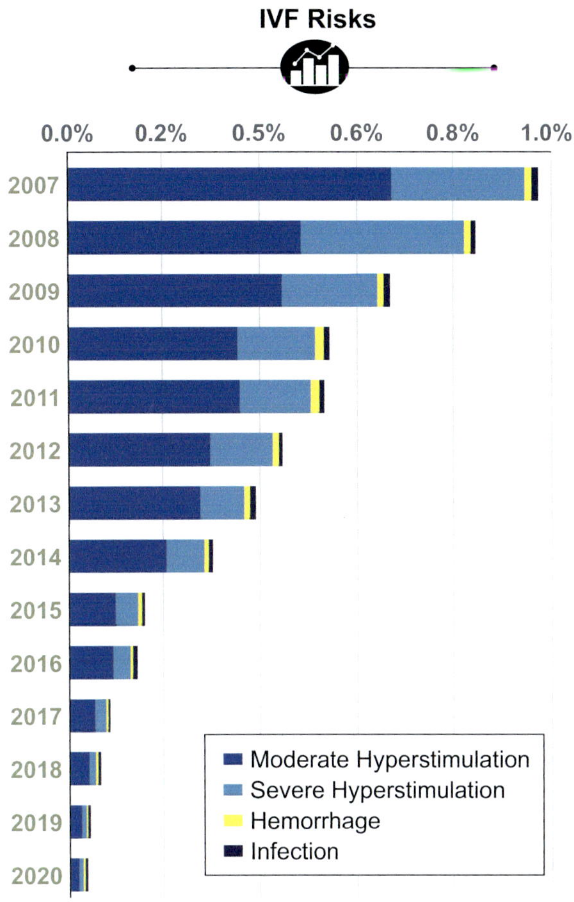

FIGURE 13.4 The risks associated with IVF in the United States (adapted from ref 11 with permission).

performed. Laboratory studies are ordered, including a CBC, PT/PTT, electrolytes, and liver enzymes. A pelvic and abdominal examination can delineate the extent of ascites. A chest Xray can be helpful if a pleural effusion is suspected.

The current standard of care is to manage moderate-to-severe ascites with vaginal ultrasound-guided paracentesis in an outpatient setting. Studies have demonstrated that this procedure expedites recovery and drastically reduces the need for hospitalization (9, 10).

Multiple Pregnancy

The rate of multiple pregnancy resulting from IVF cycles has drastically declined in recent years, from 8.4% of embryo transfers resulting in twins in 2011, to 2.3% in 2020 (11). Similarly, only 0.05% of embryo transfer cycles led to triplet pregnancies in 2020, as compared to 0.04% in 2011. This trend is a result of single embryo transfer (SET) now being considered the standard of care in most clinical scenarios. The refinement of IVF technology has markedly increased implantation rates, which means that fewer embryos can be transferred without impacting live birth rates. As most multiple pregnancies following IVF result from the implantation of more than one embryo, SET has significantly contributed to an improvement in fetal health outcomes.

Multiple pregnancies are associated with an increased risk of most complications of pregnancy including miscarriage, congenital anomalies, hypertensive disorders of pregnancy, gestational diabetes, and premature birth. The most concerning risk of a multiple pregnancy is prematurity. Babies born from a triplet pregnancy have a 20% chance of a major handicap, 17-fold increase in cerebral palsy, and 20-fold increase in death during the first year after birth (as compared to a singleton pregnancy).

Birth Defects

The possibility that IVF could increase the risk of birth defects has been a great concern for patients and clinicians. This is of particular interest since >2% of all children are now conceived following IVF (3). Although many studies have looked at malformations in IVF children, most have had limitations in sample size, and there has been a lack of a standard definition of a minor versus a major congenital malformation. However, the majority of studies point to a slightly increased risk of congenital malformations. A previous meta-analysis including seven studies compared the rate of birth defects between those conceived following ART (IVF and ICSI) with those naturally conceived (12). The pooled odds ratio was 1.40 (95% CI 1.28–1.53) and confirmed an increased risk of major birth defects in the babies conceived by ART. In a recent case-control study, the researchers confirmed a higher incidence in singleton IVF pregnancies of septal heart defects, cleft lip/palate, esophageal atresia, and anorectal atresia (13).

The increased risk of malformations may be a result of the ART procedures themselves or related to demographics and other characteristics of infertility patients. Interestingly, several studies have demonstrated that couples with infertility who ultimately achieve a pregnancy on their own are still at higher risk of birth defects (14). Similarly, there appears to be an increased risk of birth defects with ICSI as compared to conventional IVF (4); however, it is well known that men with abnormal semen parameters are at higher risk based on that diagnosis alone (15). It is probable that infertile women and men are at a slightly increased risk for children with congenital malformations whether or not they conceive with ART.

It is unclear whether there is an increased risk following ICSI or IVF itself, but, if so, the overall risk is still low when one considers the baseline major malformation rate which is 3% in the United States. This information needs to be conveyed to our patients and should be part of the informed consent process. We counsel our couples that the incidence of birth defects in naturally conceived pregnancies is 2–3% and may be increased to 3–4% in babies born following IVF treatment.

Ovarian Cancer

In the general population, every woman has a 1 in 70 chance of developing ovarian cancer during her lifetime. Known risk factors for ovarian cancer include infertility, nulliparity, and genetics. Alternatively, birth control pill use and pregnancy reduce a woman's lifetime risk of developing ovarian cancer. It has been theorized that the number of ovulations that occur during a woman's life time increases the chance of cancer formation. Hence, there is concern that the use of fertility medications could heighten the risk. This topic has been studied extensively. The Danish cohort of 50,000 infertile patients is the largest study to date that helped to shed light on the topic. The investigators in the initial study reported a higher incidence of breast and ovarian cancer in the infertile population (16). In a follow-up study of the cohort, the investigators sought out to determine the impact of fertility medications on the risk of ovarian cancer (17). They concluded that the incidence of ovarian cancer was not increased in those infertile women who took fertility medications. These findings were supported by a review by Brinton et al. (18). Therefore, while it is fact that infertile women are at greater risk of developing ovarian cancer, this risk is not heightened with the use of fertility medications.

Conclusion

There is no question that IVF is safe and the most successful treatment for the infertile patient. Continued advancements in the field have optimized implantation rates, shifting our practice to elective single embryo transfers. This change has dramatically improved the safety of IVF. The challenge that we now face is how to improve overall access to this care.

REFERENCES

1. The Nobel Prize in Physiology or Medicine 2010 - Press release [internet]: www.nobelprize.org/prizes/medicine/2010/press-release/.
2. Edwards RG et al. Early stages of fertilization in vitro of human oocytes matured in vitro. *Nature* 1969;221(5181):632–5.
3. ASRM, IVF-assisted pregnancies constitute 2.5% of all births in 2022 [internet]: www.asrm.org/news-and-events/asrm-news/press-releasesbulletins/ivf-assisted-pregnancies-constitute/.
4. ASRM, Intracytoplasmic sperm injection (ICSI) for non-male factor indications: a committee opinion [internet], 2020: www.asrm.org/practice-guidance/practice-committee-documents/intracytoplasmic-sperm-injection-icsi-for-nonmale-factor-indications-a-committee-opinion-2020/.
5. Palermo G et al. Pregnancies after intracytoplasmic injection of single spermatozoon into an oocyte. *Lancet* 1992;340(8810):17–8.
6. Penzias A et al. Performing the embryo transfer: a guideline. *Fertil Steril* 2017;107(4):882–96.
7. Devine K. Intramuscular progesterone optimizes live birth from programmed frozen embryo transfer: a randomized clinical trial. *Fertil Steril* 2021;116(3):633–43.
8. CDC, Policy Documents [Internet]: www.cdc.gov/art/nass/policy.html.
9. Alper MM et al. Ovarian hyperstimulation syndrome: current views on pathophysiology, risk factors, prevention, and management. *J Exp Clin Assist Reprod* 2009;6:3.
10. Smith LP et al. Patients with severe ovarian hyperstimulation syndrome can be managed safely with aggressive outpatient transvaginal paracentesis. *Fertil Steril* 2009;92(6):1953–9.
11. SART, National Summary Report [internet], 2021: www.sartcorsonline.com/rptCSR_PublicMultYear.aspx.
12. Hansen M et al. Assisted reproductive technologies and the risk of birth defects–a systematic review. *Hum Reprod* 2005;20(2):328–38.
13. Reefhuis J et al. Assisted reproductive technology and major structural birth defects in the United States. *Hum Reprod* 2009;24(2):360–6.
14. Serafin D et al. Evaluation of the risk of birth defects related to the use of assisted reproductive technology: an updated systematic review. *Int J Environ Res Public Health* 2022;19(8):4914.
15. Jwa SC et al. Male subfertility and the risk of major birth defects in children born after in vitro fertilization and intracytoplasmic sperm injection: a retrospective cohort study. *BMC Pregnancy Childbirth* 2019;19(1). https://doi.org/10.1186/s12884-019-2322-7
16. Jensen A et al. Risk of breast cancer and gynecologic cancers in a large population of nearly 50,000 infertile Danish women. *Am J Epidemiol* 2008;168(1):49–57.
17. Jensen A et al. Use of fertility drugs and risk of ovarian cancer: Danish population based cohort study. *BMJ* 2009;338(7694):580–2.
18. Brinton LA et al. Ovulation induction and cancer risk. *Fertil Steril* 2005;83(2):261–74.

14

Treatment Options: IV. Fresh vs Frozen Embryo Transfer, FET Protocols

Demián Glujovsky, Denis Vaughan, and Romina Pesce

There has been a significant increase in the utilization of frozen embryo transfers (FETs) as compared to fresh embryo transfers. The Centers for Disease Control and Prevention reported that in 2019, FETs comprised 78% of all embryo transfers in the United States, compared with just 25% in 2012.[1]

Reasons for this are several-fold:

1. Reducing risks of ovarian hyperstimulation syndrome and favoring a "freeze-all" approach, allowing normalization of hormones prior to embryo transfer.
2. A purported negative impact of supraphysiologic hormone levels (primarily estradiol and progesterone) on endometrial receptivity.
3. Improvements in cryopreservation methods owing to the advent of vitrification (rapid freeze techniques).
4. Increase in blastocyst culture and single embryo transfer.
5. Increase in utilization of pre-implantation genetic testing for aneuploidy.
6. Management of workload and scheduling for the embryology laboratory and other clinical staff.

In light of these advantages, many clinics in the United States have shifted practice and now only perform frozen embryo transfer.

The decision to transfer an embryo during the fresh cycle vs freezing all embryos and performing a subsequent frozen embryo transfer is nuanced, assuming clinics can provide both options. If a decision to do a fresh transfer is made, one has to consider whether to transfer at day 3 following fertilization (cleavage-stage transfer) vs culture and transfer on day 5 (at the blastocyst stage). We will discuss this decision later in the chapter.

While frozen embryo transfer, particularly after determination of ploidy status may confer improved live birth rates per transfer, compared to fresh, one has to consider the biases that exist in this conclusion.

- Those patients who have blastocyst development are better prognosis patients compared to those who do not make blastocysts and have a cleavage-stage transfer.
- Blastocysts that are frozen are, by definition in most centers, high-quality embryos, (determined to be BB or better by the Gardner grading classification[2]) whereas in a fresh transfer, most centers will transfer a viable embryo on day 5 regardless of embryo quality (either a morula/early blastocyst or poor-quality blastocyst).
- In those patients with very high estradiol/progesterone levels in the fresh transfer, outcomes are known to be inferior; therefore, strong consideration should be given to conversion to freeze all in these patients.[3]

 DOI: 10.1201/9781003460275-14

Therefore, the ideal method of comparing fresh vs frozen outcomes should evaluate cumulative live birth rates in a randomized setting rather than outcomes on a per transfer basis.

At Boston IVF, we strongly believe that there is still a place in clinical practice for fresh transfer, as it allows for sooner transfer and the possibility of pregnancy, as well as allowing for transfer in patients who do not make high-quality blastocysts. Later in this chapter, we further discuss the evidence for fresh vs frozen transfer decision-making.

Fresh Embryo Transfer

The majority of IVF cycles performed in the United States utilize the GnRH antagonist approach (see IVF chapter for further details on protocol). The primary advantage of this protocol is that it allows for flexibility regarding the trigger type. There are three primary methods of trigger that all serve the same purpose—to induce resumption of meiosis and therefore oocyte maturation.

- Human chorionic gonadotropin (hCG trigger)
- Gonadotropin releasing hormone agonist trigger (GnRH trigger, typically leuprolide acetate in the United States)
- A combination of both (dual trigger)

The burden of evidence suggests that there is no difference in oocyte competence between these three approaches,[4] provided patients take the medication as prescribed and have the expected response. Consideration must be given that when prescribing a GnRH agonist-only trigger, approximately 5% of patients will have a suboptimal response leading to failed/poor outcomes at the time of oocyte retrieval.[5] These patients are more likely to have underlying hypothalamic dysfunction. To mitigate against this risk of failure, it is common practice to measure luteinizing hormone and progesterone (LH and P4) levels the day after trigger shot, and at Boston IVF, we expect to see LH levels >15IU/L and progesterone levels >3ng/mL. If not, consideration of administration of hCG is given.

The primary advantage of a GnRH agonist trigger is rapid luteolysis and resumption of menses 5–7 days post-oocyte retrieval, thereby reducing the risk of ovarian hyperstimulation syndrome.

Despite the obvious advantages of a GnRH agonist trigger, there is debate in the field about optimal luteal support if a GnRH agonist trigger alone is used with a planned fresh transfer. Theoretically, rapid luteolysis would have a detrimental effect on implantation unless intensive luteal support with high dose progesterone +/- estrogen is used, although data is mixed.[6] At Boston IVF, we use hCG only trigger for a planned fresh transfer. These are typically low responders where the risk of OHSS is extremely low or patients have been dosed appropriately to ensure a modest response to prioritize a fresh transfer.

In rare cases where a GnRH agonist trigger is used for a planned fresh transfer (either alone or in the context of a dual trigger), we err on the side of caution and provide intensive luteal support to mimic the programmed frozen embryo transfer protocol (50mg IM progesterone daily and 3mg PO BID estradiol, starting day after oocyte retrieval).

Ordinarily, if planned fresh transfer, trigger is with hCG and supplemental vaginal progesterone is given starting 2 days after retrieval (Endometrin® 100mg TID or Crinone 8%® 90mg daily) as there are numerous corpora lutea also producing progesterone.

Choosing When to Transfer a Fresh Embryo

There is significant debate in our field regarding the optimal time to transfer an embryo in the fresh cycle day 3 following fertilization (cleavage-stage transfer) vs culture and transfer on day 5 (at the blastocyst stage). It is thought that embryos that develop into blastocysts in culture are more likely to be viable inside the uterus and result in a successful pregnancy than a cleavage-stage embryo. *In vitro* culture beyond day 3, therefore, allows for self-selection of embryos that successfully reach the blastocyst stage.

This allows the transfer of fewer embryos and decreases the likelihood of multiples (twins, triplets, etc.). However, it is possible that culture of embryos to the blastocyst stage in the lab leads to the loss of some embryos that may have survived inside the uterus. Thus, at many centers, cleavage-stage transfer is performed in patients with few available embryos to reduce the incidence of cycle cancellation if no embryo reaches the blastocyst stage. On the other hand, transferring a blastocyst on day 5 improves uterine/embryonic synchronicity and may thereby improve outcomes.

There are experts in the field that argue that if an embryo does not make it to the blastocyst stage, this embryo is a poor-quality embryo and should not be transferred as patients may be given false hope. However, this is not the belief at Boston IVF. There is no doubt in good prognosis patients, blastocyst-transfer/freeze-all approaches are helpful; however, it is not clear for poor prognosis patients, with fever embryos.

As there is no high-quality evidence, we have designed a large multicentered study, funded by Patient-Centered Outcomes Research Institute (PCORI) to help answer this question. The protocol has been published previously.[7] As discussed prior, the primary and optimal outcome for this study is cumulative live birth for one retrieval and any subsequent transfer.

Frozen Embryo Transfer Protocols

Once embryos have been cryopreserved, either surplus following a fresh transfer or following the cryo-all approach +/- PGT-A, the next step is to prepare the uterus for transfer prior to embryo thaw.

There are two broad categories of the frozen embryo transfer (FET) cycle, programmed or natural/modified natural.

A modified natural protocol is defined as any cycle in which ovulation is triggered with hCG injection (Ovidrel® 250mg or 10,000IU of hCG), followed by administration of vaginal progesterone (Crinone® 90mg daily, Endometrin® 100mg twice daily) starting 4 days after hCG trigger. Natural cycles omit the hCG trigger and wait for endogenous surge. Frozen embryo transfer occurs 7 days after hCG trigger or 6 days after an endogenous LH surge. Progesterone is continued until a negative pregnancy test result or until 8 weeks of pregnancy. Natural/modified natural cycles may be stimulated also, in cases of anovulation/oligo-ovulation and typically an aromatase inhibitor (Letrozole®) or alternatively, injectable gonadotropins may be used.

Programmed cycles use oral estradiol 3mg twice daily and/or a transdermal estradiol patch 100mcg every third day with or without the use of gonadotropin-releasing hormone agonist until the endometrial thickness was at least 7mm. Progesterone replacement is in the form of vaginal progesterone (Crinone® 90mg twice daily or Endometrin® 200mg twice daily) or IM progesterone (progesterone in oil 50mg daily). Intramuscular progesterone is administered alone or in combination with vaginal progesterone. If administered in combination, patients receive either Crinone® 90mg twice daily or Endometrin® 200mg twice daily, along with IM progesterone 50mg every third day. Frozen embryo transfer occurred 5 days (approximately 120 hours) after progesterone initiation. Both estrogen and progesterone are continued until a negative pregnancy test result or until 10 weeks of pregnancy.

While natural cycles have the benefit of fewer medications, avoiding an IM progesterone injection, they have the disadvantage of more monitoring appointments and unpredictability regarding timing of transfer, which can be challenging for both patient and clinic.

Many clinics in the US only offer programmed FET cycles for this reason.

At Boston IVF, we give patients the option to do either, as long as both are clinically reasonable.

Determining how endometrial preparation should be performed is a critical aspect of ART cycles. By examining the effectiveness of fresh and frozen embryo transfers, we can make informed decisions tailored to individual patients. Furthermore, investigating different protocols for endometrial preparation in FET cycles allows us to optimize the chances of successful embryo implantation. Understanding the potential obstetrical and perinatal risks associated with each method enhances our ability to provide comprehensive care and support to patients throughout their reproductive journey. The central question is: What does the available evidence suggest?

Comparing Fresh vs Frozen Embryo Transfers

Key Points

- In normo-responders, there are probably no differences in LBR when comparing fresh and frozen embryo transfers. However, in high responders, the LBR may be higher with freeze-all strategies.
- The freeze-all strategy has probably a lower risk of OHSS than a fresh embryo transfer.
- The frozen embryo transfers may have a higher risk of some obstetrical complications such as hypertensive disorders of pregnancy and large-for-gestational-age babies.
- Although cost-effectiveness is difficult to evaluate, most studies showed that the freeze-all strategy may not be cost-effective as a routine approach.

Reproductive Outcomes and Adverse Effects

In 2021, Zaat et al published a systematic review that included eight randomized controlled trials (RCTs) with 4,712 women in the meta-analysis and focused the effectiveness analysis on cumulative rates.[8] Their findings indicated that there are probably little or no differences in cumulative live birth rates between a fresh embryo transfer and the "freeze-all" strategy (1.08, 95% CI 0.95 to 1.22; moderate certainty of the evidence), but the risk of OHSS may be lower in the "freeze-all" strategy (OR 0.26, 95% CI 0.17 to 0.39; low certainty of the evidence).

In 2019, Bosdou published a systematic review comparing the first fresh embryo transfer vs a "freeze-all" strategy, with results stratified by the ovarian response (normo and high responders).[9] They found that there may be a higher probability of live birth in the frozen ET group in high responders (RR 1.18, 95%CI 1.06–1.31; low certainty of the evidence). Conversely, there are probably little or no differences in live birth rates in normo-responders (RR 1.13, 95%CI 0.90–1.41; moderate certainty of the evidence). They also showed that the risk of moderate/severe OHSS is probably lower in the frozen ET group when compared with the fresh ET group both in high (RR 0.19, 95%CI 0.10–0.37; moderate certainty of the evidence) and normal responders (RR 0.39, 95%CI 0.19–0.80; moderate certainty of the evidence).

Also in 2019, Roque et al published a systematic review on the same topic, stratifying the results by the ovarian response, the embryo-stage transfer, the freezing method, and the route of progesterone administration.[10] A similar result was published in this review, showing that there may be a higher LBR in elective frozen ET in high responders (RR = 1.16, 95%CI 1.05–1.28, low certainty of the evidence) but little or no differences in normo-responders (RR = 1.04, 95%CI 0.97–1.11, low certainty of the evidence). Additionally, the risk of OHSS may be lower in elective frozen ET (RR = 0.42, 95%CI 0.19–0.96, low certainty of the evidence).

In 2022, Maheshwari et al published an RCT (n = 619) that was not included in the previous reviews.[11] They compared elective frozen embryo transfers vs fresh embryo transfers. It included women under 42 years old, with at least three good-quality embryos on day 3. Although no definitive differences were found in LBR due to a wide confidence interval, it showed that an elective frozen transfer does not improve it (RR 0.83, 99% CI 0.65 to 1.06). This study was uncertain to show if any of them is better in terms of OHSS (RR 0.44, 95% CI 0.15 to 1.30) and miscarriage rate (RR 1.09, 99% CI 0.72 to 1.66). In the UK context, the elective freeze approach was unlikely to be cost-effective.

Given the complex nature of ART data, which involves multiple levels (such as patients undergoing multiple cycles with or without frozen embryo transfers) and considering the variations in clinical effectiveness and safety between the two strategies, conducting a health economic assessment becomes a challenging task. In 2023, Venetis et al published an economic evaluation of the "freeze-all" strategy in comparison to the traditional fresh embryo transfer.[12] They analyzed five studies, of which two were cost-effectiveness analyses performed based on RCTs, showing that the freeze-all strategy has a low probability of being cost-effective from a patient and NHS (healthcare payer) perspective. These authors concluded that there is a scarcity of comprehensive health economic evaluations, with only a few offering sufficient evidence on the cost-effectiveness of routinely delaying fresh embryo transfers (freeze-all) in non-PCOS patients with normal responses. These limited studies suggest that such a strategy may not be cost-effective in those patients. Nevertheless, further research is needed to examine the health–economic implications of this approach in diverse populations and various healthcare settings (note that economic evaluations are always dependent on the country where they are based and extrapolations to other settings should be avoided or done with caution).

Obstetrical and Perinatal Outcomes

In 2018, Maheshwari et al published a systematic review with a cumulative meta-analysis including 26 observational and randomized studies comparing obstetric and perinatal outcomes.[13] The certainty of the evidence is low for all the outcomes. Frozen embryo transfers may be associated with a lower probability of preterm delivery in singletons (0.90; 95%CI 0.84–0.97), low birth weight (0.72; 95%CI 0.67–0.77), and small for gestational age (0.61; 95%CI 0.56–0.67) compared to fresh embryo transfers. However, frozen embryo transfers may be associated with an increased risk of hypertensive disorders of pregnancy (1.29; 95%CI 1.07–1.56), large for gestational age (1.54; 95%CI 1.48–1.61), and high birth weight (1.85; 95%CI 1.46–2.33).

The review published by Zaat et al in 2021,[8] in which only RCTs were included, analyzed obstetrical and perinatal outcomes too. In agreement with the review just mentioned, and based on low certainty of evidence for most of the outcomes, these authors found that the "freeze-all" strategy may increase the risk of hypertensive disorders of pregnancy (Peto OR 2.15, 95%CI 1.42 to 3.25; low certainty of the evidence), large-for-gestational-age baby (Peto OR 1.96, 95%CI 1.51 to 2.55; low certainty of the evidence), and small but higher birth weight of the children born (mean difference 127g, 95% CI 77.1 to 177.8; moderate certainty of the evidence). However, there is uncertainty about small-for-gestational-age (Peto OR 0.82, 95% CI 0.65 to 1.05; low certainty of the evidence) and for preterm birth (Peto OR 1.15, 95% CI 0.89 to 1.50; low certainty of the evidence).

Similar results were found by Roque et al,[10] showing that pre-eclampsia is probably higher in elective frozen embryo transfers (RR = 1.79, 95%CI 1.03–3.09; moderate certainty of the evidence).

In summary, the low certainty evidence shows that both strategies (fresh embryo transfers and frozen embryo transfers) are similar in cumulative and first live birth rates, especially in normo-responders. However, in high-responders, live birth rate in the first embryo transfer may be higher with a "freeze-all strategy." Besides, moderate and severe OHSS is probably lower in "freeze-all" strategy in comparison to a fresh embryo transfer, both in normo and high-responders. However, hypertensive disorders of pregnancy and large-for-gestational-age babies may be higher in a "freeze-all strategy." While the rest of the obstetrical and perinatal outcomes still show controversial results in different studies, this is probably related to heterogeneity in settings and populations.

Comparing Different FET Protocols

In 2020, Glujovsky et al updated a systematic review that had been previously published in Cochrane.[14] They included 31 RCTs (5,426 women) and showed how heterogeneous an endometrial preparation could be and how difficult it is to analyze the evidence in that context. The authors found that although the certainty of the evidence is very low to evaluate if a natural cycle improves the LBR and CPR in comparison to a programmed cycle, one RCT showed that a natural cycle probably reduces the cancellation rate (OR 0.60, 95%CI 0.44 to 0.82; moderate certainty of the evidence). On the other hand, when comparing a programmed cycle to a stimulated cycle using clomiphene citrate, letrozole, or FSH, the stimulated cycle may improve the CPR (OR 1.63, 95%CI 1.12 to 2.38; low certainty of the evidence). Additionally, GnRH analogs may offer a benefit over no intervention, and one RCT suggested that GnRH antagonists may improve CPR compared to GnRH agonists (OR 0.62, 95%CI 0.42 to 0.90). However, there is uncertainty regarding the impact of using aspirin or steroids in this procedure.

Wu et al published a systematic review with network meta-analysis in 2021.[15] They included 26 RCTs and 113 cohort studies. Most of the certainty of the evidence is low to very low. Consistent with previous meta-analyses, they found no endometrial preparation superior to others. They found programmed cycles may have higher pregnancy-induced hypertension (OR 1.82, 95%CI 1.37 to 2.38), postpartum hemorrhage (OR 2.08, 95%CI 1.61 to 2.78), and very preterm birth (OR 2.08, 95%CI 1.45 to 2.94).

In contrast to this, Boston IVF has examined perinatal outcomes in detail, retrospectively, in collaboration with Beth Israel Deaconess Medical Center. We did not find any differences in perinatal outcomes between programmed and natural cycles.[16] Boston IVF also participated in a large, multicentered, randomized, controlled trial (NATPRO) to help answer this question. At the time of publication, this trial has completed recruitment, and we eagerly await the forthcoming results.

In conclusion, analyzing the protocols for preparing the endometrium is a complex task, and the evidence from the numerous published studies is currently of limited quality. No single protocol has emerged as definitively superior. Researchers should strive to enhance the quality of future studies to generate more reliable and useful evidence.

Important Pitfalls for the Practitioner

- The choice between a fresh or freeze-all embryo transfer strategy lacks definitive evidence for a one-size-fits-all approach.
- High responders may benefit from a freeze-all strategy, improving effectiveness and mitigating the risk of ovarian hyperstimulation syndrome. However, it's essential to engage patients in discussions about potential obstetrical complications.
- Various endometrial preparation protocols exist, none of which are distinctly superior. A shared decision-making process is crucial, enabling thorough discussions on the advantages and disadvantages of each option.
- There is not enough good-quality evidence to decide if a natural cycle is more effective or worse than a programmed cycle.
- Although stimulated cycle using GnRH antagonists may improve CPR, there is no evidence that it improves LBR.
- Low-quality evidence showed that programmed cycles may have higher pregnancy-induced hypertension, postpartum hemorrhage, and very preterm birth than natural cycles.

REFERENCES

1. Centers for Disease Control and Prevention. 2019 Assisted Reproductive Technology Fertility Clinic and National Summary Report [internet]: US Dept of Health and Human Services, 2021: https://archive.cdc.gov/www_cdc_gov/art/reports/2019/pdf/2019-Report-ART-Fertility-Clinic-National-Summary-h.pdf.
2. Gardner DK et al. Culture and transfer of viable blastocysts: a feasible proposition for human IVF. *Hum Reprod Update*. 1997;3:367–82.
3. Bosch E et al. Circulating progesterone levels and ongoing pregnancy rates in controlled ovarian stimulation cycles for in vitro fertilization: analysis of over 4000 cycles. *Hum Reprod*. 2010;25(8):2092–100.
4. Beebeejaun Y et al. Triggering oocyte maturation in in vitro fertilization treatment in healthy responders: a systematic review and network meta-analysis. *Fertil Steril*. 2024:S0015-0282(24)02389-6.
5. Meyer L et al. Risk factors for a suboptimal response to gonadotropin-releasing hormone agonist trigger during in vitro fertilization cycles. *Fertil Steril*. 2015;104(3):637–42.
6. Humaidan P et al. Luteal phase supplementation after gonadotropin-releasing hormone agonist trigger in fresh embryo transfer: the American versus European approaches. *Fertil Steril*. 2015;103(4):879–85.
7. Neuhausser WM et al. Non-inferiority of cleavage-stage versus blastocyst-stage embryo transfer in poor prognosis IVF patients (PRECiSE trial): study protocol for a randomized controlled trial. *Reprod Health*. 2020;17(1):16.

8. Zaat T et al. Fresh versus frozen embryo transfers in assisted reproduction. *Cochrane Database Syst Rev.* 2021;2(2):CD011184.
9. Bosdo JK et al. Higher probability of live-birth in high, but not normal, responders after first frozen-embryo transfer in a freeze-only cycle strategy compared to fresh-embryo transfer: a meta-analysis. *Human Reprod.* 2019;34(3):491–505.
10. Roque M et al. Fresh versus elective frozen embryo transfer in IVF/ICSI cycles: a systematic review and meta-analysis of reproductive outcomes. *Human Reprod Update.* 2019;25 (1): 2–14.
11. Maheshwari A et al. Elective freezing of embryos versus fresh embryo transfer in IVF: a multicentre randomized controlled trial in the UK (E-Freeze). *Human Reprod.* 2022;37(3):476–87.
12. Venetis C et al. Freeze-all embryos during treatment with assisted reproduction: health economic aspects. *Best Practice Res Clin Obstet Gynaecol.* 2023;86:102303.
13. Maheshwari A et al. Is frozen embryo transfer better for mothers and babies? Can cumulative meta-analysis provide a definitive answer? *Human Reprod Update.* 2018;24(1):35–58.
14. Glujovsky D et al. Endometrial preparation for women undergoing embryo transfer with frozen embryos or embryos derived from donor oocytes. *Cochrane Database Syst Rev.* 2020;10(10):CD006359.
15. Wu H et al. Endometrial preparation for frozen-thawed embryo transfer cycles: a systematic review and network meta-analysis. *JF Assist Reprod Genet.* 2021;38(8):1913–26.
16. Farrell AS et al. Perinatal outcomes are similar in programmed and modified natural frozen embryo transfer cycles. *Reprod Biomed Online.* 2024;49(5):104347.

15

Donor Oocyte Use in IVF

Brian M. Berger

Over the past 40 years, the use of assisted reproductive technologies has changed the choices available for older women. These choices include donor egg *in vitro* fertilization (DE IVF), which is now a standard treatment offered by most IVF centers. Initially, women who benefited from DE IVF included those with premature ovarian failure, ovarian failure due to either chemotherapy or radiation, and women with gonadal dysgenesis. Since the 1980s, a second and much larger group includes women with diminished ovarian function and age-related infertility. Other candidates include women who have previously failed multiple IVF attempts and women carrying transmittable genetic abnormalities that could affect their offspring.

Increasing Number of DE IVF Cycles

There are many reasons for the increase in the number of women who are candidates for egg donation such as those with diminished ovarian function. Surveys have shown that many women choose to delay childbearing and rear their children only after establishing a stable relationship and financial security. There are also increasing numbers of late and second marriages, and more women now wish to finish their education and establish a career before trying to start a family.[1,2] In 2021, over 450 IVF programs reported on the use of donor oocytes to the American Society for Reproductive Medicine/Society for Assisted Reproductive Technology Registry. Donor eggs (fresh and frozen) were used in approximately 12% of all ART cycles performed. The number of cycles performed using embryos from *fresh* donor eggs decreased from 10,954 in 2012 to 1,552 in 2021, while the number of cycles performed using embryos from frozen donor eggs or donated embryos increased from 8,893 in 2012 to 26,700 in 2021. The live birth rate using fresh embryos from fresh donor eggs, fresh embryos from frozen donor eggs, and frozen embryos from donor eggs was 49.5%, 44.1%, and 44.5%, respectively.[3, 4]

Ethics of DE IVF

Several publications have addressed the important ethical considerations and social issues related to egg donation in postmenopausal women. Generally, there are three main objections related to this treatment: (i) the physical risk to the older woman during pregnancy;[5] (ii) the rights of the children born to older women;[6] and (iii) the use of scarce health care resources that might deprive younger patients of treatment. Other issues which have been raised against treating older patients include the views of donors about using their oocytes for treating older women and the psychological effect of giving birth beyond the age of 50, which is unknown at present.[5] Those who are in favor of treating older patients argue that, by careful selection of patients, the risk of complications is reduced to a minimum and most older women wanting children are quite willing to accept the small risk of complications. There is also an argument about the definition of what constitutes advanced maternal age, especially given that the life expectancy of both men and women has increased considerably.[6]

DOI: 10.1201/9781003460275-15

Steps to Completing a Cycle of DE IVF

The process of completing a DE IVF cycle has five distinct steps (see Table 15.1). The patients are instructed to first set up an appointment with their physician to discuss the medical aspects of DE IVF. Spouses or partners must accompany the recipient to this appointment.

The Donor Egg Team

At Boston IVF, we have a designated DE Team which is responsible for working with all recipients. The team helps to ensure that the recipient and her partner (if applicable) and the egg donor have been properly screened and helps to coordinate the treatment cycle. First the recipients are instructed to attend an Egg Recipient Seminar with the program coordinator. At this seminar, comprehensive information about egg donation is given and all questions regarding the process are answered. We also have the patients meet with the financial coordinator. They will learn about what their insurance policy may cover and the eligibility testing that may be required, and to learn about the out-of-pocket expenses.

FDA Regulations and Egg Donation

In 2004, the FDA published the final rules to strengthen regulation of human tissue and expanded the regulations to include human cells, tissues, and cellular and tissue-based products.[7, 8] The regulations apply to reproductive tissues such as eggs, embryos, and semen. The FDA began requiring various establishments to register with the agency and list the products that are manufactured. These establishments include those that recover, process, store, label, package, or distribute the products, or that screen or test donors. More than 350 reproductive establishments, including semen banks and fertility clinics, are registered with the FDA. Reproductive establishments, including IVF centers, were required to comply with donor eligibility requirements, which became effective in May 2005. These requirements establish screening and testing criteria for donors of human cells, tissues, and cellular and tissue-based products to help prevent the transmission of communicable diseases. People who are donating to their own sexual partners are not required to be screened or tested.

For egg donors, the collection of a donor specimen for testing must occur up to 30 days before recovery of the oocytes or egg retrieval[8] (see Table 15.2). In contrast, for sperm donors (fresh specimens), the center may collect the donor specimen up to 7 days before or after the sperm is donated[8] (see Table 15.3).

Required testing must be performed by an FDA-certified laboratory. Centers must also use an appropriate FDA licensed, approved, or cleared donor screening test if available. A donor whose specimen tests reactive on a non-Treponemal screening test for syphilis and negative on a specific Treponemal confirmatory test may nevertheless be considered eligible, as long as all other required testing and screening are negative. A donor whose specimen tests reactive on a Treponemal confirmatory test is not eligible.

TABLE 15.1

Five Steps to Completing a Fresh Donor Egg Cycle

1. Completion of the recipient eligibility screening process
2. Determination of insurance eligibility/financial clearance
3. Selection or identification of a potential donor
4. Screening of the potential donor
5. Cycle coordination

TABLE 15.2

FDA Required Testing for Communicable Disease Agents or Diseases in Oocyte Donors[8]

- Human immunodeficiency virus (HIV), types 1 and 2
- Hepatitis B virus (HBV)
- Hepatitis C virus (HCV)
- Treponema pallidum (syphilis)
- Chlamydia trachomatis
- Neisseria gonorrhea

TABLE 15.3

FDA Required Testing for Communicable Disease Agents or Diseases for Sperm Donors[8]

- Human immunodeficiency virus (HIV), types 1 and 2
- Hepatitis B virus (HBV)
- Hepatitis C virus (HCV)
- Treponema pallidum (syphilis)
- Chlamydia trachomatis
- Neisseria gonorrhea
- Human T-lymphotropic virus, types 1 and 2
- Cytomegalovirus

The Egg Recipient Evaluation

All recipients are tested according to FDA regulations as described previously. In addition, the recipients will have a uterine cavity evaluation via a hysterosalpingogram, sonohysterogram, or hysteroscopy. Routine prenatal blood work will be done, and the partner will have a semen analysis. All recipients are required to schedule an appointment with a social worker. Once again, the spouse/partner must attend this appointment. This consultation allows them to explore the psychological issues involved in egg donation. If recipients are working with an egg donor who is known by or related to them (Known Donor or KD), we require that they meet once with a social worker as a couple, the donor and her spouse (if applicable) meet with the social worker once as a couple, and then all parties meet again for a joint consultation. After the testing is completed, the intended parents will schedule an appointment with their physician who will review the results of the recipient evaluation and will write orders for the treatment cycle.

To prevent miscommunication and confusion, we only allow the screening of one potential egg donor at a time. Recipients are also told that they are financially responsible for services rendered to the donor, even if she is not accepted as a donor following her medical screening.

Anonymous Egg Donation

Boston IVF allows anonymous donors to be recruited by approved egg donor agencies only. We will not permit recipients to recruit their own donors through the Internet or through any other means. This policy is necessary to ensure that anonymity is preserved and that the necessary legal contracts are properly in place. Recipients are given tremendous guidance in selecting an appropriate egg donor (see Table 15.4). Egg donors should be healthy, between the ages of 21 and 35,[9–11] and free of infectious diseases. All egg donors, whether anonymous or known, must be screened to ensure that their motivation appears reasonable and voluntary. Egg donation presents a number of unique medical, legal, and emotional issues, which need to be carefully considered.

TABLE 15.4

Features to Seek in a Donor Egg Agency

Qualities	Importance
Medical expertise	An agency that offers a staff member with medical training is invaluable. Medical expertise is important to make decisions about which donors the agency will accept and make available to recipients.
Legal counsel for both the donor and recipient	Legal consultation for both the donor and the recipient protects the interests of both parties by establishing a mutually acceptable legal contract. An agency should facilitate this process and should provide this service as a part of the agency package.
Short-term medical insurance policy for the egg donor	Should an egg donor experience any adverse medical event related to the egg retrieval or the medications, the recipient is financially responsible for her medical care and treatment. A good agency should offer a short-term insurance policy for purchase that covers any potential problems related to the procedure and the medications.
Professional, courteous staff	A staff that is professional and courteous will treat egg donors and recipients with respect and ensure that the needs of each are met in an efficient manner. Professional demeanor usually reflects a company that is organized and efficient.

Known Egg Donors

Known egg donors include sisters, relatives, or friends. Known egg donors must be medically and psychologically screened as rigorously as anonymous donors. Cross-generation egg donation in which a daughter donates to her mother or a mother donates to her daughter is not permitted at Boston IVF.

Legal Contracts

We require legal consultation and establishment of a legal contract with the donor, anonymous or known. The recipient couple is generally responsible for legal fees incurred by the donor, although many donor egg agencies include this fee in their administrative fees.

Initiating the Treatment Cycle

When recipients have selected a potential donor, the agency (or recipient if using a known donor) calls the Egg Donation Program Coordinator who will send them application and history forms, register the donor at Boston IVF, and schedule the donor's appointments. The donor should bring her completed forms and any previous medical records with her to her appointments. If using an agency, it is important for recipients to find out all of the costs of the agency before selecting an agency or paying a fee. Agency fees typically include the egg donor's compensation, a short-term medical insurance policy for the egg donor, and legal fees. In addition, if they select a donor who lives out of state, we require that she travels to Boston IVF twice, once for her screening appointments and once again for the monitoring and egg retrieval. At the time of the egg retrieval, she usually stays locally for one week.

Screening Donors

Boston IVF screens potential egg donors thoroughly according to FDA regulations. An eight-page phone screen is first performed, and a decision is made on whether or not to schedule a screening appointment. The Boston IVF physician, social worker, and the DE Program Coordinator work as a team to determine whether a donor candidate is appropriate. We perform an expanded genetic carrier screening that tests for over 100 recessive diseases. If a donor completes her screening and is approved by the medical director, the DE Program Coordinator is responsible for synchronizing the recipient's cycle with the egg donor's cycle.

Cycle Coordination

Donors

Implantation and Success in DE IVF

The process of implantation remains poorly understood, but two factors are clearly required, endometrial receptivity and synchronization of embryo and endometrial development. In the natural cycle, these factors are induced by the simultaneous development of the follicle and the surrounding hormonal events involving ovulation. In the DE IVF treatment, these events are, by definition, separated and need to be controlled and synchronized by a sequence of ovarian down-regulation and endometrial preparation. Because of these factors, controlled timing of follicle growth and egg maturation and ovulation in the donor, along with adequate stimulation of the endometrium with an estrogen–progesterone sequence in the recipient needs to be performed.

Donor Ovulation Induction Protocol

All donors are initially started on oral contraceptives (OCP). The OCP is started with the donor's menses and continues for 16 to 35 days. OCP pre-treatment in high responders has been shown to improve the success of the treatment and also reduces the risk of ovarian hyperstimulation syndrome.[12–14]

For the past 15 years, we have used a regimen consisting of FSH/low-dose hCG and a GnRH antagonist. This protocol allows us maximum flexibility in treatment and also allows us to almost eliminate the incidence of ovarian hyperstimulation (<0.2%). We perform frequent estradiol measurements in the beginning of the cycle in order to adjust the stimulation and also to ensure that the donor is responding adequately. We have also successfully utilized a protocol in which early adjustments in FSH dose are implemented based on the estradiol measurement on days 3 and 5.[15,16] We have found that modification of the initial and subsequent FSH dose yields similar clinical outcomes in oocyte donors with a significantly lower basal antral follicle count (BAFC). In donors with a high BAFC (>30), this management strategy also minimizes the risk of OHSS (1/249).[17] All donors are triggered with Lupron® 80 mg unless they have contraindications such as hypothalamic amenorrhea (in which case an hCG trigger is used). A confirmatory P4 and LH are performed the day after ovulation to document efficacy.

Recipients

Down-Regulation of Recipients

If the recipient is planning a fresh/coordinated embryo transfer, prior to the uterine preparation protocol, down-regulation of the cycle is usually performed based on studies that have clearly indicated that adequate down-regulation of the menstrual cycle beforehand is beneficial. Borini et al.[18] studied the effect of long-term down-regulation on pregnancy and implantation rates in 122 cyclic patients who received donor oocytes. Recipients who were either menopausal or cyclic but had long-term down-regulation had significantly higher pregnancy and implantation rates. Apart from the improved pregnancy and implantation rates after long-term down-regulation, these data not only demonstrate an important role of the endometrium in implantation but also suggest that a period of amenorrhea improves the pregnancy rate.

In cyclic patients with natural menstrual cycles, suppression of the cycle is accomplished with a GnRH agonist analogue (Lupron®). Lupron® has the added advantage that it can be used for several months at a time without causing any permanent changes to the reproductive system or detrimental effect on the success of the cycle. This ensures a degree of flexibility that allows egg donation to function successfully.

Estrogen Replacement for Recipients

Lutjen et al.[19] first reported egg donation to a recipient with premature ovarian failure in 1984. They used a steroid replacement regimen for the recipient consisting of estrogen valerate (Progynova®; Schering, Sydney, Australia) and progesterone suppositories (Utrogestan®; Piette, Brussels, Belgium). Since then, many different regimens of estrogen and progesterone replacement have been tried successfully, differing in both the method of administration and timing.

There are many reports dealing with the recommended type and dosage of estrogen and progesterone supplementation in artificial endometrial preparation before the transfer of embryos. We know from oocyte donation programs that maximum flexibility is necessary to synchronize the recipient until oocytes are available. The aim is an open so-called "window of implantation" with a highly receptive-appearing endometrium at the time of embryo transfer. Many studies have examined the effects of different estrogen replacement regimens. Most have shown that the length of estrogen administration could be varied and delayed. In fact, successful implantation was observed in an extreme situation even after 100 days of unopposed estradiol valerate administration.[20, 21] Ovulatory patients in this study received a GnRH analogue simultaneously. Break-through bleeding increasingly appeared according to the duration of estrogen replacement. These clinical observations provide evidence that the concept of "prolonged follicular phase" estrogen replacement for ovum donation can be maintained, at least as long as 15 weeks. Because of the high incidence of break-through bleeding after 9 weeks (>44%), the authors recommended stopping estrogen replacement after this time. Yaron et al.[22] extended uterine preparation with estradiol as long as 5 weeks without significantly decreased pregnancy rates.

It was suggested that shorter and lower dosage protocols of estradiol priming of the endometrium could result in higher abortion rates. This indicates an optimal endometrial proliferation which is necessary to enable optimal development of progesterone receptors and subsequent transformation into an endometrium receptive to the transferred embryo.[22] Neither endometrial thickness nor serum estradiol was able to predict optimal receptivity and, therefore, outcome in oocyte donation.

At Boston IVF, we continue estrogen replacement until 10 weeks estimated gestational age.

Progesterone Replacement for Recipients

Historically, much controversy has surrounded the issue of progesterone replacement in DE IVF cycles. Unfortunately, prospective studies comparing different types and durations of progesterone supplementation before transfer of DE IVF embryos with regard to treatment outcome were lacking until recent years. With regard to timing of progesterone, several retrospective studies have shed light on the implantation window. In one study, 4–5 days of progesterone administration were optimal for embryo transfer, comparing results after transfers between day 2 and day 7 of progesterone administration. Rosenwaks[23] reported best results after transfers on days 3–5 of progesterone supplementation.

Prapas et al.[24] performed an interesting retrospective study on the association between the "window of embryo transfer" and the duration of progesterone therapy. They transferred day 2 embryos (4–6-cell) after 2, 3, 4, 5, and 6 days following initiation of endometrial exposure to progesterone. Their results indicate that the window of implantation depends on the duration of progesterone treatment. It begins ~48 h after starting progesterone administration and lasts for ~4 days. Highest pregnancy rates were achieved after 5 days (48.3%), with lower rates after 4 days (40%), 6 days (20.4%), and 3 days (12%). No pregnancies were observed after 2 days of progesterone administration.

- Note: Progesterone is a critical factor in the late follicular phase of fresh IVF cycles. There is much debate on the question of whether a subtle, late follicular phase, pre-hCG rise of progesterone above a certain threshold (1.2 ng/ml) has an impact on the outcome of treatment in IVF cycles.[25] For fresh/autologous IVF, our guideline at Boston IVF is to cancel the fresh transfer and convert to a cryo-all cycle when the P4 measurement rises above a threshold of over 1.2 ng/ml.
- In the past, we used both vaginal and intramuscular progesterone combination replacement regimens for recipients since a retrospective study we performed did not see a significant

difference in success rates.[26] However, more recent randomized prospective data has shown a significant difference when intramuscular progesterone is used either alone or in conjunction with vaginal progesterone versus vaginal progesterone alone.[27] Accordingly, we recommend either administering intramuscular progesterone 50 mg daily or every 3 days along with twice daily vaginal gel. As with the estrogen replacement, we continue progesterone replacement until 10–12 weeks estimated gestational age.

Recipient Monitoring

In most cases, for synchronized fresh DE cycles, recipients are monitored once or twice with an ultrasound to measure the endometrial thickness, along with a P4 measurement. This typically occurs on days 5–7 of the donor's stimulation cycle and allows us to adjust the medications in the event that the lining is not adequate (≥7 mm).[28, 29]

Egg Banking

Since the introduction of an efficient method of oocyte vitrification by Kuwayama in 2005, there has been a growing body of clinical evidence demonstrating the potential of this procedure with applications in donor oocyte programs, and in particular, for donor egg banking.[30] This procedure has been demonstrated to be safe, and over 900 oocyte cryopreservation babies born with no apparent increase in congenital anomalies.[31] Forman et al. confirmed that oocyte vitrification does not increase the risk of embryonic aneuploidy or diminish the implantation potential of blastocysts created after intracytoplasmic sperm injection.[32] Furthermore, a prospective randomized sibling–oocyte study comparing embryo development in fresh versus vitrified oocytes in patients undergoing cycles with their own oocytes found no statistical differences between fertilization rates or embryo development/quality in the two groups.[33] In the past, there was much debate in the reproductive endocrinology community regarding the current status and clinical applicability of oocyte cryopreservation. Whereas sperm and embryo freezing had been used with good pregnancy success rates for a long enough time to gain widespread acceptance, oocyte freezing previously suffered from being labeled "experimental." This changed in January 2013, when the American Society of Reproductive Medicine (ASRM) announced that oocyte cryopreservation was no longer experimental.[34] Improved methods for oocyte preservation and demand for donor oocytes have led to the emergence of a new phenomenon in the United States and worldwide; commercial egg banks and networks that provide cryopreserved oocytes to intended recipients of egg donation have grown in number.

There are a number of potential benefits of using frozen eggs from an egg bank, but the primary benefit is cost efficiency. On average, the cost of a single cycle using an egg bank is less than 50% of a fresh donor egg IVF cycle. Other advantages include expedited treatment since the eggs are already retrieved and frozen/banked at the center. Frozen eggs can also be shipped from various centers, and there are a number of egg bank networks that routinely share eggs amongst different centers in order to create expanded choices for recipients as well as ethnic and racial diversity of egg donors from various regions in the United States. Additional advantages of cycles using an egg bank are an expedited treatment timeline with the average cycle length ranging from two to three months as opposed to upwards of four months with fresh donor egg cycles. Lastly, there are fewer canceled cycles with egg bank treatments, since the number of available eggs is already predetermined.

Replacement Protocols Versus Natural or Ovulation Induction

For egg bank and/or frozen embryos from donor eggs, treatment protocols for preparation of egg recipients can additionally be divided into replacement versus natural/ovulation induction protocols. Replacement protocols (EEP) as detailed earlier generally involve replacement with oral estrogen followed by luteal replacement with a combination of intramuscular progesterone and vaginal progesterone (see Replacement for Recipient section). If the recipient has adequate ovarian reserve and continues to be able to ovulate, a natural or ovulation induction cycle is typically easier and more patient-friendly with similar success rates to replacement protocols. A major advantage of natural or ovulatory cycles is that they preclude the need for painful intramuscular progesterone replacement since the patient's endogenous progesterone production is substantial, although we typically continue to supplement progesterone with vaginal progesterone.

Conclusion

Significant advances in technologies, such as better cryopreservation techniques, embryo freezing, and egg banking, have improved donor egg success rates and provided greater access to patients who wish to use this technology. The frozen donor egg bank segment is expected to grow significantly over the next decade, driven by advancements in vitrification technology, the growth of egg bank networks, as well as increased demand by an aging reproductive population. Furthermore, the improved cost-effectiveness of frozen donor eggs compared to traditional fresh donor egg IVF makes this option appealing to many couples.

Key Points

- Originally reserved for women with premature ovarian failure, gonadal dysgenesis, or ovarian damage from chemo/radiation, DEIVF is now widely used for age-related infertility, diminished ovarian reserve, recurrent IVF failures, and carriers of genetic conditions.
- Societal trends have substantially increased eligibility and demand.
- Core ethical debates focus on physical risks of pregnancy in older women and rights and welfare of children born to older mothers.
- FDA regulations mandate thorough screening and testing of all egg donors.
- Commercial egg banks have broadened donor selection.

REFERENCES

1. Bloom DE, Trussell J. What are the determinants of delayed childbearing and permanent childlessness in the United States? *Demography.* 1984;21(4):591–611.
2. Joseph KS et al. The perinatal effects of delayed childbearing. *Obstet Gynecol.* 2005;105(6):1410–1418.
3. Centers for Disease Control and Prevention. 2021 Assisted Reproductive Technology Fertility Clinic and National Summary Report. US Dept of Health and Human Services; 2023.
4. National Center for Environmental Health. National Report on Human Exposure to Environmental Chemicals [internet], U.S. Department of Health and Human Services, Centers for Disease Control and Prevention; 2022 (updated 2024): https://dx.doi.org/10.15620/cdc:133100.
5. Benagiano G. Pregnancy after the menopause: a challenge to nature? *Hum Reprod.* 1993;8(9):1344–1345.
6. Olshansky SJ et al. A potential decline in life expectancy in the United States in the 21st century. *N Engl J Med.* 2005;352(11):1138–1145.
7. Eligibility determination for donors of human cells, tissues, and cellular and tissue-based products. *Final Rule Fed Regist.* 2004;69(101):29785–29834.
8. Human cells, tissues, and cellular and tissue-based products; donor screening and testing, and related labeling. Interim final rule; opportunity for public comment. *Fed Regist.* 2005;70(100):29949–29952.
9. Shulman A et al. The best donor. *Hum Reprod.* 1999;14(10):2493–2496.
10. Cohen MA et al. Donor age is paramount to success in oocyte donation. *Hum Reprod.* 1999;14(11):2755–2758.
11. Financial incentives in recruitment of oocyte donors. *Fertil Steril.* 2004;82(Suppl 1):S240–244.

12. Damario MA et al. Dual suppression with oral contraceptives and gonadotrophin releasing-hormone agonists improves in-vitro fertilization outcome in high responder patients. *Hum Reprod.* 1997;12(11):2359–2365.
13. Barmat LI et al. A randomized prospective trial comparing gonadotropin-releasing hormone (GnRH) antagonist/recombinant follicle-stimulating hormone (rFSH) versus GnRH-agonist/rFSH in women pretreated with oral contraceptives before in vitro fertilization. *Fertil Steril.* 2005;83(2):321–330.
14. Morris RS et al. Predictive value of serum oestradiol concentrations and oocyte number in severe ovarian hyperstimulation syndrome. *Hum Reprod.* 1995;10(4):811–814.
15. Berger BM et al. A standardized protocol with minimal monitoring for controlled ovarian stimulation of egg donors results in improved pregnancy rates. *Fertil Steril.* 2004;82:S121.
16. ASRM. Prevention of moderate and severe ovarian hyperstimulation syndrome: a guideline. *Fertil Steril.* 2024;121(2):230–245.
17. Berger BM, Ezcurra D. Treatment modification based on basal antral follicle count maintains high pregnancy rates while preventing OHSS in egg donor IVF. *Fertil Steril.* 2009; 92:S3.
18. Borini A et al. Improvement of pregnancy and implantation rates in cyclic women undergoing oocyte donation after long-term down-regulation. *Hum Reprod.* 1995;10(11):3018–3021.
19. Lutjen P et al. The establishment and maintenance of pregnancy using in vitro fertilization and embryo donation in a patient with primary ovarian failure. *Nature* 1984;307(5947):174–175.
20. Navot D et al. The window of embryo transfer and the efficiency of human conception in vitro. *Fertil Steril.* 1991;55(1):114–118.
21. Remohi J et al. Long oestradiol replacement in an oocyte donation programme. *Hum Reprod.* 1995;10(6):1387–1391.
22. Yaron Y et al. Uterine preparation with estrogen for oocyte donation: assessing the effect of treatment duration on pregnancy rates. *Fertil Steril.* 1995;63(6):1284–1286.
23. Rosenwaks Z. Donor eggs: their application in modern reproductive technologies. *Fertil Steril.* 1987;47(6):895–909.
24. Prapas Y et al. The window for embryo transfer in oocyte donation cycles depends on the duration of progesterone therapy. *Hum Reprod.* 1998;13(3):720–723.
25. Bosch E et al. Circulating progesterone levels and ongoing pregnancy rates in controlled ovarian stimulation cycles for *in vitro* fertilization: analysis of over 4000 cycles. *Hum Reprod.* 2010; 25; 2092–2100.
26. Berger BM, Phillips JA. Pregnancy outcomes in oocyte donation recipients: vaginal gel versus intramuscular injection progesterone replacement. *J Assist Reprod Genet.* 2012;29: 237–242.
27. Devine K et al. Vitrified blastocyst transfer cycles with the use of only vaginal progesterone replacement with Endometrin have inferior ongoing pregnancy rates: results from the planned interim analysis of a three-arm randomized controlled noninferiority trial. *Fertil Steril.* 2018;109:266–275.
28. Shapiro DB et al. Progesterone replacement with vaginal gel versus IM injection: cycle and pregnancy outcomes in IVF patients receiving vitrified blastocysts. *Hum Reprod.* 2014;29:1706–1711.
29. Zenke U, Chetkowski RJ. Transfer and uterine factors are the major recipient-related determinants of success with donor eggs. *Fertil Steril.* 2004;82(4):850–856.
30. Kuwayama M et al. Highly efficient vitrification method for cryopreservation of human oocytes. *Reprod Biomed Online.* 2005;11:300–308.
31. Noyes N et al. Over 900 oocyte cryopreservation babies born with no apparent increase in congenital anomalies. *Reprod Biomed Online.* 2009;18:769–776.
32. Forman EJ et al. Oocyte vitrification does not increase the risk of embryonic aneuploidy or diminish the implantation potential of blastocysts created after intracytoplasmic sperm injection: a novel, paired randomized controlled trial using DNA fingerprinting. *Fertil Steril.* 2012;98:644–649.
33. Rienzi L et al. Embryo development of fresh "versus" vitrified metaphase II oocytes after ICSI: a prospective randomized sibling-oocyte study. *Human Reprod.* 2010; 25: 66–73.
34. ASRM. Mature oocyte cryopreservation: a guideline. *Fertil Steril.* 2013;99(1):37–43.

16

Reproductive Surgery

Pietro Bortoletto and Dan Griffin

Reproductive Surgery

Before there was *in vitro* fertilization (IVF), there was reproductive surgery. Fertility-sparing surgery came first (i.e., myomectomy), followed quickly by surgery as primary treatment for infertility (i.e., tubal surgery), and eventually surgery to enhance fertility (i.e., septoplasty). The advent of IVF greatly expanded our ability to first treat structural causes of infertility and subsequently evolved to treat non-structural causes of infertility and has dramatically improved the efficiency of human reproduction. As the dramatic gains in clinical outcomes following IVF over the last decade have plateaued, the role of reproductive surgery is underscored as vital to optimizing outcomes for patients attempting to conceive and preserving this potential for the future. In this chapter, we will cover some of the most common indications for fertility enhancing/restoring surgery.

Intrauterine Polyps and Adhesions

Endometrial polyps are localized hyperplastic overgrowths of endometrial glands and stroma. The first line imaging study is a transvaginal ultrasound that can help assess other uterine or adnexal pathologies. A hysterosalpingogram can also assess the endometrial cavity; however, it may not be able to identify small abnormalities within the cavity. Saline sonohysterogram is an excellent tool to assess intrauterine pathology including polyps or intrauterine adhesive disease. The gold standard for assessing the endometrial cavity is a diagnostic hysteroscopy. For patients that have an endometrial polyp, the best surgical option is a hysteroscopy with polypectomy. A randomized trial in 2005 showed a significant improvement in pregnancy rates with intrauterine insemination (IUI) treatment after polypectomy compared to the expectant management group (63% after polypectomy vs. 28% with expectant management) (1). Intrauterine adhesions or scar tissue in the endometrial cavity have been associated with infertility as well as recurrent pregnancy loss. If patients have intrauterine adhesions, a hysteroscopy with lysis and excision of adhesions to restore normal anatomy is recommended. Severe intrauterine adhesions can have a high recurrence rate and a repeat surgical procedure may be needed. Treatment of intrauterine adhesions has been shown to improve fertility.

Uterine Fibroid Surgery

It is generally accepted that uterine cavity disrupting fibroids (FIGO 0, 1, 2, and 3) negatively impact reproductive potential. Once pregnant, the presence of cavity distorting fibroids is associated with increased rates of abnormal placentation, early pregnancy loss, placental abruption, malpresentation, placenta previa, and even growth restriction. Retrospective data suggests that resection of cavity distorting fibroids may ameliorate the risks—hysteroscopic myomectomy being the primary mode of resection.

 DOI: 10.1201/9781003460275-16

For FIGO 3 fibroids and beyond, a minimally invasive approach is generally considered the preferred surgical route. With regard to its role as not only fertility preserving but also as a fertility enhancing intervention, several non-controlled studies have suggested that laparoscopic myomectomy for cavity distorting fibroids is associated with lower rates of pregnancy loss compared to no surgery. Furthermore, several large systematic reviews have reported pooled pregnancy rates of 49% to 57% following laparoscopic myomectomy. However, no randomized trials have been performed to evaluate the role of minimally invasive myomectomy for fertility enhancement. The heterogeneity of uterine fibroids and patient characteristics present a challenge for ascertaining the impact of fibroids on fertility. Until well controlled trials are designed and performed, we are left with causal inference to suggest that removal of cavity-distorting fibroids are a potentially useful intervention for women trying to conceive.

One area of ongoing debate is the role of myomectomy for fibroids above 3–4 centimeters in size, to enhance fertility. Even without cavity distortion, intramural fibroids may impair endometrial and myometrial blood supply, increase uterine contractility, and modify the local hormonal and paracrine milieu of the endometrium. One hypothesis in support for their removal is the increased levels of TGF-β3 released by large intramural fibroids that can alter BMP-2 and HOXA-10 expression (2). HOXA-10, a critical messenger in regulating endometrial receptivity, is consistently lower in the presence of submucosal myomas, suggesting that large intramural fibroids, even without cavity distortion, may be having similar detrimental effects. More studies are needed to fully understand the risk benefit of invasive myomectomy of non-cavity deforming uterine fibroids. The decision to perform myomectomy for fertility enhancement must be individualized, weighing the risks of surgery, delay in treatment, and increased obstetric morbidity with potential fertility enhancing benefits.

Endometriosis and Adenomyosis Surgery

Endometriosis is defined as the presence of endometrial glands and stroma outside of the uterine cavity. It is estimated that approximately 15% of reproductive-aged women have endometriosis. This number rises to 25% to 50% in women with infertility. There are several mechanisms which have been proposed to cause infertility in women who have endometriosis. One clear mechanism is the presence of adhesive disease and distortion of the normal tubo-ovarian relationship. Adhesions from endometriosis affect the ability of the tube to pick up the oocyte properly. Endometriosis alters the peritoneal environment and creates an inflammatory state within the peritoneal cavity, which may impact sperm transport, fertilization, fallopian tube, and embryo function. Several inflammatory cytokines have shown to be increased in patients with endometriosis including IL-6 and TNF-α (3). Alterations in humoral immunity including an increase in IgA and IgG antibodies as well as increased lymphocytes have been reported in the endometrium of women with endometriosis. This may contribute to decreased endometrial receptivity and impaired implantation. Endometriosis has been associated with ovulatory dysfunction including luteal phase defects. Endometriosis may also be associated with poor oocyte or embryo quality. Due to the varying stages of endometriosis and the multiple mechanisms in which it may lead to subfertility, there are different treatment options which are used to achieve a pregnancy.

For superficial lesions, destruction with ablation compared to excision was shown to be similarly effective for the treatment of pelvic pain in a randomized controlled trial; however, with deep infiltrating endometriosis, complete excision is required given the depth of the lesions and their often close proximity to surrounding organs. For infertility secondary to endometriosis, the benefits of surgical diagnosis and destruction of disease are less clear. When Marcoux et al. randomly assigned infertile patients with mild endometriosis to diagnostic laparoscopy or surgical destruction, they identified that destruction of disease increases the chance for an unassisted pregnancy (4). However, when these results were combined with a similarly designed randomized study published two years later, the number of patients with known endometriosis that are needed to treat with surgical destruction for an unassisted live birth is 12. Yet, for asymptomatic patients with unexplained infertility, assuming a 30% incidence of endometriosis found at diagnostic laparoscopy, 40 such patients would need to undergo laparoscopy for one additional unassisted live birth, a number that has resulted in a recommendation against diagnostic laparoscopy in these cases with IVF as the preferred alternative to maximize fertility. Endometriosis has been shown to have a negative impact on implantation and pregnancy rates with IVF. In lieu of surgery, medical management with leuprolide and letrozole prior to doing an embryo transfer have been shown to significantly improve implantation rates, pregnancy rates, and live birth rates (56% with treatment compared to 34% without treatment) (5).

Adenomyosis is defined as the presence of endometrial glands and stroma within the myometrium. Studies have reported a wide range of prevalence in patients undergoing hysterectomy (10–60%). In patients with endometriosis and infertility, the prevalence of co-existent adenomyosis is up to 79%. Fertility-sparing surgery for dysmenorrhea and menorrhagia secondary to adenomyosis became increasingly utilized after reports of successful wedge resections were published in the 1950–60s. Fertility-sparing surgery for adenomyosis is less commonly performed compared to other gynecologic pathologies in part due to limitations in accurate diagnostic modalities, though recent advances in imaging techniques may help to better identify appropriate surgical candidates. In addition, the lack of clear tissue planes associated with both the focal and diffuse forms of this condition inherently result in a more complicated resection compared to a myomectomy. Despite these challenges, surgical pioneers, primarily out of Japan, have developed multiple new approaches in the last few decades in an effort to maximize the amount of adenomyosis removed while preserving fertility. Two notable methods that have been proposed with the goal of complete adenomyosis excision include the asymmetric dissection method and the triple-flap method. Long-term follow-up of the 2,123 uterine adenomyomectomy cases published from 13 centers in Japan has identified 449 pregnancies resulting in 361 live birth deliveries (6). However, the large uterine incision that is necessary with these surgical methods increases the risk of uterine rupture in a future pregnancy to 3–6%, compared to a baseline of 0.005% in a non-scarred uterus and <1.0% in a uterus after a prior myomectomy or hysterotomy scar (6).

Adnexal Surgery

The chronic inflammatory damage caused by endometriomas leads to progressive tissue fibrosis, which can result in displacement and necrosis of ovarian follicles and subsequent decline in oocyte quality and ovarian reserve. Endometriomas may also decrease ovarian reserve by inciting premature follicular development and atresia, accelerating ovarian insufficiency. A recent study by Kitajima et al. showed that endometriomas may cause premature activation of granulosa cells, leading to increased follicular atresia and reduced quality of remaining primordial follicles (7).

Several techniques have been described for extirpation of endometriomas. Unlike other cysts, endometriomas are invasive and associated with significant underlying tissue fibrosis, as mentioned earlier. Laparoscopic drainage and ablation represent the early surgical approach but were associated with unacceptably high rates of recurrence. Cystectomy, where the cyst wall is stripped either in part or as a whole, was a natural evolution but one that required significantly more surgical expertise. When compared to ablation, cystectomy was associated with a significantly detrimental impact to both antral follicle count and anti-Müllerian hormone levels (8). Of utmost importance is the prioritization of a first, and only, complete surgical resection of the ovarian endometrioma, as re-operating for recurrent cyst is associated with significantly higher loss to ovarian reserve than a single procedure alone (9). Newer variations of the laparoscopic approach that have made use of hydrodissection and CO_2 laser vaporization have been shown to be potentially safer, ovarian cortex preserving techniques. Sclerotherapy, with one of several sclerosing agents such as ethanol or lidocaine, is another minimally invasive option that can be performed transvaginally via REIs already familiar with transvaginal needle procedures. Its role seems to be confined to poor surgical candidates whose ovarian cysts preclude safe oocyte retrieval.

Tubal Surgery

With modern-day minimally invasive approaches for tubal reversal, women aged 15 to 30 years, 30 to 33 years, and 34 to 49 years could expect pregnancy rates of 73, 64, and 46 percent, respectively (10). In addition to age, the type of sterilization performed (84% with clips vs. 41% with electrocautery procedure) and the amount of residual tube (≥4 cm vs. <4 cm) are both important prognosticators of reproductive success (11). Tubal surgery was the only viable treatment option to circumvent tubal disease until the late 1990s when live birth rates from IVF improved from 14% to 31.6%. When considering the role of tubal surgery in the era of ART, it is important to consider several factors such as ovarian reserve, coexisting infertility diagnosis, number of children desired, as well as patient preference, religious beliefs, and access to ART. Compared to IVF, cumulative live birth rates over 5 years were comparable to those who had undergone tubal reanastomosis (52% vs. 60%), except in women under the age of 37, for whom tubal reanastomosis was associated with higher cumulative live birth rates (72.2% vs. 52.4%) (12). For patients with proximal occlusion, hysteroscopic tubal cannulation may be performed. This procedure is able to re-establish tubal patency 85% of the time; however, a third of tubes will re-occlude after this procedure. For patients with a hydrosalpinx, it is recommended the tube be removed or proximally occluded prior to proceeding with IVF, as this significantly increases pregnancy rates with IVF. When considering the role of tubal surgery in the era of ART, it is important to consider several factors such as ovarian reserve, coexisting infertility diagnosis, number of children desired, as well as patient preference, religious beliefs, and access to ART.

Müllerian Anomalies

Müllerian anomalies represent a complex collection of developmental defects occurring in up to 5% of the general population. They are increasingly more common in individuals with infertility (8.0%) and in those with a history of pregnancy loss (13.3%); they have the highest prevalence in individuals with a history of both (24.5%). A wide spectrum of anomalies can occur based on the stage at which Müllerian development ceases in utero, ranging from mild (e.g., a partial uterine septum) to severe, with complete absence of the cervix, uterus, and fallopian tubes (e.g., Müllerian agenesis). The components of the reproductive tract involved and, importantly, whether an obstruction of the tract is involved correlates with the timing of presentation, the constellation of associated symptoms, and the necessity for either medical or surgical management.

Beyond management of uterine fibroids, endometriosis, and adnexal pathology, reproductive surgeons manage complex Müllerian anomalies. Perhaps one of the more common anomalies managed by the REI is the uterine septum. Women with septate uteri are at an increased risk of infertility, recurrent miscarriage, and preterm birth (13). Retrospective data has suggested that incision may improve pregnancy outcomes (13). A recent multicenter RCT, the TRUST trial failed to demonstrate an improvement in reproductive outcomes for women undergoing septum incision (14). The study's broad inclusion criteria, generous definition for uterine septum, and the time it took to enroll 80 patients (eight years) have been viewed as significant limiting factors for generalizability of their results. Until such a time where more rigorously designed trials are available, uncertainty remains as to the perceived benefit of septum incision. The surgical management of more complex Müllerian anomalies are typically performed to ameliorate pain and restore and preserve fertility in the cases of obstructive anomalies.

Vaginal anomalies may also be encountered and may occur as a solitary finding or in combination with uterine anomalies. For those individuals with vaginal agenesis, neovagina creation can be accomplished using vaginal stretching, replacement, or augmentation procedures. Formation of a neovagina via stretching with the use of dilators was first described in 1938 by reproductive endocrinologist Robert Frank of New York. For those in whom dilation is unsuccessful, surgical vaginal stretching using the Vecchietti procedure is exceptionally successful with vaginal lengths of 8–9 cm routinely achieved. This technique relies on the use of an "olive" placed at the perineum with an abdominal tensioning device that applies cranioventral tension over a period of 4–7 days. Beyond stretching procedures, neovaginas may be created with replacement tissues. The McIndoe and Davydov procedures rely on either a split thickness skin graft or peritoneum, respectively. Innovations in novel tissues such as buccal mucosa and tilapia fish skin allow for augmenting existing tissues in ways that further enhance tissue properties and functionality.

Uterus Transplantation

Absolute uterine factor infertility (AUFI) affects <5% of reproductive-aged women. For those with AUFI, IVF with a gestational carrier represented the only way to achieve biologically related offspring. However, the use of gestational carriers are largely illegal worldwide, costly when they are legal, and do not afford women the opportunity of carrying a pregnancy themselves. Uterus transplantation emerged as a potential way to overcome this and offer a new treatment paradigm for patients with AUFI.

While the first uterus transplant was performed in Saudi Arabia in 2000 (history of a hysterectomy related to postpartum hemorrhage), it would be nearly 14 years later before the first live birth was achieved in Sweden by the group lead by Mats Brännström. In the years that followed, attempts were made to reduce surgical morbidity to living donors by harvesting organs from both deceased and brain-dead donors, both resulting in live births. It is estimated that over 60 uterus transplants have been performed with over 20 live births as of May 2020. Of the uterus transplants in the US since 2016 (n = 33), one-year graft survival was 74% (23 of 31 recipients) and 19 of 33 recipients (58%) had delivered 21 live-born children. The median (range) gestational age at birth of neonates was 36 weeks 6 days (30 weeks 1 day to 38 weeks), and the median (range) birth weight was 2860 (1310–3940) g (median [range], 58th [6th–98th] percentile). As morbidity to the recipient and obstetric/neonatal outcomes improve, it has been suggested that there will be increasing interest in the use of uterus transplantation to afford an opportunity of pregnancy to those with AUFI, including those with a history of hysterectomy, individuals with androgen insensitivity syndrome, severe Asherman syndrome, and transgender female patients.

Radiofrequency Ablation (RFA)

Radiofrequency ablation (RFA) for uterine leiomyoma attempts to induce coagulative necrosis within a fibroid to achieve reduced fibroid volume and thus fibroid-related symptoms. Currently, two devices are available in the United States—Acessa (Hologic) and Sonata (Gynesonics) systems which utilize a laparoscopic and transcervical approach, respectively. However, the devices are only labeled for use in symptomatic uterine fibroids in patients who do not desire future fertility. RFA is an interesting technique in that it does not require myometrial incisions or suture but similarly does not allow for tissue diagnosis or removal of myoma tissue. A paucity of data exists on reproductive outcomes in reproductive-aged women desiring future fertility. A recent systematic review by Polin et al. identified a total of 50 pregnancies following 923 RFA patients (10 transcervical and 40 laparoscopic) (15). Amongst these, there were 6 spontaneous abortions (12%) and 44 full-term pregnancies (88%) with only 2 recorded complications, placenta previa and post-partum hemorrhage with expulsion of a degenerated myoma. No uterine ruptures, invasive placentation, or preterm deliveries were reported. More data is needed to ensure efficacy and safety of RFA for women with uterine fibroids desiring future fertility. Until such data exists, their role in reproductive-aged women is limited.

Key Points

- Reproductive surgery has the potential to restore fertility as well as enhance treatment outcomes from assisted reproduction.
- There is a paucity of data on reproductive surgery outcomes with regard to fertility and long-term obstetric implications.
- The use of assisted reproductive technologies for fertility preservation ahead of surgical intervention may be of significant benefit.

REFERENCES

1. Pérez-Medina T et al. Endometrial polyps and their implication in the pregnancy rates of patients undergoing intrauterine insemination: a prospective, randomized study. *Hum Reprod Oxf Engl* 2005;20(6):1632–5.
2. Rackow BW, Taylor HS. Submucosal uterine leiomyomas have a global effect on molecular determinants of endometrial receptivity. *Fertil Steril* 2010;93(6):2027–34.
3. Bedaiwy MA et al. Prediction of endometriosis with serum and peritoneal fluid markers: a prospective controlled trial. *Hum Reprod Oxf Engl* 2002;17(2):426–31.
4. Marcoux S et al. Laparoscopic surgery in infertile women with minimal or mild endometriosis. Canadian collaborative group on endometriosis. *N Engl J Med* 1997;337(4):217–22.
5. Steiner N et al. Effect of GnRH agonist and letrozole treatment in women with recurrent implantation failure. *Fertil Steril* 2019;112(1):98–104.
6. Osada H. Uterine adenomyosis and adenomyoma: the surgical approach. *Fertil Steril* 2018;109(3):406–17.
7. Kitajima M et al. Enhanced follicular recruitment and atresia in cortex derived from ovaries with endometriomas. *Fertil Steril* 2014;101(4):1031–7.
8. Zhang Y et al. Impact of cystectomy versus ablation for endometrioma on ovarian reserve: a systematic review and meta-analysis. *Fertil Steril* 2022;118(6):1172–82.
9. Muzii L et al. Second surgery for recurrent endometriomas is more harmful to healthy ovarian tissue and ovarian reserve than first surgery. *Fertil Steril* 2015;103(3):738–43.
10. Trussell J et al. Sterilization failure, sterilization reversal, and pregnancy after sterilization reversal in Quebec. *Obstet Gynecol* 2003;101(4):677–84.
11. Yoon TK et al. Fertility outcome after laparoscopic microsurgical tubal anastomosis. *Fertil Steril* 1997;67(1):18–22.
12. Boeckxstaens A et al. Getting pregnant after tubal sterilization: surgical reversal or IVF? *Hum Reprod Oxf Engl* 2007;22(10):2660–4.
13. Rikken JF et al. Septum resection for women of reproductive age with a septate uterus. *Cochrane Database Syst Rev* 2017;1:CD008576.
14. Rikken JFW et al. Septum resection versus expectant management in women with a septate uterus: an international multicentre open-label randomized controlled trial. *Hum Reprod Oxf Engl* 2021;36(5):1260–7.
15. Polin M, Hur H-C. Radiofrequency ablation of uterine myomas and pregnancy outcomes: an updated review of the literature. *J Minim Invasive Gynecol* 2022;29(6):709–15.

17

Polycystic Ovary Syndrome

Rita M. Sneeringer and Kristen Page Wright

Introduction

Polycystic ovary syndrome (PCOS) is the most common endocrinopathy of reproductive-age women and the most frequent cause of anovulatory infertility. As a syndrome, it is a collection of specific signs and symptoms rather than a well-defined disorder. As such, it can include variable clinical presentations. Depending on the criteria used for diagnosis, the prevalence ranges from 9% to 18%.[1] Emerging evidence suggests that the cause of PCOS is multifactorial due to a combination of genetic predispositions and environmental factors such as obesity, environmental pollutants, diet, lifestyle, and alterations in the gut microbiome.[2] PCOS is associated with long-term health complications, including diabetes, obesity, heart disease, and endometrial hyperplasia or cancer. Accurate diagnosis allows for directed treatment and prevention of comorbidities. Diagnostic criteria, clinical presentation, potential pathophysiology, and evidence-based treatments are summarized here.

Diagnosis

Stein and Leventhal first described the syndrome of PCOS in 1935 as the combination of polycystic ovaries and amenorrhea. Since then, the definition and, hence, diagnosis of PCOS has evolved. Much controversy exists due to the varied presentation. In the past decades, several different diagnostic criteria have been developed for the classification of PCOS (Table 17.1). The initial diagnostic criteria were developed during a consensus meeting at the NIH in 1990. The NIH criteria required both chronic anovulation as well as clinical and/or biochemical signs of hyperandrogenism.[3] Notably, polycystic ovaries were not required for the diagnosis of PCOS. In 2003, a consensus workshop held jointly by the European Society of Human Reproduction and Embryology (ESHRE) and the American Society for Reproductive Medicine (ASRM) in Rotterdam revised the diagnostic criteria. For the Rotterdam criteria, two out of the following three symptoms are required: oligo-ovulation and/or anovulation, clinical and/or biochemical signs of hyperandrogenism, and polycystic ovaries.[4] The Rotterdam criteria broadened the clinical spectrum of PCOS by including two additional groups of women who did not previously meet the NIH definition: women with only hirsutism and polycystic ovaries but regular menstrual cycles; and women with oligomenorrhea and polycystic ovaries but without hyperandrogenism. Finally, in 2006 the Androgen Excess Society (AES) Task Force developed consensus guidelines that placed a greater emphasis on the elevated androgens that characterize this syndrome. In the AES criteria, PCOS can be diagnosed following documented hyperandrogenism (hirsutism and/or hyperandrogenemia) and ovarian dysfunction (oligo-ovulation and/or anovulation and/or polycystic ovaries).[5] Women with ultrasound appearance of polycystic ovaries and ovulatory dysfunction in the absence of hyperandrogenism would not meet the AES criteria for the diagnosis of PCOS. Further, the AES and NIH criteria are quite similar with some minor modifications to include women with hyperandrogenism and polycystic ovaries in the absence of menstrual irregularity.

 DOI: 10.1201/9781003460275-17

TABLE 17.1

Diagnostic Criteria for PCOS and Associated Variable Phenotypes

Criteria	Hyperandrogenism (clinical or biochemical)	Menstrual irregularity/ anovulation	Polycystic-appearing ovaries on ultrasound
NIH	✓	✓	
Rotterdam	✓	✓	
	✓		✓
		✓	✓
	✓	✓	✓
Androgen Excess Society	✓	✓	
	✓		✓
	✓	✓	✓

Recognizing the confusion with multiple classifications systems, the NIH, in 2012, held an evidence-based methodology workshop on PCOS where experts agreed to the 2003 Rotterdam criteria. Additionally, they identified specific subtypes of PCOS, including 1) androgen excess and ovulatory dysfunction, 2) androgen excess and PCO ovarian morphology, 3) ovulatory dysfunction and PCO ovarian morphology, and 4) androgen excess, ovulatory dysfunction and PCO ovarian morphology. The Rotterdam criteria has now been endorsed by the Australian Guideline Committee,[6] the National Institute for Health in the US,[7] the US Endocrine Society Practice Guideline,[8] The European Society for Endocrinology position statement,[9] and the World Health Organization.[10]

Importantly, the Rotterdam criteria, in addition to the NIH and AES criteria, require the exclusion of other etiologies of menstrual irregularities and hyperandrogenism. Possible other diagnoses include adrenal or ovarian androgen-secreting neoplasm, hyperprolactinemia, syndromes of severe insulin resistance, thyroid dysfunction, congenital adrenal hyperplasia, Cushing's syndrome, and acromegaly. Typically, the measurement of thyroid stimulating hormone, prolactin, glucose, insulin, and an androgen panel (DHEA-S, testosterone, and 17-OH progesterone) is sufficient to exclude other major causes if normal levels are noted. Specific testing for Cushing's syndrome and acromegaly is done if suspected based on history or phenotypic changes noted on physical exam (e.g., striae, round face, dorsal fat pad, central obesity, uncontrolled hypertension, increased glove or shoe size). For patients that have either severe or rapid onset of hyperandrogenic symptoms, an alternative diagnosis should be suspected as this is atypical for PCOS. Virilization (clitoromegaly, male-pattern frontal balding, or increased musculature) may also suggest tumor development. An androgen-secreting tumor would typically contribute to serum testosterone levels greater than 150–200 ng/dl or DHEAS levels above 700 μg/dL in premenopausal women. Congenital adrenal hyperplasia is suspected if 17-OH progesterone level is elevated. Further assessment with an ACTH stimulation test should be performed when a morning 17-OH progesterone level performed in the follicular phase is >200 ng/dL.

Additional testing that is consistent with the diagnosis of PCOS but is not part of any criteria includes an elevated LH/FSH ratio (>3:1), elevated AMH, and hyperinsulinemia. These factors have been linked to PCOS, possibly secondary to underlying etiology, but are not necessary for the diagnosis of PCOS. It is also important to emphasize that PCOS is a syndrome, a collection of features rather than a definitive disease that may represent multiple underlying disorders.

Clinical Presentation and Evaluation

Patients with PCOS usually present to care for three primary reasons: menstrual disturbances, hyperandrogenism, and infertility. Additional hallmarks of PCOS include obesity and metabolic disorders such as diabetes. There can also be a strong family history. A few distinct subgroups may present without the "typical phenotype" including women with lean PCOS and adolescents. The clinical characteristics of PCOS and suggested evaluation are described in Table 17.2.

TABLE 17.2

Suggested Evaluation of PCOS/Chronic Anovulation

History and physical
Menstrual history, galactorrhea
BMI, blood pressure, waist circumference, hirsutism, acanthosis nigricans, thyroid
Striae, round face, dorsal fat pad, hypertension, central obesity (Cushing's symptoms)
Enlarged hands and feet, prominent facial features (acromegaly)
Confirm the diagnosis of PCOS
Ultrasound of the ovaries and endometrial stripe
Androgens (mildly elevated) and sex hormone binding globulin
Consider luteal progesterone
Exclude other endocrinopathies/causes of chronic anovulation
hCG (pregnancy)
Total testosterone (ovarian/adrenal tumor)
DHEA-S (adrenal tumor)
Morning 17-OH progesterone (congenital adrenal hyperplasia)
FSH/LH (ovarian failure)
TSH (thyroid disorder)
Prolactin (hyperprolactinemia)
Dexamethasone suppression test (Cushing's syndrome, only if suspected)
IGF-1 (acromegaly, only if suspected)
Evaluate for Comorbidities of PCOS
HgbA1C (diabetes/glucose intolerance)
Endometrial biopsy for prolonged anovulation (endometrial hyperplasia/cancer)
Lipid profile (hyperlipidemia, metabolic syndrome)

Menstrual disturbances are found in the majority of PCOS patients. The type of menstrual disorder can vary, but the underlying etiology is the same, anovulatory cycles. Most patients present with oligo-ovulation or anovulation leading to oligomenorrhea or amenorrhea. However, some women appear to have spontaneous menses with abnormal flow. This excessive bleeding could be the result of an absent luteal phase causing heavy, prolonged bleeding due to unopposed effects of estrogen. Thus, for women who have any irregularity of their menses (cycles <21 days or >35 days, highly variable cycle length, or abnormal flow), PCOS is a potential diagnosis. Additional testing, such as a luteal progesterone level, can help to determine if cycles are anovulatory. A progesterone level of >3 ng/mL is confirmatory of ovulation.

Ultrasound assessment may reveal polycystic ovaries which are associated with chronic anovulation and can be a sign of the ovarian dysfunction in PCOS. However, this finding is not specific and can be seen in patients with multiple etiologies for anovulation. Further, polycystic ovaries can be a normal isolated finding in approximately one-third of ovulating women without metabolic sequelae typical for PCOS.[11] Therefore, it is important to correlate the presence of polycystic ovaries with other clinical findings. The specific parameters for the diagnosis of PCO-appearing ovaries, according to the Rotterdam criteria, are as follows: ≥20 follicles in each ovary that measure 2–9 mm or ovarian volume ≥10 cc (Figure 17.1). Ultrasound evaluation is not valid if a dominant follicle is present.

Anti-Müllerian hormone (AMH) level correlates with number of antral follicles and is frequently elevated in women with PCOS. An elevated AMH of >3.8 ng/mL is suggestive of PCOS; however, there is significant overlap between ovulatory women and women with PCOS.[10, 12] An elevated AMH alone in the absence of other diagnostic criteria is not sufficient for a diagnosis of PCOS.

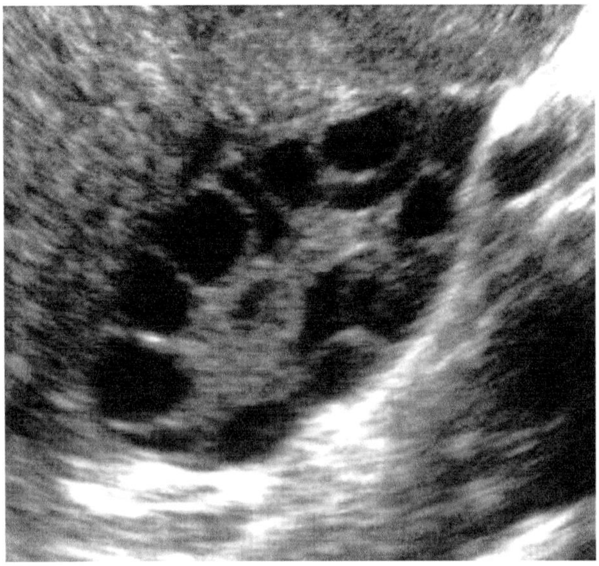

FIGURE 17.1 PCO Morphology Parameters: ≥12 follicles per ovary that measure 2–9 mm or ovarian volume ≥10 cc. The ultrasound evaluation is not valid if a dominant follicle is present. PCO morphology can be seen in only one ovary. PCO morphology alone is not sufficient for the diagnosis of PCOS and can be a normal finding of 20% of fertile women.

Hyperandrogenism is the other major component of PCOS. Hirsutism (excessive hair growth) is dependent.[12–14] A standardized scoring system, such as the Ferriman–Gallwey score, can be a helpful tool in evaluating hirsutism (Figure 17.2). This scale assesses the density and distribution of hair growth on multiple areas of the body. Generally, a summation score of greater than 8 is consistent with hirsutism. Acne, oily skin, and male-pattern alopecia are less specific features and should not be considered

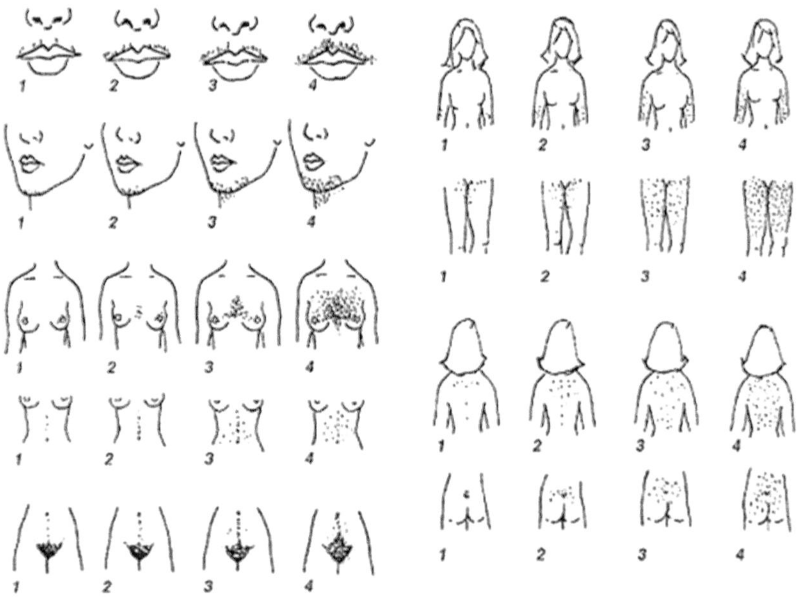

FIGURE 17.2 Ferriman–Gallwey Score for the clinical assessment of hirsutism. A summation score of 8 is consistent with hirsutism (from ref 14 with permission).

clinical evidence of hyperandrogenemia.[15] Biochemical markers of hyperandrogenism include elevated testosterone or DHEA-sulfate levels.

In addition to the diagnostic symptoms, many patients with PCOS have metabolic abnormalities that should be recognized in order to mediate future health risks. Insulin resistance, and, hence, hyperinsulinemia is an important finding in many PCOS patients and is suspected particularly among patients with acanthosis nigricans on physical exam. Acanthosis nigricans is a pigmented, velvety skin lesion that is noted most commonly on the back of the neck, axilla, and groin. PCOS patients are at an increased risk for glucose intolerance or diabetes with up to 45% of patients affected[16] and approximately 16% of patients developing glucose intolerance annually.[17] Centripetal obesity is found in the majority of patients with PCOS and is considered part of the typical phenotype. It likely exacerbates the risk of other comorbidities. The metabolic syndrome characterized by abdominal obesity, hypertension, high triglycerides, inflammatory factors, and increased thrombophilic factors is twice as likely to occur in patients with PCOS and is associated with an increased risk of cardiovascular disease.[18] Clearly, these associated metabolic conditions have significant long-term consequences, and all patients with PCOS should be screened with regular assessment of glucose tolerance testing, blood pressure, waist/hip measurement, body mass index, and lipid panel (including triglycerides, total cholesterol, and HDL). Fasting glucose, fasting insulin levels, and/or HbA1C testing can be considered in lieu of glucose tolerance testing.[10]

Reproductive potential is impacted greatly by anovulation. Issues of subfertility and infertility are central to the presentation of PCOS patients, as are concerns about pregnancy outcomes and health risks to their offspring. Women with PCOS are more likely to use assisted reproductive technology than women without the diagnosis. Furthermore, women with PCOS are at increased risk for first trimester miscarriage with rates of 30–50% compared to 10–15% in the general population.[19] The exact reason for this is not known but may be linked to insulin resistance. In addition, obstetric risks, including pregnancy-induced hypertension, gestational diabetes, and pre-term birth are increased among patients with PCOS. These obstetric risks are also further exacerbated by obesity.

A higher incidence of endometrial abnormalities secondary to chronic anovulation is found in some patients with PCOS. Endometrial hyperplasia and carcinoma can occur; the incidence of endometrial cancer is four times higher in women with PCOS compared to women without PCOS.[22] Pathology evaluation of the endometrium is warranted in anovulatory patients regardless of age. However, an endometrium of <5 mm noted on vaginal ultrasound exam is rarely associated with endometrial hyperplasia, and, therefore, an endometrial biopsy is not necessary in this circumstance.

PCOS can be associated with a significant psychological impact that is often overlooked. The feminine identity and body image are primarily affected, as patients suffer from obesity, acne, oily skin, excess hair growth, as well as infertility and several other health care issues. The data is limited, but evidence exists that PCOS patients are more prone to also develop several psychiatric disorders, including major depression, anxiety, low self-esteem, negative body image, and psychosexual dysfunction.[21, 22] As a result, patients whose lives and moods are significantly affected by the syndrome might also have a tougher time complying with lifestyle and treatment recommendations, all issues that need to be recognized and explored by clinicians.

Some patients do not fit the usual profile of PCOS. A special subset of patients are the lean PCOS patients. They represent between 10–50% of all PCOS patients[23] and present a challenging clinical conundrum. Despite having a normal BMI, these patients have greater insulin resistance compared to weight-matched controls.[24] They also manifest various metabolic abnormalities such as dyslipidemia,[25] pro-thrombotic tendency, and increased pro-inflammatory markers. Unfortunately, their diagnosis is often delayed or missed altogether because they do not exhibit the typical obese PCOS phenotype.

Adolescents are a second atypical group and there is no overall consensus how to diagnose PCOS in adolescence. A majority of young women have anovulatory menstrual cycles during the first 1–3 years after menarche, and hirsutism is less common in adolescence as this feature tends to develop over time. Biochemical markers of hyperandrogenemia and increased ovarian volume on ultrasound may, therefore, be more sensitive markers for the diagnosis of PCOS in adolescents.[15] Often the diagnosis is delayed or oral contraceptives are initiated without a complete evaluation for PCOS. However, adolescents still have significant risks of metabolic comorbidities that could be mediated by early intervention and prevention strategies. This includes initiating weight management before severe obesity develops. Thus, it is important to complete a clinical assessment on adolescent patients that exhibit possible features of PCOS with re-evaluation recommended three years post-menarche.[26]

Pathophysiology/Etiology

The exact etiology of PCOS is likely multifactorial due to a combination of genetic and environmental factors. Several theories have been proposed, two of which have significant supporting research. These include theories of LH dysregulation and hyperinsulinemia. As PCOS is a heterogeneous disorder with varied presentations, it is possible that both theories are correct but simply apply to different populations of patients. Alternatively, they could represent components of the same complex, physiologic pathway. Specific research findings and potential explanations for the clinical presentation of PCOS for each theory are described.

The dysregulation of LH in PCOS patients has been reported in multiple studies and may account for many of the clinical symptoms of PCOS. Increased pulsatile GnRH secretion leads to increased LH pulse frequency. The primary cause of increased GnRH is unclear; it could be an intrinsic abnormality of the pulse generator or secondary to other factors such as chronically low levels of progesterone (from anovulation) and/or hyperinsulinemia.[27–29] Women with PCOS have reduced hypothalamic sensitivity to ovarian sex steroids[30] and enhanced pituitary sensitivity to GnRH, which likely contributes to the increased LH secretion and pulse amplitude. The increased LH secretion relative to FSH stimulates ovarian androgen (testosterone and androstenedione) production leading to clinical hyperandrogenism. Anovulation results from insufficient selection of a dominant follicle in the setting of hyperthecosis.

Other research suggests hyperinsulinemia as the primary insult through direct and indirect effects.[25] Insulin augments LH stimulation of ovarian androgen production and inhibits hepatic sex hormone binding globulin (SHBG) production, which increases free androgen and estrogen levels. IGF-1 acts directly on the ovary to stimulate androgen production. Insulin at sufficiently high levels may cross-react with ovarian IGF receptors, enhance IGF action by up-regulating IGF receptors, and inhibit IGF-binding protein (IGFBP)-1 production, leading to increased IGF-1.[27] The end result of insulin action on the ovary is the preferential production of androgens with higher free levels due to reduced SHBG. This explains how PCOS patients have hyperandrogenic symptoms despite normal androgen levels. The strong correlation of PCOS with hyperinsulinemia (see clinical presentation previously discussed) supports hyperinsulinemia as a possible central etiology.

Other physiologic effects are less-well described but may also play a role. For example, a reduction in ovarian aromatase activity has been proposed as a contributing factor to hyperandrogenism in PCOS, although this issue remains controversial.[27]

Management

Several effective treatment strategies are available for patients with PCOS, including lifestyle modifications, medications, non-medical treatments, and surgical intervention. Given the multifaceted approach to management, a multidisciplinary team is usually needed for the best results. In addition, treatment should be tailored to a patient's specific needs, with attention to reproductive goals. Several treatments are contraindicated in patients who are pursuing fertility. The optimal management of PCOS incorporates healthy changes that can be maintained for a lifetime.

Lifestyle Interventions

Lifestyle changes should be the first-line approach for any PCOS patient, particularly those with obesity. Most importantly, lifestyle intervention should address weight loss or prevention of weight gain through dietary modifications and regular exercise. A body weight reduction of 5–10% has been shown to exert a significant benefit on major psychological, reproductive (menstrual regulation, ovulation, fertility), and metabolic (hirsutism, insulin resistance, risk factors for diabetes and cardiovascular disease) outcomes.[31] In addition, body mass index is a clear prognostic factor for infertility treatments with reduced pregnancy rates among obese PCOS patients compared to normal weight PCOS patients. Consultation with a nutritionist who is familiar with the specific challenges of PCOS is recommended. In addition, regular exercise with a structured routine of at least 30 minutes a day can reduce cardiovascular risk associated with PCOS.

Bariatric surgery is sometimes considered in women with PCOS and obesity who are unsuccessful at weight loss after diet and exercise adjustments. Current guidelines state that bariatric surgery can be considered for women with BMI >40 kg/m2 or BMI >35 kg/m2 in the presence of obesity-related comorbidities such as type 2 diabetes. Bariatric surgery improves many features of PCOS including anovulation rate, hirsutism, insulin resistance, and sexual libido. However, small-for-gestational-age infants and pre-term birth have emerged as complications associated with births after bariatric surgery due to the resulting malabsorptive nutritional state of the mother. It is, therefore, unclear whether bariatric surgery improves overall maternal and fetal outcomes. Women with PCOS who become pregnant after bariatric surgery should be considered high risk and should be followed by a multidisciplinary health care team including a dietician.[10] Additionally, pregnancy should be avoided during periods of rapid weight loss and for at least 6–12 months after bariatric surgery.

Several medications to combat obesity and insulin resistance have recently emerged that may be helpful for women with PCOS. The glucagon-like peptide-1 agonists (GLP-1) and dual glucose-dependent insulinotropic polypeptide (GIP) and GLP-1 agonists are currently indicated for individuals with obesity and/or type II diabetes and have proven very effective in achieving weight loss. Whether these medications are also effective in ameliorating some of the symptoms of PCOS remains to be seen. It is important to note that these medications are contraindicated during pregnancy and current recommendations are to discontinue these medications eight weeks prior to attempting conception.

Medical Therapies

Several medical therapies effectively treat the symptoms of PCOS (Table 17.3). The choice of medications depends on the specific symptoms and their severity. Medical therapies are often optimal when combined with lifestyle interventions or non-medical therapies.

The symptoms of menstrual irregularity and hyperandrogenism can be improved through use of the oral contraceptive pill (OCP). The maximal benefit is achieved with combined estrogen–progestin pills, since these formulations take advantage of the first pass effect in the liver. As a result, levels of hepatic proteins, including sex hormone binding globulin, are significantly increased, thus reducing free circulating androgen concentrations. After initiation of OCP therapy, the regulation of the menstrual abnormality is usually immediate, but improvement in hyperandrogenic symptoms may not be appreciated for 4–6 months. Additionally, OCPs protect the endometrium from hyperplasia by providing progesterone exposure. For all patients that have prolonged anovulation, some form of progesterone exposure is needed. For most, OCPs offer the most convenient solution. For patients with contraindications to oral estrogen, progesterone administration alone for at least 10 days per month can be prescribed. Alternative routes of administration of progesterone such as the progestin containing IUD, progesterone implant, and Depo-Provera injection will effectively protect the endometrium from hyperplasia but are less useful for improving symptoms of hyperandrogenism.

Several other medical treatments for hirsutism are also available for severe symptoms or symptoms not responsive to OCPs[32] (Table 17.3). As many of these medications work via an anti-androgen mechanism, which could be teratogenic, they are often combined with the use of OCPs. Hirsutism medical therapies include spironolactone, flutamide, finasteride, ketoconazole, and eflornithine. The choice of type of treatment must consider the side-effect profile. Spironolactone (25–100 mg twice daily) acts as an androgen receptor blocker, preventing the action of androgens at the hair follicle. It is also a diuretic and should be avoided in patients with renal impairment due to increased risk of hyperkalemia. Flutamide (125–250 mg/day) is non-steroidal anti-androgen which is a teratogen and has been associated with hepatotoxicity rarely. Finasteride is a 5-alpha-reductase inhibitor that prevents the formation of a potent androgen (DHT) that is the primary binding androgen at the hair follicle receptor. Finasteride is also a teratogen

TABLE 17.3

Summary of Medical Treatments for PCOS. Combined Therapy with OCPs and Anti Androgens Are Often Utilized for Higher Efficacy with Contraception for the Teratogen Risk

Medication and dose	Mechanism	Indications	Contraindications and side effects
Oral contraceptives	Suppress ovulation and ovarian androgen production	Menstrual irregularity (prevention of endometrial disease); contraception; hirsutism	Increased risk of thrombosis (low)
Spironolactone (50–100 mg twice daily)	Androgen receptor blocker and diuretic	Hirsutism	Hepatic toxicity; renal dysfunction; potential teratogen; hyperkalemia (rare); hypotension; menstrual irregularity; polyuria
Finasteride (2.5–5.0 mg daily)	5 α reductase inhibitor	Hirsutism	Teratogen (can be absorbed through skin/do not handle); potential renal or hepatic toxicity (rare)
Flutamide (250–500 mg daily)	Anti-androgen	Hirsutism	Hepatic toxicity (rare but could be severe); teratogen; yellow urine
Ketoconazole (400 mg daily)	Steroidogenesis inhibitor	Hirsutism	Adrenal insufficiency; hepatotoxicity
Eflornithine (13.9% cream twice daily)	Ornithine decarboxylase inhibitor	Hirsutism	Skin sensitivity
Clomiphene (50–150 mg x 5d)	SERM/partial estrogen agonist at the pituitary	Ovulation induction	Multiple gestations (<10%); pituitary edema (rare) with visual changes; headache; hot flashes; mood lability
Letrozole (5–7.5 mg x 5d)	Aromatase inhibitor	Ovulation induction	Contraindicated with hepatic disease; headaches; hot flashes
Metformin (500–2000 mg daily)	Biguanide; insulin sensitizing agent	Ovulation induction (not first-line) Diabetes prevention	Contraindicated with renal or hepatic disease; lactic acidosis (higher risk if renal disease); diarrhea

but is associated with less renal or hepatic toxicity. Ketoconazole is an antifungal that inhibits steroid synthesis. Its use is limited by side effects of hypo-adrenalism and hepatotoxicity. Eflornithine is a topical treatment that is an irreversible inhibitor of ornithine decarboxylase, an enzyme that is important for the growth of hair. Optimal results are achieved when combined with mechanical removal of hair (see further discussion). The treatments for hirsutism offer moderate results over long-term treatment. For most of the medications, response is often not noticeable until after months of treatment. Patients pursuing fertility are poor candidates for medical therapy given the potential for birth defect. They may choose alternative non-medical therapies.

For patients with documented insulin resistance or glucose intolerance, insulin sensitizing agents have been central to medical therapy. Metformin is a biguanide that acts by improving peripheral insulin sensitivity. It is currently FDA-approved for the treatment of type 2 diabetes mellitus (T2DM), but it has also been used extensively in the treatment of PCOS. Multiple studies have demonstrated an improvement in ovulation, menstrual cyclicity, and hirsutism with the initiation of metformin therapy.[33] In addition, metformin improves the cardiovascular and metabolic profiles of these patients, mainly reducing their risk of Type 2 DM.[34] The recommended starting dose is 500 mg of the slow-release tablets once daily, followed by a gradual increase over weeks to months up to 2 g daily, if tolerated. Major side effects of metformin include GI upset (diarrhea). Lactic acidosis is a significant but rare complication of metformin use and is almost exclusively encountered in patients with renal disease.

Myo-inositol can also be a useful medication to treat the hyperinsulinemia associated with PCOS. Inositols are incorporated into cell membranes as phosphatidyl-MI, which is a precursor of inositol triphosphate (InsP3). InsP3 is a second messenger for insulin and FSH, and defects in this pathway can cause insulin resistance. There are two inositol stereoisomers, myo-inositol and D-chiro-inositol. D-chiro-inositol is involved in glycogen synthesis and storage, while myo-inositol is involved in regulating hormones such as TSH, FSH, and insulin. Small studies utilizing myo-inositol 2 g/day have demonstrated improvement in the metabolic parameters associated with PCOS such as lowering testosterone levels and improving insulin resistance.[35] However, it is uncertain whether myo-inositol treatment definitively improves pregnancy rates in women undergoing infertility treatment.[36] Myo-inositol is considered a nutritional supplement in the US and is, therefore, not regulated by the FDA.

For treatment of anovulatory infertility due to PCOS, ovulation induction with clomiphene citrate (CC) was originally described and is still used today. CC is a non-steroidal selective estrogen-receptor modulator (SERM) that acts on the pituitary to increase endogenous production of FSH. The most recent joint ESHRE/ASRM recommendations suggest CC for up to six ovulatory cycles. When administered to anovulatory PCOS patients, it results in a 60–80% ovulation rate and a 30–40% pregnancy rate. The dose of CC is usually started at 50 mg for 5 days in the follicular phase and increased up to 150 mg as needed to achieve ovulation. The main side effects associated with CC include multiple gestation (5–10%), hot flashes, and mood changes. Visual changes due to pituitary edema are rarely encountered but warrant immediate discontinuation of the medication for symptom resolution.

Aromatase inhibitors such as letrozole have replaced CC as a first-line treatment for ovulation induction for women with PCOS. Aromatase inhibitors decrease serum estradiol concentrations, which decreases negative feedback to the pituitary, thereby increasing FSH. A multicenter, randomized, controlled trial conducted by the Reproductive Medicine Network compared CC to letrozole in women with PCOS and demonstrated that letrozole resulted in higher ovulation rates and higher live-birth rates than CC with no difference in pregnancy loss rate.[38] Importantly, the mean BMI in this study was 35 kg/m2, and letrozole resulted in improved live-birth rates in all BMI quartiles, with a more pronounced effect in patients with BMI >30 kg/m2. Treatment with letrozole is also associated with a reduction in multiple gestation risk because letrozole is associated with improved monofollicular ovulation compared to CC.[39] The dose of letrozole is usually started at 2.5 mg for 5 days in the follicular phase and increased up to 7.5 mg as needed to achieve ovulation. The most common side effects with letrozole are fatigue and headache. Letrozole is not currently FDA approved for ovulation induction. An analysis of the risk of birth defects in a large multicenter trial demonstrated no increased risk of birth defects in babies that were conceived via letrozole compared to CC.[38]

Metformin has also been shown to increase ovulation in PCOS patients in several small observational studies. However, it is not as effective as clomiphene or letrozole for pregnancy and live birth. A randomized controlled trial by the Reproductive Medicine Network compared the efficacy of metformin and clomiphene.[40] Although patients with metformin did ovulate, this did not translate to a comparable rate of live birth. Thus, metformin as a single agent for the treatment of infertility is not recommended. A subanalysis of this study confirmed the significant role of obesity in the prognosis of patients undergoing fertility treatments. For all groups, increased body mass index was correlated with a reduced chance of a live birth.[41] There are conflicting reports as to whether metformin is useful as an adjuvant to CC in improving live-birth rates, but it may be useful in women with insulin resistance.

For women with resistance to oral medications, use of injectable gonadotropins can be used to achieve ovulation; however, the risk of multiple birth pregnancy is ~30%, and the risk of high order multiple birth pregnancy is 5–10%. Gonadotropins bypass negative feedback inhibition to the pituitary, and multifollicular development is common. Low-dose stimulation protocols are generally employed to mediate this risk, but even with careful monitoring, multiple birth pregnancy can occur. Gonadotropins can be used more safely during *in vitro* fertilization (IVF) where single embryo transfer is now the norm for most patients. Women with PCOS are at increased risk of ovarian hyperstimulation syndrome (OHSS) at IVF, and women with a high AMH and/or antral follicle count are at highest risk. However, advances in IVF protocols, including the use of leuprolide (Lupron) for ovulation trigger and embryo freeze all cycles, have significantly reduced this risk.

Non-medical Therapies

Cosmetic procedures are frequently utilized for the treatment of hirsutism and are quite effective. These include bleaching, shaving, plucking, waxing, depilatory creams, electrolysis, light-assisted hair removal, and laser. Electrolysis and laser photothermolysis are among the most effective but also the most expensive treatments. Laser therapy is most effective in patients with darker hair and lighter skin, where selective hair follicle damage is favored. These treatments can be used in combination with medical therapies.

Surgical Interventions

The surgical treatment for ovulation induction in patients with PCOS involves multiple ovarian punctures, i.e., "ovarian drilling" or ovarian wedge resection, which is removal of part of the ovary. Prior to the advent of artificial reproductive technology (ART), these types of surgeries were the only treatment that was offered to the PCOS patient, with ensuing post-surgery ovulation rates reported as high as 70–80%. More recently, with laparoscopic advances, this procedure has progressed to laparoscopic ovarian diathermy (LOD) or laser. The main indication for surgical intervention is clomid or letrozole resistance in anovulatory PCOS patients. When compared with clomid–metformin combination treatment, LOD resulted in comparable ovulation and pregnancy rates.[42] In addition to the usual surgical risks, this procedure may cause adnexal adhesions, and there is concern that destroying part of the ovary can reduce ovarian reserve in the long term by accelerating the depletion of follicles.

Summary

PCOS is a complex clinical syndrome that is characterized by hyperandrogenism and ovulatory dysfunction. For accurate diagnosis, other endocrinopathies must be excluded. Presentations can vary significantly, but often include comorbidities of obesity, glucose intolerance, and other metabolic derangements. Anovulatory infertility is another hallmark of this disorder. Management is directed toward specific symptoms experienced and includes lifetime monitoring for risk factors. A multidisciplinary approach with the inclusion of lifestyle modifications is the key to optimal health outcomes for PCOS patients.

Key Points

- PCOS is the most common cause of irregular menses with a population prevalence of 9% to 18%.
- PCOS is associated with metabolic disturbances and long-term health complications, including diabetes, obesity, heart disease, and endometrial hyperplasia or cancer.
- Diagnosis of PCOS includes two out of the following three criteria: 1) menses >35 days in length, 2) clinical and/or biochemical signs of hyperandrogenism, and 3) polycystic-appearing ovaries on ultrasound.
- Several medical therapies are available for the treatment of PCOS symptoms, and progesterone replacement is important for prevention of endometrial hyperplasia.
- Letrozole is first-line therapy for ovulation induction in women with PCOS who desire pregnancy.

REFERENCES

1. March WA et al. The prevalence of polycystic ovary syndrome in a community sample assessed under contrasting diagnostic criteria. *Hum Reprod* 2010; 25(2):544–51.

2. Singh S et al. Polycystic ovary syndrome: etiology, current management, and future therapeutics. *J Clin Med* 2023;12(4):1454.
3. Zawadski JK, Dunaif A. Diagnostic criteria for polycystic ovary syndrome; towards a rational approach. In: Dunaif A, Givens JR and Haseltine F (eds), *Polycystic Ovary Syndrome*. Blackwell Scientific, Boston, 1992: 377–84.
4. The Rotterdam ESHRE/ASRM-Sponsored PCOS Consensus Workshop Group. Revised 2003 consensus on diagnostic criteria and long-term health risks related to polycystic ovary syndrome (PCOS). *Fertil Steril* 2004; 81(1):19–25.
5. Azziz Ret al. Position statement: criteria for defining polycystic ovary syndrome as a predominantly hyperandrogenic syndrome: an Androgen Excess Society guideline. *J Clin Endocrinol Metab* 2006;91(11):4237–45.
6. Teede HJ et al. Assessment and management of polycystic ovary syndrome: summary of an evidence-based guideline. *Med J Aust* 2011;195:S65–112.
7. Johnson T et al. Evidence-based Methodology Workshop on Polycystic Ovary Syndrome. National Institutes of Health, 2012.
8. Legro RS et al. Diagnosis and treatment of polycystic ovary syndrome: an endocrine society clinical practice guideline. *J Clin Endocrinol Metab* 2013;98:4565–4592.
9. Conway G et al., Group EPSI. The polycystic ovary syndrome: a position statement from the European society of endocrinology. *Eur J Endocrinol* 2014;171:1–29.
10. Balen AH et al. The management of anovulatory infertility in women with polycystic ovary syndrome: analysis of the evidence to support the development of global WHO guidance. *Hum Reprod Update* 2016:1–22. https://doi.org/10.1093/humupd/dmw025
11. Johnstone EB et al. The polycystic ovary post-Rotterdam: a common, age-dependent finding in ovulatory women without metabolic significance. *J Clin Endocrinol Metab* 2010; 95(11): 4965–72.
12. Dewailly D et al. Definition and significance of polycystic ovarian morphology: a task force report from the Androgen Excess and Polycystic Ovary Syndrome Society. *Hum Reprod Update* 2014;20:334–52.
13. Yildiz BO et al. Visually scoring hirsutism. *Hum Reprod Update* 2010;16(1):51–64.
14. Ferriman D, Gallwey JD. Clinical assessment of body hair growth in women. *J Clin Endocrinol Metab* 1961;21:1440–7.
15. Fauser BC et al. Consensus on women's health aspects of polycystic ovary syndrome (PCOS). *Hum Reprod* 2012;27(1):14–24.
16. Ehrmann DA et al. Prevalence of impaired glucose tolerance and diabetes in women with polycystic ovary syndrome. *Diabetes Care* 1999;22(1):141–6.
17. Legro RS et al. Changes in glucose tolerance over time in women with polycystic ovary syndrome: a controlled study. *J Clin Endocrinol Metab.* 2005;90(6):3236–42.
18. Apridonidze T et al. Prevalence and characteristics of the metabolic syndrome in women with polycystic ovary syndrome. *J Clin Endocrinol Metab.* 2005r;90(4):1929–35.
19. Kamalanathan S et al. Pregnancy in polycystic ovary syndrome. *Indian J Endocrinol Metab* 2013;17(1):37–43.
20. Johnson JE et al. Risk of endometrial cancer in patients with polycystic ovarian syndrome: a meta-analysis. *Oncol Lett* 2023;25(4):168.
21. Rassi Aet al. Prevalence of psychiatric disorders in patients with polycystic ovary syndrome. *Compr Psychiatry* 2010;51(6):599–602.
22. Deeks AA et al. Anxiety and depression in polycystic ovary syndrome: a comprehensive investigation. *Fertil Steril* 2010;93(7):2421–3.
23. Morales AJ et al. Insulin, somatotropic, and luteinizing hormone axes in lean and obese women with polycystic ovary syndrome: common and distinct features. *J Clin Endocrinol Metab* 1996;81:2854–64.
24. Dunaif A et al. Profound peripheral insulin resistance, independent of obesity, in polycystic ovary syndrome. *Diabetes* 1989;38:1165–74.
25. Ehrmann, D.A. Medical progress: polycystic ovary syndrome. *N Engl J Med* 2005;352:1223–36.
26. Peña AS et al. Adolescent polycystic ovary syndrome according to the international evidence-based guideline. *BMC Med* 2020;18(1):72.
27. Eagleson CA et al. Polycystic ovarian syndrome: evidence that flutamide restores sensitivity of the gonadotropin-releasing hormone pulse generator to inhibition by estradiol and progesterone. *J Clin Endocrinol Metab* 2000;85:4047–52.

28. Salehi M et al. Pathogenesis of polycystic ovary syndrome: what is the role of obesity? *Metab Clin Exp* 2004;53:358–76.
29. Daniells TJ,.. Berga SL. Resistance of gonadotropin releasing hormone drive to sex steroid-induced suppression in hyperandrogenic anovulation. *J Clin Endocrinol Metab* 1997;82:4179–80.
30. Hall JE et al. Insights into hypothalamic-pituitary dysfunction in polycystic ovary syndrome. *J Endocrinol Invest* 1998;21:602–11.
31. Huber-Buchholz MM et al. Restoration of reproductive potential by lifestyle modification in obese polycystic ovary syndrome: role of insulin sensitivity and luteinizing hormone. *J Clin Endocrinol Metab* 1999; 84:1470–4.
32. Moghetti P, Toscano V. Treatment of hirsutism and acne in hyperandrogenism. *Best Pract Res Clin Endocrinol Metab* 2006;20(2):221–34.
33. Tang T et al. Insulin-sensitising drugs for women with polycystic ovary syndrome, oligo amenorrhea and subfertility. *Cochrane Database Syst Rev* 2010;20(1). https://doi.org/10.1002/14651858.cd003053.pub4
34. Knowler WC et al., Diabetes Prevention Program Research Group. Reduction in the incidence of type 2 diabetes with lifestyle intervention or metformin. *N Engl J Med* 2002;346(6):393–403.
35. Kalra B et al. The inositols and polycystic ovary syndrome. *Indian J Endocrinol Metab* 2016;20(5):720–4.
36. Showell MG et al. Inositol for subfertile women with polycystic ovary syndrome. *Cochrane Database Syst Rev* 2018;12:CD012378.
37. Palomba S et al. Management strategies for ovulation induction in women with polycystic ovary syndrome and known clomifene citrate resistance. *Curr Opin Obstet Gynecol* 2009;21:465–73.
38. Legro RS et al. Network NRM Letrozole versus clomiphene for infertility in the polycystic ovary syndrome. *N Engl J Med* 2014;371:119–129.
39. Franik S et al. Aromatase inhibitors for subfertile women with polycystic ovary syndrome: summary of a Cochrane Review. *Fertil Steril* 2015;103:353–5.
40. Legro RS et al. Clomiphene, metformin, or both for infertility in the polycystic ovarian syndrome. *N Engl J Med* 2007;356(6):551–66.
41. Rausch ME et al. Predictors of pregnancy in women with polycystic ovarian syndrome. *J Clin Endocrinol Metab* 2009;94(9):3183–4.
42. Abu Hashim H et al. Combined metformin and clomiphene citrate versus laparoscopic ovarian diathermy for ovulation induction in clomiphene-resistant women with polycystic ovary syndrome: a randomized controlled trial. *J Obstet Gynaecol Res* 2011;37(3):169–77.

18

Recurrent Pregnancy Loss

Benjamin Lannon, Lauren Murphy, and Alexandra Huttler

The evaluation and management of couples with recurrent pregnancy loss (RPL) can often be challenging for both the clinician and patient. For the patient, the devastation caused by a single pregnancy loss, let alone repeated losses, is emotionally draining and further burdensome due to uncertain causality and prognosis. The clinician is faced with addressing the psychosocial needs of the patient while embarking on a complex and sometimes ambiguous series of tests and treatment options that may not guarantee the desired outcome of a healthy live birth. Caring for the RPL patient requires responsiveness to the evolving diagnostic and treatment algorithms for RPL while focusing on the individual needs and therapy goals of the patient.

Defining Recurrent Pregnancy Loss

Traditionally, RPL has been defined by three or more losses. The Practice Committee of the American Society of Reproductive Medicine (ASRM) defines recurrent pregnancy loss as two or more failed clinical pregnancies.[1] This definition is also supported by the recently updated guidelines from the European Society of Human Reproduction and Embryology (ESHRE) with the following exception: The ASRM definition is restricted to clinically recognized pregnancy losses, with pregnancy confirmed by ultrasonography or histopathologic examination, while ESHRE guidelines include losses of non-visualized pregnancies after 6 weeks gestation.[1, 2] In efforts to minimize the unnecessary hardship to patients who may suffer otherwise preventable pregnancy loss, most clinicians and the ASRM favor initiating clinical evaluation after two first-trimester losses, despite recognition of the effort and cost associated with a full RPL diagnostic evaluation. It is important to note that many of the potential etiologies of RPL are not absolute, so the occurrence of interval live births does not preclude a diagnosis of RPL. Certainly, each case of RPL should be considered individually, and recommendations should be based on the needs of the specific couple including their history of loss, prior live births, or other obstetric complications rather than focus purely on the number of miscarriages.[3]

Incidence

In young women, 15–20% of clinically recognized pregnancies and upwards of 50% of all pregnancies undergo spontaneous loss. These figures increase substantially with maternal age to as high as 40% and 85%, respectively, in women 40 years and older. The prevalence of RPL is difficult to determine given the ambiguity in its definition and inconsistent reporting and documentation of early pregnancy losses. It is estimated that 5% of women experience two consecutive losses, with 1% experiencing three or more.[1]

 DOI: 10.1201/9781003460275-18

Etiology

A number of etiologies have been proposed for RPL, and they may present alone or in combination. When counseling patients with RPL, it is helpful to present the potential etiologies in broad terms including anatomic factors, genetic variations, endocrinopathies, thrombophilias, autoimmune phenomena, and infectious etiologies. Despite these various potential causes, the majority of cases of RPL, around 50%, remain unexplained,[1] a feature of this condition which is met with further frustration and helplessness for patients. In addition, due to the non-specific nature of many of these etiologies, there is potential to attribute the cause of RPL to an incidental finding.

An important consideration in the evaluation of RPL is the age of the patient, as the rate of spontaneous miscarriage increases with maternal age. This is not included in the formal definition of RPL, and other causes of RPL can occur at any age. However, the clinician must assess the role of declining oocyte quality and age-related spontaneous aneuploidy rates when beginning an assessment. Another consideration is the timing of the miscarriage. If due to a specific etiology, RPL tends to occur at the same gestational age. Factors associated with embryonic loss, <10 weeks gestation, are different than those presenting with late RPL (between 10 to 16 weeks' gestation).[4] Likewise, there are obstetric factors, such as cervical insufficiency, that may contribute to late second-trimester loss or extreme preterm delivery that are not included in this topic.

Anatomic Factors

Anatomic factors contributing to RPL are divided into congenital and acquired factors, and together account for 15–25% of RPL. Congenital anomalies, including septate, bicornuate, unicornuate, and didelphic uteri, are found more commonly in women with RPL than the general population. Septate uterus is the most prevalent anomaly and is the anomaly most tightly linked to reproductive failure, with an associated pregnancy loss rate as high as 79%.[5] An association between arcuate uterus and RPL is uncertain.[5] However, the specific contribution of these findings to RPL is difficult to quantify due to the varying diagnostic and management techniques reported in the literature. The pathophysiology is thought to be primarily a vascular phenomenon where there is reduced perfusion of the uterine septum and abnormal development of the overlying endometrium.[4]

Acquired uterine factors such as fibroids, polyps, and Asherman's syndrome may also contribute to RPL. These factors may have some impact on embryonic implantation or uterine receptivity. The contribution of these pathologies to abnormal implantation, placentation, and pregnancy growth are speculative but are likely similarly related to aberrant vascularization and insufficient endometrial support of the pregnancy, combined with alterations in the intrauterine immunological milieu favoring inflammation rather than growth.

Genetic Factors

In sporadic pregnancy loss, chromosomal abnormalities account for at least 50% of clinically diagnosed spontaneous abortions and perhaps upwards of 60–75% of all pregnancy losses. In RPL, 25–51% of fetal losses are demonstrated to be aneuploid.[3]

In sporadic pregnancy loss due to aneuploidy, age is certainly the major determining factor with the chance of loss increasing directly with age from a 15–20% prevalence in women less than 35 years of age to 40% in women over 40 years. This is attributable to the accumulated risk of acquired meiotic segregation errors which lead to oocyte and embryonic aneuploidy. Interestingly, the correlation of age-related aneuploidy is similar in the sporadic and recurrent pregnancy loss populations,[1] suggesting that some cases of RPL, particularly in women over the age of 35 years, are due to probability alone or that additional factors, independent of age and aneuploidy, are also important in RPL.

Parental structural chromosome abnormalities are observed in 2.5–8% of RPL.[3] Translocations account for the majority of these cases and include balanced reciprocal translocations, in which two different segments of parental autosomes are exchanged, and balanced Robertsonian translocations, in which the long arms of two acrocentric chromosomes (chromosomes 13, 14, 15, 21, 22) join to form a single new chromosome. Chromosomal inversions and other parental karyotypic abnormalities are seen as well. In some series, translocations are more commonly found in the female partner of a couple with RPL and are more likely to result in loss than male-derived translocations. Couples with a translocation may present with a history of prior live birth, RPL at an early age, or a family history of RPL. Segregation genetics would suggest predictable rates of unbalanced, balanced, and normal chromosomes in conceptuses. Yet in reality, the distribution is skewed, and a relatively lower rate of balanced and normal pregnancies are observed than would be expected resulting in a higher embryo and pregnancy loss rate. Nevertheless, both miscarriages and normal pregnancies are possible outcomes in cases of parental structural chromosomes, and a history of recurrent losses interspersed with normal full-term pregnancies should instigate parental chromosome testing.

Endocrinopathies

The primary endocrinopathies associated with RPL are thyroid dysfunction, hyperprolactinemia, diabetes mellitus, and polycystic ovarian syndrome (PCOS).

A euthyroid state is critical for optimal function in reproduction and pregnancy, and poorly controlled thyroid disease has been associated with poor pregnancy outcome and RPL. The prevalence of abnormal thyroid function may be 3–7% in the RPL population.[3] Further, even a subtle hypofunction of the thyroid, as in subclinical hypothyroidism, or euthyroidism in the presence of thyroid autoimmunity (the presence of thyroid peroxidase and thyroglobulin antibodies) may be associated with failed placentation and RPL.[6] While not confirmed, the etiology may relate to the increased demands of thyroid hormone in pregnancy, the resulting impact on placental growth, and a potentially detrimental effect of thyroid antibodies on the placenta.[6] A recent review of the literature elucidates the role of thyroid hormone and thyroid antibodies in gamete function, embryogenesis, embryo implantation, and placentation. Abnormal thyroid function may impact any of these key reproductive processes and ultimately lead to pregnancy complication or failure. However, the underlying pathobiology as well as specific treatment regimens remain unclear.[6]

Abnormal prolactin levels can be associated with RPL, potentially relating to an association with autoimmunity or alternatively as a marker of hypothalamic-pituitary dysfunction in the setting of neuroendocrine stress.[1] Hyperprolactinemia alters the hypothalamic pituitary-ovarian axis with resultant impaired folliculogenesis and oocyte maturation and/or a shortened luteal phase.[1]

A connection between glycemic control and insulin resistance on maintaining an ongoing healthy pregnancy has been established. Well controlled diabetes mellitus does not seem to increase the risk of pregnancy loss. However, poor control is associated with RPL, and this may be related to the impact of hyperglycemia towards worsening underlying vascular disease or impact of insulin resistance on fibrinolysis during placentation, although the mechanism of impact of insulin resistance on pregnancy loss remains unknown.[2] The prevalence of previously undiagnosed frank diabetes is expected to be low (< 1%) in the RPL population.[3] Higher rates of pregnancy loss in patients with PCOS lends further evidence that insulin resistance, alone or combined with hyperandrogenism, may have a negative impact on placental growth and maintenance of pregnancy, and among patients with RPL the prevalence of PCOS is as high as 50%.[2]

The impact of deficient production of progesterone in the luteal phase has been hypothesized as a cause of RPL, though substantial data to prove a causality between progesterone deficiency or adequacy and pregnancy outcome has not been established.[2]

Autoimmune Phenomena

Antiphospholipid antibodies are the most significant autoimmune phenomena associated with RPL, present in between 18–20% of cases.[1, 3] Antiphospholipid antibodies have been associated with both recurrent embryonic and fetal (>10 week) loss. In addition, they have been connected to other obstetric complications such as preeclampsia and fetal growth restriction, as well as venous thromboembolism

(VTE).[1] Specific diagnostic criteria for the antiphospholipid antibody syndrome are listed in a later section, as well as indications for testing. There is likely an overlap between patients with isolated positive antibodies and unrelated sporadic miscarriage, and, therefore, testing should only be performed when the clinical history is supportive of true RP.[1] Likewise, given the potential for additional obstetric and maternal complications, treatment guidelines should be followed. The role of other antibody and rheumatologic testing such as phosphatidyl inositol, ANA, and specific lymphocyte testing is uncertain.

Celiac disease is another autoimmune disorder that has been associated with several obstetric complications. A recent cohort study revealed a higher percentage of spontaneous abortions in women with celiac (50.6% vs. 40.6%), compared to controls. It is unclear if these results are mitigated by a gluten-free diet.[7]

Immunomodulatory Factors

Immune modulation at the interface between the embryo and the maternal decidua is a critical factor in successful implantation and maintenance of pregnancy. Major shifts in the population of uterine natural killer (NK) cells are observed during the menstrual cycle with a preponderance of the $CD56^{bright}CD16^{-}$ NK cell subtype at the time of implantation, which is distinct from NK cell profile of $CD56^{dim}CD16^{+}$ cells which predominate in peripheral blood, and it is believed that the uterine NK cells play an essential supportive role in implantation. Regulatory T cells (T_{reg}), macrophages, dendritic cells, and innate lymphoid cells also are important in the uterine decidua and maintenance of pregnancy. Though widely hypothesized, it has not been clearly established whether abnormalities or modulation of uterine NK cells, T_{reg} cells, or other immune dysfunction are responsible for recurrent pregnancy loss.[8]

Inherited Thrombophilias

Thrombophilia is defined as any disorder associated with an increased risk of thrombosis and VTE. A number of inherited thrombophilias have been connected with RPL and other obstetric complications. Specific inherited thrombophilias linked to adverse obstetric outcomes and pregnancy loss include Factor V Leiden mutation, prothrombin gene mutation, anti-thrombin III deficiency, protein C deficiency, and protein S deficiency. While early data suggested that methylene tetrahydrofolate reductase mutations and hyperhomocysteinemia caused VTE, more recent data has not validated this causality. Perhaps the most controversial of the etiologies, the association, causality, and treatment of inherited thrombophilias in patients with RPL is a source of debate in the field.[9] Some studies demonstrate no increased prevalence of heritable thrombophilias in the RPL population.[3] The thrombosis of uteroplacental vessels underlies the theoretical pathobiology of these conditions and they are typically associated with late RPL, and the role of thrombophilias in early pregnancy and embryonic loss (<10 wks) is unclear.[9] Likewise, the degree of risk for RPL and efficacy of treatment have been debated in the literature and in practice, with routine testing of women with RPL for inherited thrombophilias not currently recommended by the ASRM.[1, 9]

Infectious Etiologies

Based on associations with sporadic miscarriage, identification and treatment of certain microorganisms has been proposed in the evaluation of RPL. However, no studies have clearly identified infectious agents as a cause for RPL and, therefore, screening for chlamydia, mycoplasma, and ureaplasma species is not recommended.[1]

Chronic endometritis, characterized by a plasma cell infiltrate in the endometrium, is associated with various pathogenic organisms. Research is suggestive of a variable prevalence of 7–58% in women with RPL, which has not been found to significantly differ from patients without RPL.[2] Treatment of chronic endometritis with antibiotics has not been evaluated in rigorous trials and, therefore, additional research is required before screening for, and treatment of, chronic endometritis in the RPL population can be recommended.

Lifestyle and Exposures

Lifestyle stress has been frequently implicated anecdotally and scientifically as an etiology for pregnancy loss and RPL. It is believed that stress-induced increases in adrenocorticosteroids or stress-induced decreased immunity may negatively impact the ability to maintain a pregnancy. Dietary factors including high caffeine intake of the equivalent of over three cups of coffee a day or low antioxidant serum levels are associated with RPL. Tobacco smoking and other toxic environmental exposures have also been associated with RPL. While the data is not conclusive, a possible link between these lifestyle factors cannot be completely excluded.[2]

Insufficient levels of Vitamin D may also be associated with recurrent pregnancy loss. This may be mediated by Vitamin D's role in cellular immune function in which Vitamin D inhibits the T cell activation of NK cells. In a retrospective study of women with RPL, almost half were found to have hypovitaminosis D. In addition, *in vitro* studies of these women revealed altered immune function with an increase in NK cell activity.[2]

Sperm Factors

The sperm genome and sperm DNA integrity are known to be critical factors in embryo development and the maintenance of pregnancy, and high levels of sperm DNA fragmentation may be associated with poorer embryo quality and lower rates of conception and embryo survival. Increasing paternal age is associated with higher levels of DNA fragmentation and higher pregnancy loss rates. A recent meta-analysis of 16 cohort studies suggests that pregnancy loss may be increased two-fold with increased sperm DNA fragmentation and that normal loss rates may be restored by applying methods to preselect normal sperm followed by intracytoplasmic sperm injection (ICSI).[10]

Other

Several additional rare or less well-defined conditions may be associated with spontaneous miscarriage and possibly RPL. These include obesity, diminished ovarian reserve, and teratospermia.

Evaluation and History

For patients and clinicians alike, the uncertainty of the etiology and inability to predict recurrence of RPL creates a strong incentive to identify a specific cause. While an extensive battery of testing could be performed, likely the best approach is to limit diagnostics to identify etiologies where causality and therapy options have been established by evidence-based research. The initial approach includes a thorough medical history and physical exam with attention to details of timing and outcomes of prior pregnancies and miscarriages, presence of uterine and pelvic factors, and evidence of associated medical conditions.

Personal and Familial History

The personal history questionnaire should include symptoms and diagnoses related to endocrinopathies, autoimmune disorders, coagulopathies, obesity, and infections, lifestyle, and environmental exposures. The reproductive history should include past uterine instrumentation, pelvic infection, total number of pregnancies, and outcomes. Pregnancy loss history should specify sequential or sporadic timing of pregnancy, the gestational age at diagnosis, whether fetal cardiac activity was documented, management, comorbidities, and fetal chromosome data if available. Familial history should include a thorough screening for RPL, stillbirth or other fetal loss, as well as mental retardation, endocrinopathies, autoimmune disorders, coagulopathies, and obesity.

Physical Exam

Specific focus on the physical exam should be placed on identifying signs of thyroid disease, diabetes, lupus, rheumatoid arthritis, other autoimmune disorders, and pelvic anatomy.

Diagnostic Testing

It is recommended to initiate a diagnostic evaluation of RPL after two consecutive pregnancy losses. This approach is favored over waiting for the classic definition of three consecutive losses, in part to minimize further distress to a patient should a treatable etiology be identified. Further, the probability of identifying a pathophysiological factor through testing is similar (40%) in patients with two and with three consecutive losses.[1, 3]

Uterine Examination

A hysterosalpingogram (HSG) is the preferred single uterine cavity study. If available, a saline and air contrast sonohysterosalpingogram is equally effective. This will allow accurate diagnosis of uterine anomalies, as well as detect intracavitary masses or lesions with a positive predictive value of upwards of 85%. If HSG findings are not definitive, or if more specific testing is desired, a saline infused sonography (SIS) is recommended to detect intracavitary lesions with a positive predictive value of 95%. If definitive diagnosis is desired or intracavitary lesions are suspected based on prior radiological studies, hysteroscopy in the office or operative setting should be performed. If a congenital uterine anomaly is suspected based on HSG or SIS, a 3D ultrasound or pelvic MRI can be performed.

Genetic Testing

A chromosomal analysis on both partners is recommended to assess for potential parental structural chromosomal abnormalities. In the patient with RPL undergoing surgical evacuation of products of conception, an analysis of fetal chromosomes could prove extremely helpful, particularly as evidence of sporadic aneuploidy may be definitively diagnostic and obviate additional testing. This testing may also be of psychological value to the patient. However, cytogenetic assessment revealing an abnormal karyotype should not universally prevent investigation of other causes of RPL. The routine and traditional method of chromosome analysis is a metaphase spread karyotype on cultured parental blood lymphocytes or cultured chorionic villi cells. An additional option is employing newer technologies such as single nucleotide polymorphism (SNP) microarray or next generation sequencing (NGS), which, in the cases of aneuploidy, identify the paternal or the maternal line as the source for the acquired or inherited defect.

Endocrine Testing

The panel of endocrine testing to screen for potential endocrinopathies associated with RPL includes tests to assess for underlying thyroid disease, hyperprolactinemia, diabetes, and diminished ovarian reserve.

Specifically, this serological testing panel includes thyroid stimulating hormone (TSH), with or without free thyroxine (FT4), anti-thyroid peroxidase antibodies and anti-thyroglobulin antibodies, prolactin (PRL), fasting glucose or HgbA1C and cycle day 3 follicle stimulating hormone (FSH) and estradiol, and/or anti-Müllerian hormone (AMH).

Diagnostic Testing for Antiphospholipid Syndrome (APS)

In order to fulfill the laboratory testing criteria for antiphospholipid syndrome (APS), it is required to demonstrate positive serum antiphospholipid at significant levels on two or more occasions and at least

12 weeks apart. Positive testing for antiphospholipid antibodies includes the detection of lupus anticoagulant (LAC), medium to high titers of anticardiolipin IgG or IgM antibodies, and titers of anti-B2 glycoprotein-1 antibodies upwards of the 99th percentile.[1] Anti-phosphatidylserine levels may also be measured, but the correlation with RPL is less well established and these antibodies are not included in the diagnostic criteria for APS.

Screening for Inherited Thrombophilias

The decision to include screening for inheritable thrombophilias in RPL is not straightforward. Causality between these conditions and adverse pregnancy outcomes early in gestation has not been established, and the cost-effectiveness of ordering the thrombophilia testing panel in the RPL evaluation is questionable. Based on current opinions from ASRM and ACOG, routine screening for inherited thrombophilias in women with RPL is not recommended. Nevertheless, one may consider inclusion of this laboratory screening in RPL, particularly when additional risk factors for coagulopathy are supported by the patient's personal or familial history or in patients with recurrent late fetal loss (>10 weeks) or with evidence of placental ischemia, infarction, or thrombosis. Testing should be limited to screening for abnormalities associated with thromboembolic events, and these include testing for Factor V Leiden gene mutation, prothrombin G20210A gene mutation, protein C and protein S deficiency via functional activity assays, and anti-thrombin III levels. Insufficient evidence exists to link hyperhomocysteinemia or methylene tetrahydrofolate reductase deficiency with RPL or VTE and, therefore, testing for these is not currently recommended.

Sperm Factors

The typical semen analysis including sperm concentration, motility, and morphology does not appear to correlate with RPL. Recent studies have looked at the role of more advanced sperm testing, including DNA fragmentation or epigenetic analysis in RPL. While these tests may offer further insight into qualitative sperm factors, and some guidelines suggest consideration of sperm DNA fragmentation in the diagnostic workup, they are not currently recommended in the standard evaluation of RPL.[1, 2]

Management

Anatomic Factors

An improvement in obstetrical outcome following surgical correction of uterine anomalies has been best established in cases of uterine septi. Uterine septi are the most commonly diagnosed congenital uterine anomalies associated with early pregnancy loss and have been found to confer a risk of RPL of up to 79%.[5] Hysteroscopic metroplasty has been shown to decrease the chance of pregnancy loss to <15% and increase the chance of live birth from <20% to 35–80%.[5] In cases of incidental diagnosis of uterine septi, it is not unreasonable to consider hysteroscopic resection for prevention of pregnancy loss, though this approach is not universally advocated. Patients with Asherman's syndrome similarly benefit from surgical intervention via hysteroscopic adhesiolysis, which increases the chance for live birth and reduces rates of first and second-trimester losses. The outcomes after hysteroscopic adhesiolysis are associated with severity of disease. The term pregnancy rate after surgical intervention may be upwards of 81% and 66% for mild (American Fertility Society [AFS] Stage I) and moderate (AFS Stage II) disease, respectively. Given the partially irrecoverable losses to endometrial function in Asherman's syndrome, relatively high rates of pregnancy failure and relatively low chance for live birth (32% or less) are observed in patients with severe disease (AFS Stage III) after successful surgical resection.[11] In cases of polyps and fibroids, the link between etiology is less well established and decreased pregnancy loss rates have been demonstrated, but not consistently, in studies examining the impact of open myomectomy, hysteroscopic myomectomy, and hysteroscopic polypectomies on RPL.[4]

Genetic Factors

Preimplantation genetic testing for aneuploidy (PGT-A) is an option for couples with RPL due to aneuploidy. Advances in embryo genetic screening platforms, trophectoderm biopsy, and embryo vitrification have allowed marked increases in utilization and accuracy of this technology. The concept is to biopsy embryos at the blastocyst stage (embryo day 5–7) and test the cells for euploidy or aneuploidy by analyzing all 23 pairs of chromosomes via NGS platforms. Embryos are typically frozen, and then euploid embryos are transferred in subsequent endometrial preparation cycle(s). While complete outcomes data for PGT-A technologies suggest improved live birth rate, lower miscarriage rate, and shorter time to pregnancy in women over the age of 37 years, data pertaining specifically to the RPL population are lacking. Of the limited studies examining outcomes with PGT-A in RPL, most are retrospective and limited prospective studies are available to date. PGT-A may, in fact, improve outcomes in RPL patients who successfully achieve a euploid embryo for transfer. However, when all cycle starts are considered, PGT-A may not improve the live birth rate per attempt given the high rate of PGT-A cancellation due to insufficient embryo yield or blastulation; in cases of low embryo yield, PGT-A may actually extend the time to pregnancy and live birth compared to those patients expectantly managed.[11] In fact, a recent randomized controlled trial suggested no improvement in ongoing pregnancy or live birth rates with PGT-A in women aged 25–40 years; however, it is important to note that women with a history of more than miscarriage were excluded from this study.[12] Biological and technical limitations of PGT-A include cellular mosaicism, the embryo's inherent ability to undergo some self-correction to demote aneuploid cells away from essential embryonic development pathways, and assay platform accuracy and precision. Nevertheless, the benefit of employing PGT-A in cases of RPL may include shortened time to pregnancy in patients with high oocyte and embryo yields, increased implantation rates, and decreased pregnancy loss rates. The psychological reassurance of transferring euploid rather than untested embryos is another benefit of PGT-A for RPL patients. Cost effectiveness studies have demonstrated a potential benefit of PGT-A when PGT-A is simply added to preexisting indications for IVF and when maternal age is 35 to 37 years or older, but PGT-A combined with IVF may prove to be cost prohibitive for the patient or couple conceiving spontaneously without difficulty or in couples with advanced maternal age or previously demonstrated high rates (>65%) of embryonic aneuploidy.[13] Nevertheless, both RPL patients who chose PGT-A and those who opt for expectant management face a favorable prognostic outlook, with a 63–71% chance of live birth without intervention. This data has been reproduced widely and supports the benefits of natural selection as a viable option for RPL management.[14]

In cases of male factor infertility, advanced paternal age, and increased sperm DNA fragmentation, the application of ICSI combined with various methods of preselection of normal sperm may improve embryo quality, increase the rates of ongoing pregnancy, and lower rates of miscarriage.[15]

Endocrinopathies

The extent to which endocrine dysfunction directly contributes to early pregnancy loss is not known. However, correction of underlying clinical or subclinical endocrinopathies is intuitive, not only in hopes of minimizing the risk of early pregnancy loss, but also to optimize general endocrine health as a person embarks on a pregnancy. Hyperthyroid disease should be fully evaluated for underlying pathology including nodules, cancer, and Graves' disease and treated appropriately. In clinical hypothyroidism, levothyroxine treatment has been well established as a means to minimize adverse pregnancy outcomes of miscarriage and preterm birth. While not firmly established, levothyroxine treatment of autoimmune and subclinical hypothyroidism may also improve pregnancy outcomes and reduce pregnancy loss and recurrent pregnancy loss.[6] Levothyroxine dosing is based on weight and effect to achieve a TSH is above 0.4 mIU/L and less than 2.5 mIU/L. Given the increased thyroid hormone demands of pregnancy, increasing the levothyroxine dose by 33% during early pregnancy is appropriate.[6] In a large, randomized trial, the use of levothyroxine in euthyroid women with thyroid peroxidase antibodies did not result in a higher rate of live births than placebo.[16]

Dopamine agonists, bromocriptine or cabergoline, may be used to normalize elevated prolactin levels and discontinued once pregnancy occurs. Both medications appear to be non-teratogenic in pregnancy.

As more pregnancy safety data becomes available, many providers favor bromocriptine use for treatment of hyperprolactinemia when pregnancy is anticipated.

Glucose intolerance and diabetes may be managed by diet and exercise and pharmacologically as needed to achieve normal fasting glucose levels and HbA1c levels prior to conception.

Thrombophilias

At this time, a connection between inherited thrombophilias and early pregnancy loss has not been firmly established nor has a reduction in subsequent losses been demonstrated with use of anticoagulation. While still an area of debate, most guidelines, including ACOG's, dissuade from anticoagulation prophylaxis in cases of early RPL with underlying inheritable thrombophilia due to the relative risk of treatment complication and the lack of proven benefit.[1, 2, 9] A recent systematic review of trials of low molecular weight heparin in women with placenta-mediated pregnancy complications failed to show a reduction of risk. The obstetric outcomes included preeclampsia, late pregnancy loss, placental abruption, and birth of a small-for-gestational-age neonate.[17]

Autoimmune Phenomena

Substantial data has supported the benefits of anticoagulation in cases of APS and prior adverse pregnancy outcomes including RPL. Based on randomized control trials and meta-analyses of available literature, the largest reduction in risk for RPL or other adverse pregnancy outcomes has been observed with a combination of heparin and aspirin. Therefore, at the present time, patients with APS should begin prophylactic dosing of unfractionated or low molecular weight heparin plus low dose aspirin with the diagnosis of pregnancy.[1] The use of intravenous immunoglobulin or other immunomodulators for suspected autoimmune mediated pregnancy loss is not recommended as a consistent benefit has not been demonstrated.[1, 2]

Immunotherapies

In attempts to foster implantation and to promote immunological tolerance of the embryo at the level of the maternal decidua, various immunotherapies including intravenous immunoglobulin (IVIG), granulocyte-macrophage colony stimulating factor (GM-CSF), and intralipids (intravenous lipid emulsion) have been evaluated but none have consistently demonstrated increases in ongoing pregnancy or live birth. At the present time, there is insufficient evidence to recommend immune-modulating therapies for treatment of unexplained RPL.[2]

Counseling

RPL can be an emotionally and psychologically devastating condition for many patients. The uncertainty of etiology and potential for recurrence can be truly unsettling and may prevent individuals from attempting to conceive. It is equally likely for patients, in desperation, to adopt any number of superstitious behaviors or request unfounded testing or treatments. While many of these activities may provide some comfort, they also have potential for harm. It is essential to provide a careful explanation of what evidence exists for particular recommendations as well as identifying the patient's specific concerns and anxieties. It is also highly recommended that a mental health professional be available for additional counseling.

Prognosis

Fortunately, the majority of patients with RPL will achieve their goal of having a healthy child, with an overall chance of subsequent successful pregnancy of 65%. The challenge, no doubt, is helping patients through the difficult process of getting to that goal, while supporting those patients who must endure the potentially devastating impact of being in the 35% who are not successful.

Key Points

- Recurrent pregnancy loss (RPL) is defined as two or more failed pregnancies, and workup should be initiated after two first-trimester losses.
- There are various etiologies of RPL, but 50% of cases do not have an identifiable cause.
- Contributors to RPL include anatomic, genetic, endocrine, autoimmune, clotting, infectious, and sperm factors, and the diagnostic workup should evaluate for these factors.
- Management of RPL includes treatment of identifiable and modifiable contributing factors such as anatomic, genetic, or clotting abnormalities, and may include use of *in vitro* fertilization with genetic testing.

REFERENCES

1. Practice Committee ASRM. Evaluation and treatment of recurrent pregnancy loss: a committee opinion. *Fertil Steril* 2012;98(5):1103–11.
2. ESHRE Guideline Group on RPL et al. ESHRE guideline: recurrent pregnancy loss: an update in 2022. *Hum Reprod Open* 2023;2023(1):hoad002.
3. Jaslow CR et al. Diagnostic factors identified in 1020 women with two versus three or more recurrent pregnancy losses. *Fertil Steril* 2010;93(4):1234–43.
4. Branch DW et al. Clinical practice. Recurrent miscarriage. *N Engl J Med* 2010;363(18):1740–47.
5. Practice Committee ASRM. Evidence-based diagnosis and treatment for uterine septum: a guideline. *Fertil Steril* 2024;122(2):251–65.
6. Vissenberg R et al. Pathophysiological aspects of thyroid hormone disorders/thyroid peroxidase autoantibodies and reproduction. *Hum Reprod Update* 2015;21(3):378–8.
7. Moleski SM, et al. Increased rates of pregnancy complications in women with celiac disease. *Ann Gastroenterol* 2015;28(2):236–40.
8. Sharma S. Natural killer cells and regulatory T cells in early pregnancy loss. *Int J Dev Biol* 2014;58(0):219–29.
9. ACOG practice bulletin 197: inherited thrombophilias in pregnancy. *Obstet Gynecol* 2018;132(1):e18–34.
10. Robinson L et al. The effect of sperm DNA fragmentation on miscarriage rates: a systematic review and meta-analysis. *Hum Reprod* 2012;27(10):2908–17.
11. Murugappan G et al. Intent to treat analysis of in vitro fertilization and preimplantation genetic screening versus expectant management in patients with recurrent pregnancy loss. *Hum Reprod* 2016;31(8):1668–74.
12. Munné S et al. Preimplantation genetic testing for aneuploidy versus morphology as selection criteria for single frozen-thawed embryo transfer in good-prognosis patients: a multicenter randomized clinical trial. *Fertil Steril* 2019;112(6):1071–79.e7.
13. Fritz MA, Speroff L. *Clinical Gynecologic Endocrinology and Infertility*, 8th edn. Philadelphia: Lippincott Williams & Wilkins, 2011; 1191–220.
14. Stephenson MD, Sierra S. Reproductive outcomes in recurrent pregnancy loss associated with a parental carrier of a structural chromosome rearrangement. *Hum Reprod* 2006;21(4):1076–82.
15. Robinson L et al. The effect of sperm DNA fragmentation on miscarriage rates: a systematic review and meta-analysis. *Hum Reprod* 2012;27(10):2908–17.
16. Dhillon-Smith RK et al. Levothyroxine in women with thyroid peroxidase antibodies before conception. *N Engl J Med* 2019;380:1316–25.
17. Roger MA et al. Low-molecular-weight heparin and recurrent placenta-mediated pregnancy complications: a meta-analysis of individual patient data from randomized controlled trials. *Lancet* 2016;388(10060):2629–41.

19

Diminished Ovarian Reserve and Premature Ovarian Insufficiency

Samuel A. Pauli and Emily A. Seidler

Introduction

Diminished ovarian reserve (DOR) and premature ovarian insufficiency (POI) represent significant challenges in reproductive medicine, impacting fertility and overall well-being. DOR refers to a decline in either egg quantity or egg quality of the remaining egg pool, often associated with advanced maternal age but can be seen at any reproductive age. Further on the spectrum, POI refers to premature menopause before age 40. These conditions, especially DOR, are seen frequently in a reproductive medicine setting, and require a comprehensive understanding of their etiology, diagnosis, and management. In this chapter, we delve into the intricate aspects of DOR and POI, exploring their pathophysiology, clinical manifestations, diagnostic strategies, and therapeutic interventions to provide clinicians with invaluable insights for effective patient care and counseling.

Various factors contribute to DOR, including genetic predispositions, environmental influences, and lifestyle factors such as smoking and obesity. Understanding the underlying mechanisms of DOR is crucial for clinicians to develop effective strategies for diagnosis and management of fertility treatment, such as IVF (*in vitro* fertilization).

In contrast, premature ovarian insufficiency (POI) represents a distinct entity characterized by the onset of menopause before the age of 40, associated with menstrual cycle irregularity or absence, and elevated FSH (follicle stimulating hormone) levels. The etiology of POI is multifactorial, with genetic predispositions, autoimmune factors, and iatrogenic interventions such as chemotherapy or pelvic radiation therapy implicated in its pathogenesis [1]. POI profoundly impacts women's reproductive choices and necessitates comprehensive evaluation and tailored interventions to address potential fertility preservation or treatment and hormone replacement therapy.

Navigating the complexities of DOR and POI requires a multidisciplinary approach encompassing clinical expertise, advanced diagnostic modalities, and evidence-based interventions. Recent advancements in assisted reproductive technologies (ART), including oocyte cryopreservation and IVF, offer promising options for women facing DOR and POI [2]. Moreover, ongoing research aimed at elucidating the molecular pathways underlying ovarian aging and dysfunction hold the potential to revolutionize therapeutic interventions and enhance fertility outcomes for affected individuals. In this chapter, we explore the contemporary landscape of DOR and POI, synthesizing current knowledge and emerging trends to empower clinicians with the tools necessary to optimize patient care and reproductive outcomes.

DOI: 10.1201/9781003460275-19

Understanding DOR and POI: Definitions, Prevalence, and Causative Factors

Understanding DOR and POI is paramount in addressing the complexities of female reproductive health. DOR signifies a decline in ovarian follicle quantity and quality, often associated with advanced maternal age, though it can also manifest in younger women. The prevalence of DOR in infertility practices has risen due to societal trends toward delayed childbearing. In a study by Sunkara et al. [3], it was found that women aged 35 and older accounted for a significant proportion of patients seeking assisted reproductive technologies (ART) due to age-related decline in fertility. This highlights the importance of recognizing DOR as a significant concern in contemporary reproductive medicine.

More severely, POI refers to the loss of ovarian function before the age of 40, leading to hormonal imbalances and infertility. The prevalence of POI varies across populations, affecting approximately 1% of women by the age of 40 [1]. While genetic predispositions play a role in POI, environmental factors such as exposure to toxins, autoimmune diseases, and iatrogenic interventions like chemotherapy may contribute significantly to its pathogenesis [2]. The increasing awareness of POI underscores the need for early detection and comprehensive management to mitigate its adverse effects on reproductive health and overall well-being.

Several causative factors contribute to the development of DOR and POI. Genetic predispositions, including mutations in genes involved in ovarian development and function, have been implicated in both conditions. Environmental factors such as smoking, excessive alcohol consumption, and obesity have also been associated with decreased ovarian reserve and earlier onset of menopause. Additionally, autoimmune disorders, such as autoimmune thyroiditis and systemic lupus erythematosus, can target ovarian tissue, accelerating ovarian aging and diminishing fertility potential.

Understanding the definitions, prevalence, and causative factors of DOR and POI lays the foundation for effective clinical management and patient counseling. By elucidating the intricate interplay between genetic, environmental, and lifestyle influences, clinicians can adopt a proactive approach toward preserving fertility and optimizing reproductive outcomes in women affected by these conditions.

Pathogenesis of DOR and POI

Patients often want to understand the underlying cause of their DOR or POI. While the most common cause of DOR is advancing age, up to 70% of POI is idiopathic or unknown. The pathogenesis of DOR and POI involves intricate molecular and physiological mechanisms that impact ovarian function and follicular dynamics. Genetic factors play a significant role in both conditions, with mutations in genes responsible for ovarian development, folliculogenesis, and hormone signaling pathways implicated in their pathogenesis. Mutations in genes encoding for key regulators of follicle development, such as FMR1 and FOXL2, have been associated with DOR and POI [4]. In addition, X chromosome anomalies including 45,X Turner syndrome and Turner syndrome mosaicism are associated with POI. Genetic aberrations likely disrupt the delicate balance of ovarian follicle maturation and hormone production, leading to diminished ovarian reserve and premature cessation of ovarian function.

Beyond genetic predispositions, environmental and lifestyle factors contribute to the pathogenesis of DOR and POI. Oxidative stress, resulting from exposure to environmental toxins, radiation, and inflammatory processes, exerts detrimental effects on ovarian follicles, accelerating their depletion and compromising ovarian function [5]. Additionally, autoimmune disorders characterized by the production of autoantibodies targeting ovarian antigens contribute to ovarian damage and dysfunction, exacerbating the progression of POI [1].

Furthermore, emerging evidence suggests a potential role of epigenetic modifications in modulating ovarian aging and dysfunction. Epigenetic alterations, including DNA methylation patterns and histone modifications, influence gene expression patterns and cellular processes essential for ovarian follicle development and function [6]. Dysregulation of epigenetic mechanisms may disrupt folliculogenesis, impair oocyte quality, and contribute to the pathogenesis of DOR and POI.

Understanding the pathogenesis of DOR and POI is essential for elucidating novel therapeutic targets and developing targeted interventions aimed at preserving ovarian function and fertility. By unraveling the complex interplay between genetic, environmental, and epigenetic factors, researchers and clinicians can pave the way for innovative approaches to mitigate the impact of DOR and POI on women's reproductive health and quality of life.

Diagnosis of DOR and POI

Diagnosing DOR and POI is crucial for guiding appropriate management strategies and counseling patients regarding their reproductive options. Accurate diagnosis relies on comprehensive evaluation, including clinical assessment, hormonal testing, and imaging modalities. This section explores the diagnostic criteria for DOR and POI, as well as the current approaches and limitations associated with their diagnosis.

Diagnostic Criteria for DOR

Diagnosis of diminished ovarian reserve relies on a combination of clinical assessment and specific laboratory parameters. The Bologna criteria, established by the European Society of Human Reproduction and Embryology (ESHRE) in 2011, provide standardized guidelines for defining poor ovarian response in assisted reproductive technology (ART) cycles [7]. According to the Bologna criteria, DOR is characterized by at least two of the following three features: advanced maternal age (typically over 35 years), previous poor ovarian response in ART cycles (defined as the retrieval of three or fewer oocytes despite high gonadotropin dosing), and an abnormal ovarian reserve test (elevated basal FSH level above 10 IU/L, low AMH level, or low antral follicle count (AFC) of fewer than 5–7 follicles).

These criteria serve as valuable tools for clinicians in identifying women with compromised ovarian reserve who may experience suboptimal response to ovarian stimulation during ART procedures. By incorporating age-related factors, past treatment history, and laboratory assessments, the Bologna criteria offer a comprehensive framework for diagnosing DOR and guiding treatment decisions in clinical practice.

Diagnostic Criteria for POI

Premature Ovarian Insufficiency diagnosis relies on clinical presentation, biochemical markers, and ovarian imaging studies. Clinical features may include vaginal dryness, dyspareunia, hot flashes, oligomenorrhea, and/or amenorrhea. Diagnostic criteria for POI is variable but generally include menstrual cycle irregularity or amenorrhea for at least four months before the age of 40, accompanied by elevated serum FSH levels above 25 IU/L on two occasions at least one month apart, and estradiol levels consistent with menopause [1]. Of note: Some criteria use higher FSH level cutoffs of 30–40 IU/L. In addition to hormonal assessments, pelvic ultrasound may reveal decreased ovarian volume and decreased follicle count, supporting the diagnosis of POI.

The evaluation of POI should also include the exclusion of other disorders, as well additional testing once the diagnosis is confirmed. Pregnancy, thyroid dysfunction, and hyperprolactinemia should be ruled out. Genetic testing includes screening for Fragile X and a karyotype to rule out Turner syndrome. Autoimmune testing includes both ovarian antibodies, adrenal antibodies, TSH, and thyroid-peroxidase antibodies (TPO). Given POI is a risk factor for bone loss and osteoporosis, we recommend a dual-energy x-ray absorptiometry [DXA] to assess long term fracture risk.

Limitations of Current Diagnostic Tests

Despite advancements in diagnostic modalities, several limitations exist in the assessment of DOR and POI. Ovarian reserve testing, including FSH, AMH, and AFC, may exhibit variability due to inter-cycle fluctuations and assay discrepancies, leading to diagnostic ambiguity (Nelson et al., 2020). Furthermore, while elevated FSH levels are indicative of diminished ovarian reserve, they may also reflect transient hormonal fluctuations, necessitating repeated testing for confirmation. Similarly, the diagnosis of POI poses challenges due to the heterogeneity of clinical presentation and the lack of standardized diagnostic criteria, leading to diagnostic delays and suboptimal patient care.

The diagnosis of DOR and POI requires a comprehensive evaluation incorporating clinical assessment, hormonal testing, and imaging studies. While existing diagnostic criteria provide valuable insights into ovarian function and reserve, clinicians must remain cognizant of the limitations associated with current diagnostic tests to ensure accurate diagnosis and optimal management of women with DOR and POI.

Therapeutic Approaches for Managing DOR and POI

Therapeutic intervention strategies for managing diminished ovarian reserve (DOR) and premature ovarian insufficiency (POI) aim to optimize fertility outcomes and alleviate associated symptoms. This section explores various therapeutic routes, encompassing both autologous interventions and donor egg *in vitro* fertilization (IVF), tailored to address the distinct challenges posed by DOR and POI.

Autologous Interventions for DOR and POI

Autologous interventions offer options for women with DOR and POI to optimize fertility potential using their own gametes. Given these entities fall on a spectrum, early recognition and diagnosis is critical in order to maximize a patient's reproductive potential and offer possible fertility preservation, depending on family-building goals.

In cases of DOR, the American Society for Reproductive Medicine (ASRM) guideline of 2018 compared pregnancy rates for poor responders undergoing IVF with mild ovarian stimulation versus conventional IVF, suggesting that mild ovarian stimulation protocols may offer comparable pregnancy rates to conventional IVF while potentially reducing the risk of ovarian hyperstimulation syndrome and minimizing patient discomfort and cost [8]. Of note, a study by Fouks et al. [9] showed that embryonic aneuploidy rates do not correlate with ovarian reserve or egg yield but rather are consistent with expected aneuploidy based largely on age.

Several adjuncts to treatment are often discussed in the context of DOR/POI, with the hope of improving ovarian function and egg yield. Following encouraging preclinical data in a mouse model, clinical evidence regarding the efficacy of coenzyme Q10 (CoQ10) supplementation in improving egg quality and fertility outcomes in women with DOR and POI remains limited [10]. While CoQ10 may exert antioxidant effects and potentially enhance mitochondrial function within ovarian follicles, robust clinical trials are needed to ascertain its clinical utility in human subjects.

Despite promising outcomes in other applications, studies investigating the use of platelet-rich plasma (PRP) injections into the ovaries have failed to demonstrate significant benefits in improving ovarian function or fertility outcomes in women with DOR or POI [11]. Despite the theoretical rationale for PRP therapy, current evidence does not support its routine use in clinical practice for the management of DOR and POI.

The use of growth hormone (GH) as an adjunctive therapy in IVF cycles remains controversial. Although GH supplementation has been proposed to enhance egg yield and response to ovarian stimulation, available data from clinical trials suggest that GH therapy does not significantly increase live birth rates in women undergoing IVF treatment [12, 13]. Furthermore, GH therapy lacks approval by the Food and Drug Administration (FDA) for use in IVF and should be approached with caution due to limited evidence supporting its efficacy and safety profile in this context.

Donor Egg IVF

Donor egg IVF represents a viable option for women with severe DOR or POI who are unable to conceive using their own oocytes. Donor egg IVF involves the retrieval and fertilization of donor oocytes, followed by embryo transfer into the recipient's uterus. This approach circumvents the limitations imposed by diminished ovarian reserve or ovarian insufficiency, offering women the opportunity to achieve pregnancy and live birth using donor gametes. Donor egg IVF boasts high success rates, particularly compared to autologous outcomes in women of advanced maternal age or with compromised ovarian function, providing a promising avenue for overcoming infertility challenges associated with DOR and POI.

In summary, while autologous interventions offer potential avenues for enhancing fertility outcomes in women with DOR and POI, the translation of these interventions into clinical practice requires further investigation and validation through well-designed prospective studies and randomized controlled trials.

Long-Term Sequelae for Patients with POI

Health Implications of POI

Premature ovarian insufficiency (POI) poses significant long-term health implications for affected individuals. Estrogen deficiency associated with POI increases the risk of cardiovascular diseases, osteoporosis, and genitourinary symptoms such as vaginal dryness and dyspareunia [1]. Women with POI may also experience psychological distress, including anxiety, depression, diminished quality of life, and impaired sexual function, stemming from concerns regarding fertility loss and hormonal changes. Furthermore, estrogen deficiency in POI is associated with an accelerated decline in bone mineral density, predisposing affected individuals to an increased risk of osteoporotic fractures later in life.

Hormone Replacement Therapy (HRT)

Hormone replacement therapy (HRT) remains the cornerstone of management for women with POI to mitigate the adverse effects of estrogen deficiency and alleviate associated symptoms. Patients with POI can experience intermittent ovarian function and ovulation with 5–10% of POI patients conceiving spontaneously. In patients wishing to avoid pregnancy, oral contraceptive pills are preferred, as the higher dose of hormones is more effective in preventing pregnancy. If pregnancy is desired, estrogen and progestin therapy is the desired treatment modality for hormone replacement. Transdermal estrogen delivery, either through patches or gels, has emerged as a preferred option over oral formulations due to its lower risk of venous thromboembolism and potentially superior bone-preserving effects [14]. Progestin supplementation is recommended in women with an intact uterus to prevent endometrial hyperplasia and mitigate the risk of endometrial cancer associated with unopposed estrogen therapy.

When considering HRT for women with POI, clinicians must weigh the benefits of symptom relief and long-term health preservation against potential risks, including cardiovascular events, venous thromboembolism, and breast cancer. Individualized treatment plans should account for patient age, cardiovascular risk factors, and personal preferences regarding hormonal therapy. Monitoring of HRT efficacy and safety should be conducted regularly, with adjustments made as needed based on clinical response and adverse effects.

Monitoring and Interdisciplinary Care

Long-term management of POI calls for a multidisciplinary approach involving gynecologists, endocrinologists, psychologists, and bone health specialists to address the diverse needs of affected individuals. Regular monitoring of bone mineral density, lipid profile, and cardiovascular risk factors is essential to detect and mitigate potential complications associated with estrogen deficiency and HRT. Psychosocial support, including counseling and support groups, can aid women in coping with the emotional impact of POI and navigating decisions regarding fertility preservation, family planning, and hormone therapy.

In summary, addressing the long-term sequelae of POI requires a comprehensive and individualized approach that prioritizes symptom management, bone health preservation, and psychological well-being. Through coordinated interdisciplinary care and evidence-based interventions, women with POI can optimize their long-term health outcomes and quality of life.

Key Points

- Diminished ovarian reserve (DOR) and premature ovarian insufficiency (POI) are frequently seen in a reproductive medicine setting and require significant counseling and a multidisciplinary approach.
- DOR and POI fall on a clinical spectrum; early diagnosis is critical in order to offer patients autologous treatment and possible fertility preservation, when appropriate.
- Autologous treatment and adjuncts may be appropriate depending on severity of DOR/POI, but no "magic bullet" or one-size-fits-all best approach has been identified.
- Donor egg IVF represents an excellent option with high success rates for patients with severe DOR/POI where autologous treatment is not possible.

REFERENCES

1. Webber L et al. ESHRE guideline: management of women with premature ovarian insufficiency. *Human Reprod* 2016;31(5):926–937.
2. Nelson SM et al. The ageing ovary and uterus: new biological insights. *Human Reprod Update* 2020;26(6):671–690.
3. Sunkara SK et al. Association between the number of eggs and live birth in IVF treatment: an analysis of 400 135 treatment cycles. *Human Reprod* 2018;33(1):193–201.
4. Simpson JL, Rajkovic A. Ovarian differentiation and gonadal failure. *Am J Med Gen Part C Sem Med Gen* 2019;181(1):64–76.
5. Cakmak et al. Antioxidant response of Chlamydomonas reinhardtii grown under different element regimes. *Phycological Res* 2015;63:202–211
6. Wang S et al. Hypermethylation of homeobox A10 predicts unfavorable prognosis in women with ovarian cancer. *Oncol Let* 2018;15(3):3303–3310.
7. Ferraretti AP et al. ESHRE consensus on the definition of 'poor response' to ovarian stimulation for in vitro fertilization: the Bologna criteria. *Human Reprod* 2011;26(7):1616–1624.
8. Practice Committee ASRM. Comparison of pregnancy rates for poor responders using IVF with mild ovarian stimulation versus conventional IVF: a guideline. *Fertil Steril* 2018;110(6):966–977.
9. Fouks Y et al. A diagnosis of diminished ovarian reserve does not impact embryo aneuploidy or live birth rates compared to patients with normal ovarian reserve. *Fertil Steril* 2022;118(3):504–512.
10. Bentov Y, Casper RF. The aging oocyte—can mitochondrial function be improved? *Fertil Steril* 2013;99(1):18–22.
11. Kim CH et al. Autologous platelet-rich plasma injection for severe ovarian insufficiency. *Korean J Reprod Med* 2016;43(2):51–55.
12. Xu B et al. (2017). Effect of growth hormone on pregnancy rates of patients undergoing IVF-ET: a meta-analysis of randomized controlled trials. *Arch Gynecol Obstet* 2017;295(3):543–552.
13. Yovich JL, Stanger JD. Growth hormone supplementation improves implantation and pregnancy productivity rates for poor-prognosis patients undertaking IVF. *Reprod Biomed Online* 2010;21:37–49.
14. Prior JC et al. Oral Contraceptives and estrogen/progestin replacement therapy: a meta-analysis of associations with coronary artery calcification. *J Women's Health* 2014;23(6):420–439.

20

Pregnancy of Unknown Location

Elise Abi Antoun, Kim Thornton, and Riwa Sabbagh

Definition

A pregnancy of unknown location (PUL) is defined as a positive qualitative or quantitative hCG test without an intrauterine or extrauterine/ectopic pregnancy seen on transvaginal ultrasound (TVUS) [1]. It is important to note that a pregnancy is confirmed on ultrasound when both a gestational and a yolk sac are visualized.

In the presence of a positive hCG, a patient can be categorized into five classes based on ultrasound findings:

1. Definite ectopic pregnancy: Presence of an ectopic gestational sac with a yolk sac.
2. Probable ectopic pregnancy: Presence of an adnexal mass or gestational sac or sac-like structure without a yolk sac.
3. PUL: Absence of a defined or probable intrauterine pregnancy (IUP) or ectopic pregnancy.
4. Probable IUP: Presence of an intrauterine gestational sac without a yolk sac.
5. Definite IUP: Presence of a gestational sac with a yolk sac and/or an embryo.

Epidemiology

The rate of PUL has been reported to range from 8% to 31% [2–4]. This wide range is likely attributed to operator experience and degree of ultrasound resolution and the ability to visualize an early pregnancy.

Clinical Presentation

Patients with PUL usually present with symptoms of early pregnancy (nausea, vomiting, fatigue, breast tenderness) and/or symptoms similar to those of an ectopic pregnancy (abdominal pain, vaginal bleeding, hemodynamic instability). However, the majority of patients with a PUL are asymptomatic.

Differential Diagnosis

The differential diagnosis of a PUL includes an intrauterine pregnancy (viable, non-viable), ectopic pregnancy, molar pregnancy, invasive mole, choriocarcinoma, ovarian malignancy, pituitary production of hCG in postmenopausal women, and presence of heterophilic antibodies.

DOI: 10.1201/9781003460275-20

Evolution of a PUL

A PUL is not a final diagnosis, and an evaluation should be completed until a diagnosis is reached. A PUL might be an intrauterine or ectopic pregnancy, but it may spontaneously resolve without its location ever being determined, which is the most common final outcome [3] (Figure 20.1). In the latter case, it can correspond to:

- A resorbed PUL (intrauterine or ectopic) if the hCG decreases spontaneously.
- A treated PUL if medical (via methotrexate) or surgical (via uterine evacuation) treatment is done with subsequent decrease in hCG and without confirmation of the location of the pregnancy on TVUS.

Evaluation

History

Obtaining a thorough history including an obstetrical and gynecologic history is important. Providers seeing patients with a PUL should ask about the date of the last menstrual period (LMP) to help date the pregnancy. They should also focus on the presence of risk factors for an ectopic pregnancy such as prior ectopic pregnancy, history of pelvic inflammatory disease, genital infections or infertility history, *in vitro* fertilization, presence of an intrauterine device, or prior tubal surgery [5–7]. Additionally, a detailed history of current symptoms such as the presence of abdominal pain and/or vaginal bleeding should be undertaken.

Physical Examination

Patients with PUL need to undergo a physical examination. It is first important to assess the patient's vital signs and assess their hemodynamic stability. Further examination should focus on an abdominal exam to assess for tenderness, guarding, and rebound. The presence of guarding and rebound is concerning for a ruptured ectopic pregnancy, which requires surgical management. A sterile speculum exam should be done to assess for active bleeding through the cervix, and a bimanual exam helps identify adnexal masses that can be concerning for an ectopic pregnancy.

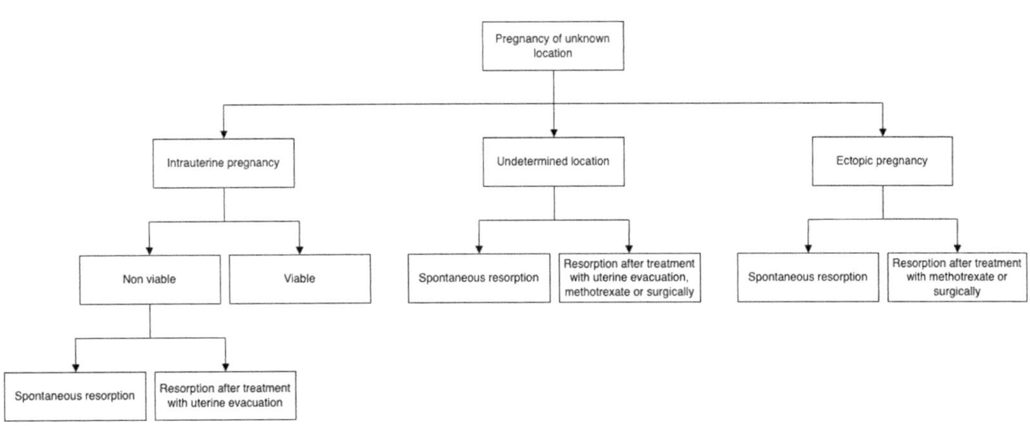

FIGURE 20.1 Evolution of a pregnancy of unknown location.

Laboratory Assessment

Obtaining a quantitative hCG level is crucial since hCG is the most commonly used hormone for the management of a PUL. It is important to obtain as a single measurement as well as serial measurements to predict the outcome of a PUL. The discriminatory zone, which is the serum hCG level at which a gestational sac should be visualized on ultrasound, should be used with caution. Discriminatory levels vary between institutions. It generally ranges between 1500–3000 IU/mL for transvaginal ultrasound and 6000–6500 IU/mL for transabdominal ultrasound. Using a higher threshold such as 2500–3000 IU/mL for transvaginal ultrasound helps decrease the risk of a false negative result but may also delay the diagnosis of an ectopic pregnancy.

Other laboratory tests may include a complete blood count (CBC), a type and screen, and liver function tests (LFTs). A CBC is done to assess for the presence of anemia, especially in the case of vaginal bleeding or if a ruptured ectopic pregnancy is suspected. A CBC can also be obtained along with LFTs to assess if the patient is an appropriate candidate for methotrexate if needed (discussed further in the chapter). A type and screen are useful to assess for the need for RhoGAM administration in Rh-negative patients. A serum progesterone has been measured to guide in the follow up of PULs; however it is unable to predict the location a PUL making its use in clinical practice limited.

Imaging

Ultrasonography is the most commonly used imaging modality in the evaluation of patients with a PUL. Transvaginal ultrasound (TVUS) is the mainstay for initial and serial imaging studies in patients with a PUL. It is preferred over a transabdominal ultrasound (TAUS) due to its ability to detect a pregnancy and fetal cardiac activity earlier.

Magnetic Resonance Imaging (MRI) can be used in select cases when visualization of soft tissues is difficult with ultrasonography because of the presence of uterine fibroids, uterine anomalies, or due to body habitus. However, gadolinium contrast should be avoided in pregnant patients due to risk of teratogenicity.

Management

Although there is no definitive management algorithm for patients with PULs, the aim should be to reach a diagnosis as early as possible. The initial approach to the management of a PUL should be based on the patient's hemodynamic stability.

Hemodynamically unstable patients may experience signs or symptoms of intra-abdominal bleeding (e.g., acute onset of severe abdominal pain, guarding, or rebound on abdominal exam, lightheadedness, dizziness), which is most likely due to a ruptured ectopic or less commonly from an early IUP loss. In this case, immediate fluid resuscitation and surgical management is required, either through a diagnostic laparoscopy or uterine evacuation. A diagnostic laparoscopy is done in the case of a suspected ruptured ectopic pregnancy for hemoperitoneum evacuation and resection of the ectopic pregnancy.

In the case of a hemodynamically stable patient, the management approach will be based upon whether the pregnancy is desired or not (Figures 20.2 and 20.3).

If the pregnancy is desired, it is recommended to obtain a repeat hCG measurement 48 hours later. In the setting of a viable intrauterine pregnancy, the hCG level rises by at least 53% [8]. However, in that case, an ectopic pregnancy cannot be completely ruled out. Interval weekly TVUS should be obtained until a final diagnosis is reached and a pregnancy is visualized. Imaging can be obtained earlier if the hCG level reaches the discriminatory zone.

If the hCG is not rising appropriately (i.e. by less than 53% in 48 hours), then a shared decision-making process should be undertaken. One possible approach is monitoring hCG levels every 48 hours and obtaining a weekly TVUS to localize the pregnancy until a final diagnosis is reached (intrauterine vs. ectopic pregnancy). Monitoring the patient's signs and symptoms is important in this scenario given the risk of rupture in the setting of an ectopic pregnancy.

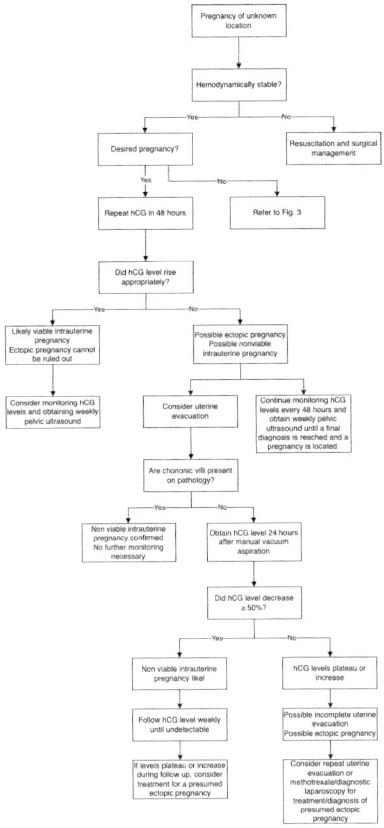

FIGURE 20.2 Treatment algorithm of a pregnancy of unknown location in the setting of a desired pregnancy.

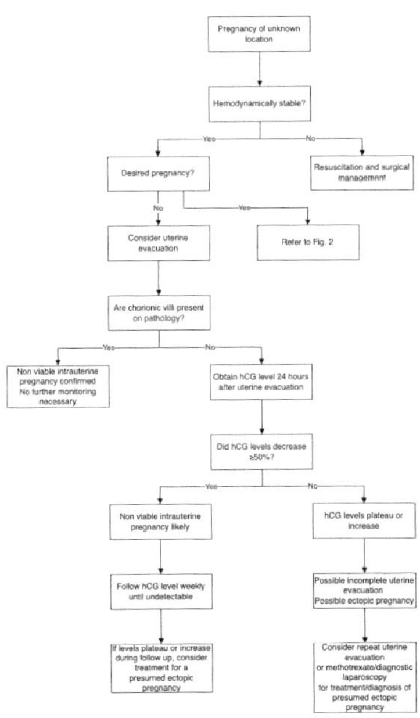

FIGURE 20.3 Treatment algorithm of a pregnancy of unknown location in the setting of an undesired pregnancy.

If hCG levels plateau, this is usually concerning for a failing intrauterine or ectopic pregnancy. Another approach includes performing endometrial sampling via manual vacuum aspiration (MVA) to help reach a final diagnosis sooner. Medical management of an ectopic pregnancy with methotrexate is not without risk and methotrexate carries significant side effects; therefore, performing an MVA can help avoid the unnecessary administration of methotrexate. The presence of chorionic villi on pathology confirms an evacuated intrauterine pregnancy and further follow-up is not necessary. If pathology is not obtained, then it is important to get a follow-up hCG level 24 hours after the procedure. Levels are considered to have plateaued if they decrease by less than 10–15% [8]. A plateau or increasing level indicates that the MVA was incomplete or the presence of an ectopic pregnancy and further treatment, with repeat MVA or methotrexate, is warranted. A decrease in the hCG level by 50% or greater indicates a high likelihood of an intrauterine pregnancy. In this case, hCG levels should be followed until undetectable. If levels plateau during the follow-up period, then treatment for a presumed ectopic pregnancy should be considered.

If the pregnancy is undesired, then further management can be expedited. A diagnostic MVA with or without laparoscopy can be performed in patients desiring active management. If chorionic villi are found in the endometrial sampling, then no subsequent follow-up is necessary. If the pathology was not sent, then hCG levels should be obtained 24 hours after the procedure. If hCG levels decrease by at least 50%, then the diagnosis is consistent with a failed intrauterine pregnancy; hCG levels should then be monitored until undetectable. If hCG levels increase or plateau either initially or during the monitoring phase, treatment with methotrexate for a presumed ectopic pregnancy should be discussed. If the patient desires expected management, treatment is similar to that of a desired pregnancy. An hCG level should be obtained at 48-hour intervals. If the hCG level is declining, the diagnosis is most consistent with a failing intrauterine pregnancy and hCG levels should be obtained until undetectable. If hCG levels plateau or start increasing, further intervention should be done via uterine evacuation or methotrexate treatment for a presumed ectopic pregnancy.

RhoGAM

The risk of allo-immunization is low before 10–12 weeks given that fetal red blood cell (RBC) exposure is below the calculated threshold to cause maternal Rh sensitization [9, 10]. However, data is insufficient on the use of RhoGAM in the setting of a PUL and its administration is institution-dependent.

Conclusion

When a pregnancy of unknown location is identified, efforts should be made to localize the pregnancy and achieve a final diagnosis. The initial assessment should focus on hemodynamic stability and resuscitation of the patient. The evaluation should include a baseline hCG level and an ultrasound to attempt to localize the pregnancy. Visualization of the pregnancy on ultrasound depends on the "discriminatory zone," and repeat hCG levels may be needed to help determine the final diagnosis. The management of a pregnancy of unknown location will depend on the patient's desire for the pregnancy. A more aggressive approach with manual vacuum aspiration of the uterine cavity and medical/surgical treatment of a presumed ectopic pregnancy can be undertaken in the case of an undesired pregnancy. On the other hand, a more conservative approach and close follow-up with repeat hCG levels and ultrasound studies can be considered in the case of desired pregnancy in a hemodynamically stable patient.

Key Points

- Pregnancy of unknown location is not a final diagnosis.
- Further evaluation is necessary to attempt to localize the pregnancy.
- Initial assessment should focus on hemodynamic stability and resuscitation.
- Imaging studies with ultrasound to localize the pregnancy are operator-dependent.

- hCG discriminatory zone is different between institutions but generally ranges between 1500–3000 IU/mL for transvaginal ultrasound and 6000–6500 IU/mL for transabdominal ultrasound
- Management of a pregnancy of unknown location is widely dependent on the desire for pregnancy.

REFERENCES

1. Barnhart K et al. Pregnancy of unknown location: a consensus statement of nomenclature, definitions, and outcome. *Fertil Steril* 2011;95(3):857–66.
2. Milman T et al. Pregnancy of unknown location. *CMAJ* 2020;192(39):E1132.
3. Hahlin M et al. The expectant management of early pregnancies of uncertain site. *Hum Reprod* 1995;10(5):1223–7.
4. Dart RG et al. Subclassification of indeterminate pelvic ultrasonography: prospective evaluation of the risk of ectopic pregnancy. *Ann Emerg Med* 2002;39(4):382–8.
5. Kamwendo F et al. Epidemiology of ectopic pregnancy during a 28 year period and the role of pelvic inflammatory disease. *Sex Transm Infect* 2000;76(1):28–32.
6. Du T et al. Comparison of ectopic pregnancy risk among transfers of embryos vitrified on day 3, day 5, and day 6. *Fertil Steril* 2017;108(1):108–116.e1.
7. Li C et al. Contraceptive use and the risk of ectopic pregnancy: a multi-center case-control study. *PLoS One* 2014;9(12):e115031.
8. ACOG practice bulletin 193: tubal ectopic pregnancy. *Obstet Gynecol* 2018;131(3):e91–e103.
9. Horvath S et al. Society of Family Planning committee consensus on Rh testing in early pregnancy. *Contraception* 2022;114:1–5.
10. Schmidt-Hansen M et al., Anti-D prophylaxis for rhesus D (RhD)-negative women having an abortion of a pregnancy up to 13(+6) weeks' gestation: a systematic review and new NICE consensus guidelines. *BMJ Sex Reprod Health* 2020;bmjsrh-2019-200536.

21

The IVF Laboratory

Denny Sakkas and C. Brent Barrett

Introduction

The treatment of infertility has been a technological challenge as far back as the 14th century, when there are accounts of Arab peoples using artificial insemination on horses. Even in the 3rd century AD, records show that Jewish thinkers were discussing the possibility of accidental or unintentional human insemination by artificial means.

The first attempts at human artificial insemination by John Hunter are believed to have occurred in 1785, with a baby born the same year. Early reports of donor insemination were published in the British Medical Journal in 1945, and in 1955, four successful pregnancies using previously frozen sperm were reported. In 1944, Rock and Menkin reported the first case of *in vitro* fertilization (IVF) and embryo development in the human. Interestingly, they made the following description about the developing fertilized embryo:

> One of these (embryo), when first seen in cleavage, consisted of one large blastomere and two smaller ones, each of the three containing a round, vesicular nucleus. The second egg from this same patient was in a similar stage, but part of the cytoplasm appeared fragmented, and soon proceeded to undergo rapid degenerative changes.

It took until the 1960s and 1970s for many of the different clinical and laboratory aspects of IVF to be improved for more routine use. In 1973, the first IVF pregnancy in the world was reported by a team in Melbourne, Australia, which resulted in early embryo death. Subsequently, in 1977 another IVF pregnancy was reported but it was an ectopic pregnancy. Finally, in 1978, the culmination of knowledge in the technologies associated with IVF led to the first IVF birth in the world by Steptoe and Edwards.

This chapter will give a broad review of current laboratory technologies and procedures that allow IVF to now be a routine clinical procedure.

Laboratory Procedures After Recovery of Oocytes

Routine IVF

Stimulation protocols and oocyte recovery techniques have been reviewed earlier in this book. Once satisfactory stimulation is achieved, the retrieved oocyte-cumulus complexes are collected from follicular aspirates using the following procedure.

DOI: 10.1201/9781003460275-21

Oocyte retrieval

All steps are performed using sterile technique. Extra caution and protective equipment should be used for infectious disease patients. Once the patient paperwork or Electronic Record File is verified, the embryologist should check for any special instructions involved with the case. Identifiers, including name, date of birth, clinic or patient number, etc., should be noted and confirmed on all laboratory items to be used. All the steps involved in the treatment of gametes and embryos must be witnessed to ensure error-free treatment.

The retrieval procedure is initiated by providing the operating room with medium for egg collection. It is recommended to use a holding medium normally containing HEPES (4-(2-hydroxyethyl)-1-piperazi neethanesulfonic acid) or sometimes MOPS 3-(N-morpholino) propanesulfonic acid. These are both organic chemical buffering agents which are used in cell culture to assist in maintaining physiological pH. This property allows them to act as a better buffering agent, in particular when the oocytes are maintained outside of an incubator and at 37°C. The medium may or may not contain heparin to limit clotting of the follicular aspirate.

Before commencing the procedure, it is imperative to verify and have witnessed the patient's name, the spelling, the patient's date of birth and name band. A checklist sheet documenting this step should be maintained. Once collection begins, the aspirate is poured from the test tube into a tissue culture dish and the contents are scanned for the presence of a cumulus-oocyte complex (COC). The following procedure should be performed at a controlled temperature of 37°C. The COCs are pipetted into a tissue culture dish containing a buffered medium or an equilibrated culture medium when working in an appropriately gassed environment. This step is repeated for all tubes received from the physician. Ideally, the COCs should be washed in rinse dishes, containing culture medium under oil, and a pre-determined number of COCs placed into each culture medium drop for holding. A commonly used medium to maintain the oocyte-cumulus complexes is human tubal fluid (HTF) medium (Irvine Scientific, Santa Ana, CA) overlaid by paraffin oil. Many clinics also perform egg retrieval directly into HTF or other egg handling medium with bicarbonate. In these practices, the retrieval can be performed in a mobile incubator where the eggs are collected and harvested in an enclosed environment of 37°C in 5.0% CO_2, 5% O_2, 90% N_2, or 5% CO_2, (Tri-gas) in air. This avoids any additional manipulation of the COCs.

The dish or dishes are then placed in an incubator, making sure that all details relating to patient's name on the dish(es) and the correct location in the incubator are verified. Once the retrieval is finished, the number of COCs, timing, and personnel who performed the procedure, etc. must be documented.

Analysis and Preparation of Semen Samples for IVF

Semen samples are routinely obtained from the male by masturbation into a sterile container. Traditionally, the male was recommended to not have ejaculated for 2–3 days prior to collection; however a number of studies are now finding that shorter abstinence periods could be beneficial to IVF cycle outcomes.

Analysis

A previous diagnostic semen analysis is normally carried out according to WHO guidelines (WHO 6th edition). This will help direct the type of treatment a couple may undergo. In general, sperm concentration, motility, and morphology are required parameters. Other diagnostic tests for the male can include an assessment of sperm nuclear DNA. Although this test has led to some controversy, it is believed to provide useful information in relation to the male's ability to achieve a conception naturally or after intra-uterine insemination, but the results relating to IVF are less convincing.[1] Sperm DNA testing is now recommended in couples experiencing recurrent pregnancy losses.[2] Another diagnostic test that can be used is the Hyaluronan (HA) Binding Test.[3] This test provides information about the maturity of the sperm. Briefly, human sperm that bind to HA exhibit attributes similar to that of zona pellucida-bound sperm, including minimal DNA fragmentation, normal shape, and low frequency of chromosomal aneuploidies.[4] Large trials conducted using this technology indicate some benefit in reducing miscarriages and in couples where the female is over 38 years old.[5, 6]

Preparation

In the majority of laboratories, the preparation of choice is by either a swim-up (SU) technique or by density gradient (DG) centrifugation. Sperm preparation for assisted conception by DG centrifugation routinely uses 0.5–1mL volumes of a 40% suspension layered over 0.5–1mL of a 90% suspension of a colloidal silica suspension in an isotonic salt solution mixed in human tubal fluid (HTF) media or a similar commercial media. Semen is overlaid on the 40% and 90% layers (Figure 21.1) and then centrifuged for approximately 20 minutes (300g). Variations of the theme exist including 40–80% bilayers, single layer preparations using only 90%, or mini-preparations. In all cases after centrifugation, the sperm in the higher percentage layer, 80% or 90% pellet, are harvested. The swim-up method requires centrifugation of the ejaculate to form a pellet followed by layering of clean medium (0.5–1ml) over the pellet. The sperm are then allowed to swim freely up into the clean portion and are then harvested. Other sperm preparation techniques that are now available are those based on microfluidics. Initial data indicates that this technology is able to provide highly enriched motile sperm and with drastically lower levels of sperm DNA fragmentation.[7] Other techniques that have been developed to improve sperm preparation include de-selection of apoptotic sperm.

Insemination and Intracytoplasmic Sperm Injection (ICSI)

Once the sample is prepared, the total motile sperm concentration is calculated using the volume and number of motile sperm. Insemination can then be performed by adding a pre-determined amount to the droplet of culture medium containing the cumulus-enclosed oocytes. Oocytes can be inseminated in groups or individually in droplets of embryo culture medium with between 50–500,000 motile sperm per ml overnight. Insemination is routinely performed between 1,300 and 1,500, allowing incubation overnight and checking of two pronuclei in the morning. The use of time lapse incubators can remove the need for this specific timing. There are some indications that embryo quality is improved when clinics have utilized a short insemination period,[8] whereby the sperm are introduced for a period of 1–4h only and then the oocytes are removed. With this approach, the oocytes are not exposed to radical oxygen species and other possible harmful factors generated by the large population of sperm overnight.

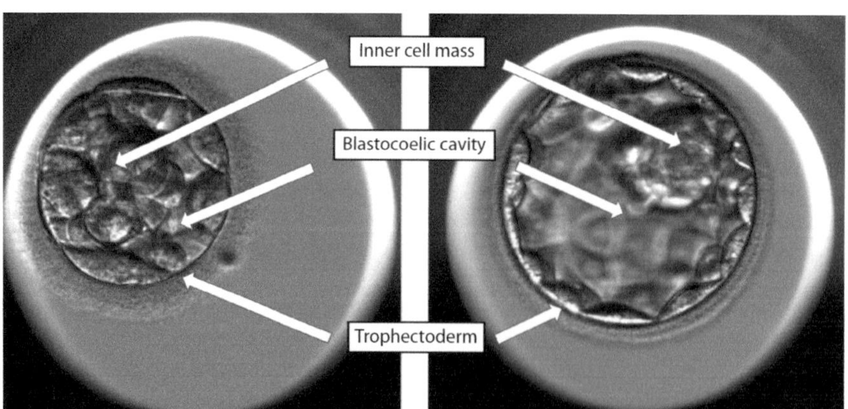

FIGURE 21.1 Blastocyst scoring characterizes the expansion of the blastocoelic cavity, the quality of the Trophectoderm (TE) and tightness of the Inner Cell Mass (ICM). The figure on the left shows the blastocoelic cavity just forming and the initial differentiation of cells identifiable by microscopy to the ICM and TE. The figure on the right shows a more advanced expanded blastocyst with clear ICM and TE.

This step is critical to be witnessed as verification must be made that the name and other identifiers on the sperm tube match that of the patient's retrieval dish containing the oocytes.

If the sperm preparation is substandard in number and/or motility or if the patient has previously been identified to be a candidate for ICSI, the following procedure is followed. In preparation for ICSI, the COCs are first placed in a medium with hyaluronidase for <2 minutes for partial removal of the cumulus cells. The remaining cumulus cells are removed by mechanical manipulation of the oocyte during further rinsing in the medium. Mechanical manipulation consists of passing the COC through a series of pipettes decreasing in size from 250–135µm. The aim is to denude the oocytes of the cumulus cells to allow complete visualization of the oocyte and polar body so that the ICSI procedure can proceed.

ICSI is sometimes now chosen as the standard method of insemination. One reason for the overuse of ICSI is a fear of fertilization failure when using conventional insemination, for non-male factor infertility patients. A number of recent studies have, however, shown that if a conventional insemination case has low or no fertilization, rescue ICSI can be used. Studies have now been published out of China using rescue ICSI when no polar bodies are extruded several hours after insemination.[9] Otherwise, day after rescue ICSI has also been shown to circumvent fertilization failure after conventional insemination and provide good pregnancy rates when blastocysts are frozen.[10] Current rates of ICSI utilization in the US and worldwide are close to 70% of cycles. This has led to investigating whether it is overused in non-male factor patients. A number of papers have shown that conventional insemination may actually yield more fertilized eggs, more euploid and higher pregnancy rates in non-male factor patients when compared to ICSI.[11] Other concerns with ICSI still remain, in particular, with respect to its safety. Current data, however, indicate that children born after ICSI have not shown any differences when compared to children born from routine IVF or natural conception.[12]

Embryo Culture and Medium Selection

At 16–18h after insemination (day 1), each oocyte is examined for evidence of fertilization (pronuclei) and placed into groups or individual droplets of sequential cleavage stage and blastocyst media or in a single step culture medium. If no pronuclei are seen and cleavage is seen the following day, we have found that if good quality blastocysts develop, they are highly viable. There are a number of papers now indicating that failure to observe two pronuclei is not a necessity if a good embryo develops.

The general constituents of the sequential and single step culture media are shown in Table 21.1 and analyzed in more detail by Morbeck et al.[13, 14] Embryos can remain in the cleavage medium until the morning of day 3 when they are changed over to blastocyst medium (Table 21.1). Embryos are then maintained in blastocyst medium until day 5, 6, or 7 depending on the day of transfer/cryopreservation /preimplantation genetic testing (PGT) decided for the treatment of the patient. Even with single step medium, the embryos can be changed over on day 3 of culture or be maintained throughout the whole culture period in the same droplets. Numerous commercial single step and sequential culture media exist which broadly follow this protocol.

TABLE 21.1

Major Constituents and Differences of Day 1–3 Cleavage Stage and Day 3–5 Blastocyst Stage Media

Sequential Cleavage Culture Media	Sequential Blastocyst Culture Media	Single Step Media
Days 1–3	**Days 3–6**	**Days 1–6**
• low or no glucose	• high glucose	• glucose
• high pyruvate and lactate	• low pyruvate and lactate	• pyruvate and lactate
• EDTA	• essential amino acids	• EDTA
• non-essential amino acids	• non-essential amino acids	• amino acids

A common constituent of modern embryo culture media are various amino acids. This is in contrast to early media, such as HTF, which were simple salt solutions. The major benefit of modern human embryo culture media has been a dramatic improvement in their ability to improve blastocyst culture. Amino acids are important regulators of many cellular functions such as chelators, osmolytes, pH buffers, antioxidants, regulators of energy metabolism and biosynthetic precursors, and energy substrates. The other main constituent is the protein source. A number of choices are available: human serum albumin (HSA), recombinant HSA or serum supplements that usually consist of a high percentage of HSA, and alpha and beta globulins. Modifications and development of new media are still lacking, but some studies are now testing the addition of factors such as antioxidants.

More effort is also being made to modernize embryo culture platforms. In particular, the use of microfluidic systems to facilitate embryo culture is being further developed.

Assessment of the Embryo

Numerous methods have been adopted to assess the embryo as it develops from the pronuclear through to the blastocyst stage. The many transformations that take place during the fertilization process make the pronucleate stage a dynamic stage to assess. The human oocyte contains the majority of the developmental materials and maternal mRNA for ensuing that the embryo reaches the 4-to-8-cell stage. The quality of the oocyte, therefore, plays a crucial role for determining embryo development and subsequent viability. Time lapse morphokinetics has now allowed us a greater appreciation of the intricate changes that occur in the first days of development.

Regardless of techniques such as time lapse and PGT, the most widely used criteria for selecting the best embryos for transfer are still based on morphology. This is still the mainstay of the embryologists' tool for selecting which embryo to transfer. Although blastocyst transfers make up the majority of cases in the US, a significant proportion of cleavage stage transfers still occur. Variations on the basic selection of the best cleaving embryo by cell number and morphology have been used. For example, it is believed that by using strict embryo criteria to select "top" quality embryos, one can achieve a high implantation potential.

Although performed less frequently, assessment of the embryos at either the pronuclear or cleavage stages can, at best, be considered an assessment of the oocyte. The quality of the oocyte is undoubtedly important, as the quality of the developing embryo is ultimately dependent on the quality of the gametes from which it is derived; but this provides limited information regarding true embryo developmental potential. Furthermore, there is the potential of a paternal effect on development that is mainly evident after the 8-cell stage when the embryonic genome is activated. Only by culturing embryos past this stage to the blastocyst does it become possible to assess true embryonic development.

The use of blastocyst culture has become the primary tool for embryo selection. A number of reasons have supported its more widespread adoption, in particular in the US. These include the triage of successful *in vitro* developing embryos at the blastocyst stage, cryopreservation by vitrification, and the rise in the use of Preimplantation Genetic Screening for aneuploidy using trophectoderm biopsy (covered in a separate chapter).

For assessing blastocysts, the simplest criteria are reflected using an alphanumeric scoring system. This takes into account three aspects of blastocyst morphology: degree of blastocoel expansion, inner cell mass (ICM) development, and trophectoderm (TE) development. The most common method is the Gardner grading system or modifications of it.

A more detailed analysis of the impact that the different assessment criteria have on viability has indicated that the trophectoderm provides greater predictive weight for embryo selection. An initial study by Aelstrohm et al.[15] concluded that the predictive strength of the trophectoderm grade was greater compared to that for the ICM for selecting the best blastocyst for embryo transfer. It has been suggested that even though ICM is important, a strong trophectoderm layer is essential at this stage of embryo development, allowing successful hatching and implantation. This has been validated by a number of studies[16, 17] which all highlighted the need for a strong trophectoderm grading in relation to pregnancy.

Time Lapse Imaging

The use of time lapse imaging and the use of morphokinetic scoring systems has also been examined to predict embryo viability. Large, randomized trials have shown that the time lapse systems alone do not dramatically improve embryo selection;[18] however, the ability to allow embryos to develop continually without removing them from the incubator is a definite advantage.[19] Retrospective data analyses found specific cleavage patterns and timings that indicate which embryos would be successful to establish pregnancies.[20]

The combination of time lapse imaging and data with artificial intelligence has opened up new opportunities for embryo assessment and prediction of embryo viability. In retrospective analysis, the introduction of algorithms appears to dramatically improve embryo selection when compared to scoring an embryo traditionally.[21–23] It certainly appears that artificial intelligence can assist in embryo grading. Illingworth et al.[24] in particular found that an algorithm provided an almost 10-fold reduction in the time required for evaluation of blastocysts cultured in the EmbryoScope™ time-lapse incubator. Further, current algorithms only incorporate a small fraction of the data acquired during development, typically utilizing less than 10 times points. Numerous trials are currently underway to establish whether AI is as effective as highly trained embryologists in ranking the viability of embryos from a patient's cohort. Preliminary data indicate that AI for blastocyst selection is most advantageous for patients under 35, i.e., those cases most likely to have several blastocysts for transfer.[25] Interestingly, rather than considering whether AI should replace the decision-making of an embryologist, it would perhaps be best to consider that AI and the embryologist are complementary and that AI could be used as part of the decision-making process rather than the sole tool. A number of trials have now been conducted comparing the pregnancy rates of time-lapse imaging systems for embryo incubation to standard incubators and also the incorporation of some initial time-lapse models for embryo selection.[26, 27] None of the studies was able to show increased chances of pregnancy when using time-lapse imaging systems for embryo culture and selection. More recently a large RCT by Illingworth et al.[24] was not able to demonstrate non-inferiority of deep learning for clinical pregnancy rate when compared to standard morphology and a predefined prioritization scheme.

Oocyte and Embryo Freezing

Cryopreservation is now an integral part of many IVF clinics throughout the world, enabling patients to utilize the maximum number of embryos generated from any one oocyte retrieval whilst protecting against ovarian hyperstimulation syndrome (OHSS) and the risk of higher order multiple births.

There are a number of different cryoprotectants currently used in cryostorage of the oocyte/embryo, e.g., dimethyl sulphoxide (DMSO), ethylene glycol (ETG), trehalose, glycerol, and propane-1,2-diol (PrOH). Cryopreservation is now predominantly performed using vitrification. Vitrification can be applied at all stages of embryo development and to the oocyte, with the preferred stage for embryos being the blastocyst stage.

Most importantly, it is evident that vitrification has now allowed live birth outcomes from frozen embryo transfers to surpass those from fresh transfers. The question now is whether clinically it makes more sense to transfer only frozen embryos rather than perform transfers in fresh cycles. The data appears to be compelling on two fronts. First, there is the deleterious effect of a stimulated uterine environment, in particular elevated progesterone levels, that appear to harm the chance of pregnancy; and second, live birth weights of children born from frozen embryo transfers are consistently better when compared to those from fresh embryo transfers. One area under consideration for frozen embryo transfers is the preparation of the endometrium, with some studies indicating that natural cycles lead to less perinatal issues than programmed cycles.

For the oocyte, the majority of data has been collected from donor oocytes whereby success rates of vitrified oocytes versus fresh oocytes have been shown to be close.[28] Oocyte vitrification for donors provides numerous advantages, including being more efficient, more economical, easier for both donors and recipients and potentially also safer, because eggs can now be quarantined for 6 months (or longer) to retest for infectious diseases in the donors. Oocyte vitrification is also allowing benefits to patients in areas such as fertility preservation for social or oncologic reasons. Data, however, does indicate that although oocyte vitrification provides many benefits, a small loss in viability compared to fresh oocytes is still evident.[29]

Vitrification Procedure

The vitrification procedure consists of three solutions that are used to achieve equilibration of the oocyte or embryo for different times. Commonly used solutions may or may not contain DMSO. One protocol, for example, involves an equilibration solution (containing the cryoprotectants DMSO and ethylene glycol with a serum supplement) and a vitrification solution (containing the same solutions but in a higher concentration). The aim of any freezing or vitrification protocol is to use the cryoprotectants to replace any water in the oocyte/embryo while still providing protection to the cell membrane and other organelles. Removal of water effectively removes any chance of crystals forming within the oocyte/embryo and creates damage.

Routinely, the oocyte/embryo is incubated in the equilibration solution for between 5–10 minutes while they are placed in the final vitrification solution for between 30–60 seconds. The timings are dependent on specific protocols recommended by manufacturers or used by individual laboratories. When removed from the vitrification solution, the embryo is normally pipetted onto a cryostorage device in minimal volume that just covers the embryo or oocyte. These devices should allow the embryo in its cryoprotectant to be vitrified at very high cooling rates.

To warm embryos prior to transfer, the reverse process is effectively applied. An initial thawing solution containing sucrose and the serum supplement is used followed by a diluted form of the same solution which contains less sucrose. Finally, the oocyte/embryo is allowed to recover in the usual culture medium for a period prior to use. Interestingly, there has recently been a movement to a more rapid warming procedure, allowing the procedure to proceed even faster. Whether quickening the steps of the vitrification procedure will also be adopted is still debatable. Finally, implementation of microfluidics to facilitate vitrification is also fast becoming a reality.

Conclusion

IVF reproductive technologies have come a long way since the first birth in 1978. The technical progression from ICSI to treat many male infertility patients, to the use of preimplantation genetic screening and vitrification, has allowed dramatic improvements in both oocyte and embryo storage and has shown how laboratory improvements can impact success. Technological advances in the IVF laboratory, including improvements in molecular analysis, novel non-invasive assessment profiles, and revolutionary microfluidic platforms (see chapter "The Future of the IVF Laboratory") are currently being used in other areas of medicine and will likely impact the IVF laboratory in the near future, leading to even further improvement in both access to treatment and the chances of patients having a normal healthy offspring.

Key Points

- The IVF laboratory will continue to evolve.
- The constant aim will be to provide normal healthy live births without the fear of harm being introduced to offspring from the *in vitro* procedures adopted.

REFERENCES

1. Bungum M et al. The predictive value of sperm chromatin structure assay (SCSA) parameters for the outcome of intrauterine insemination, IVF and ICSI, *Hum Reprod* 2004;19(6):1401–1408.
2. Schlegel PN et al. Diagnosis and treatment of infertility in men: AUA/ASRM guideline part I, *Fertil Steril* 2021;115(1):54–61.
3. Huszar G et al. Fertility testing and ICSI sperm selection by hyaluronic acid binding: clinical and genetic aspects, *Reprod Biomed Online* 2007;14(5):650–663.
4. AJakab A et al. Intracytoplasmic sperm injection: a novel selection method for sperm with normal frequency of chromosomal aneuploidies, *Fertil Steril* 2005;84(6):1665–1673.
5. Kirkman-Brown J et al. *Sperm selection for assisted reproduction by prior hyaluronan binding: the HABSelect RCT.* National Institute for Health Research, Evaluation, Trials and Studies Coordinating Centre, 2019.
6. Miller D et al. Physiological, hyaluronan-selected intracytoplasmic sperm injection for infertility treatment (HABSelect): a parallel, two-group, randomised trial, *Lancet* 2019;393(10170):416–422.
7. Parrella A et al. A treatment approach for couples with disrupted sperm DNA integrity and recurrent ART failure, *J Assist Reprod Genet* 2019;36(10):2057–2066.
8. Gianaroli L et al. Reducing the time of sperm-oocyte interaction in human in-vitro fertilization improves the implantation rate, *Hum Reprod* 1996;11(1):166–171.
9. Jiang Y et al. Cumulative live birth rate and neonatal outcomes after early rescue ICSI: a propensity score matching analysis, *Hum Reprod Open* 2023;2023(4):hoad046.
10. Batha S et al. Day after rescue ICSI: eliminating total fertilization failure after conventional IVF with high live birth rates following cryopreserved blastocyst transfer, *Hum Reprod* 2023;38(7):1277–1283.
11. Patel K et al. Compared with conventional insemination, intracytoplasmic sperm injection provides no benefit in cases of nonmale factor infertility as evidenced by comparable euploidy rate, *Fertil Steril* 2023;120(2):277–286.
12. Belva F et al. Neonatal outcome of 724 children born after ICSI using non-ejaculated sperm, *Hum Reprod* 2011;26(7):1752–1758.
13. Morbeck DE et al. Composition of single-step media used for human embryo culture, *Fertil Steril* 2017;107(4):1055–1060.e1051.
14. Morbeck DE et al. Composition of commercial media used for human embryo culture, *Fertil Steril* 2014;102(3):759–766.e759.
15. Ahlström A et al. Trophectoderm morphology: an important parameter for predicting live birth after single blastocyst transfer, *Hum Reprod* 2011;26(12):3289–3296.
16. van der Weiden RM. Trophectoderm morphology grading reflects interactions between embryo and endometrium, *Fertil Steril* 2013;100(4):e23.
17. Shear MA et al. Blasts from the past: is morphology useful in PGT-A tested and untested frozen embryo transfers? *Reprod Biomed Online* 2020;41(6):981–989.
18. Goodman LR et al. Does the addition of time-lapse morphokinetics in the selection of embryos for transfer improve pregnancy rates? A randomized controlled trial, *Fertil Steril* 2016;105(2):275–285. e210.
19. Kaser DJ, Racowsky C. Clinical outcomes following selection of human preimplantation embryos with time-lapse monitoring: a systematic review, *Hum Reprod Update* 2014;20(5):617–631.
20. Meseguer M et al. Embryo incubation and selection in a time-lapse monitoring system improves pregnancy outcome compared with a standard incubator: a retrospective cohort study, *Fertil Steril* 2012;98(6):1481–1489.e1410.
21. Loewke K et al. Characterization of an artificial intelligence model for ranking static images of blastocyst stage embryos, *Fertil Steril* 2022;117(3):528–535.
22. Tran NH et al. Deep learning enables de novo peptide sequencing from data-independent-acquisition mass spectrometry, *Nat Methods* 2019;16(1):63–66.
23. VerMilyea M et al. Development of an artificial intelligence-based assessment model for prediction of embryo viability using static images captured by optical light microscopy during IVF, *Hum Reprod* 2020;35(4):770–784.
24. Illingworth PJ et al. Deep learning versus manual morphology-based embryo selection in IVF: a randomized, double-blind noninferiority trial, *Nature Med* 2020;30:3114–3120.

25. Ueno S et al. Pregnancy prediction performance of an annotation-free embryo scoring system on the basis of deep learning after single vitrified-warmed blastocyst transfer: a single-center large cohort retrospective study, *Fertil Steril* 2021;116(4):1172–1180.
26. Bhide P et al. Clinical effectiveness and safety of time-lapse imaging systems for embryo incubation and selection in in-vitro fertilisation treatment (TILT): a multicentre, three-parallel-group, double-blind, randomised controlled trial, *Lancet* 2024;404(10449):256–265.
27. Kieslinger DC et al. Clinical outcomes of uninterrupted embryo culture with or without time-lapse-based embryo selection versus interrupted standard culture (SelecTIMO): a three-armed, multicentre, double-blind, randomised controlled trial, *Lancet* 2023;401 (10386):1438–1446.
28. Cobo A et al. Six years' experience in ovum donation using vitrified oocytes: report of cumulative outcomes, impact of storage time, and development of a predictive model for oocyte survival rate, *Fertil Steril* 2015;104(6):1426–1434.e1421–1428.
29. Cornet-Bartolomé D et al. Efficiency and efficacy of vitrification in 35 654 sibling oocytes from donation cycles, *Hum Reprod* 2020;35(10):2262–2271.

22

Preimplantation Genetic Testing

Mina Popovic

Preimplantation genetic testing (PGT) encompasses a group of diagnostic techniques used in the context of medically assisted reproduction to evaluate embryos for genetic abnormalities prior to transfer. In practice, it involves the analysis of embryonic DNA obtained through cellular biopsy and includes three main types (Figure 22.1): PGT for aneuploidies (PGT-A), PGT for monogenic disorders (PGT-M), and PGT for structural rearrangements (PGT-SR).

- **PGT-A** tests for chromosomal abnormalities (aneuploidies).
- **PGT-M** tests for specific single-gene (monogenic) mutations known to cause inherited diseases, in cases where patients have a personal or familial risk.
- **PGT-SR** tests for structural (segmental) chromosomal abnormalities, in cases where one or both partners carry a known balanced structural rearrangement in their chromosomes.

The Evolution of Preimplantation Genetic Testing

PGT has advanced significantly over the years. Its evolution has not only been driven by improvements in molecular genetic technologies but also by key innovations in laboratory culture conditions, embryo handling, and cryopreservation techniques (Figure 22.2). These developments have collectively enhanced the accuracy and reliability of PGT procedures, ultimately allowing for more refined embryo selection.

PGT originated from pioneering research conducted by Richard Gardner and Robert Edwards in the 1950s and 1960s. Their work focused on determining the sex of rabbit and cow blastocysts, laying the foundation for modern techniques in human reproductive genetics. In 1968, they introduced an innovative embryo biopsy method utilizing rabbit embryos. Using a holding pipette and fine iridectomy scissors, they removed trophectoderm (TE) cells from blastocysts, without compromising embryo viability. The TE cells were then stained for the presence of a Barr body, a dense structure formed by the inactive X chromosome in females, allowing them to successfully determine the sex of the embryos. This approach held significant implications for assisted reproduction, especially for couples at risk of passing on X-linked inherited diseases. However, despite this potential, the technical challenges of handling and analyzing human embryos at the time delayed further progress.

The first breakthrough came with the advent of the polymerase chain reaction (PCR) that made genetic analysis of a small number of cells feasible. PGT in human embryos was first introduced in the early nineties, aimed at preventing the transmission of single-gene disorders and other chromosomal abnormalities, such as translocations, from parents to their offspring. These early successes demonstrated the clinical viability of the technique and opened the door for its broader adoption. Initially, PGT also relied heavily on fluorescence in situ hybridization (FISH), performed on polar bodies or blastomeres from cleavage stage embryos. FISH assays use fluorescent nucleic acid probes complementary to DNA to visualize regions of interest. While pioneering at the time, the technology had significant limitations, as it could only analyze a subset of chromosomes over multiple rounds of hybridization. The informativity and accuracy of the results were influenced by the quality of the material, particularly the morphology

DOI: 10.1201/9781003460275-22

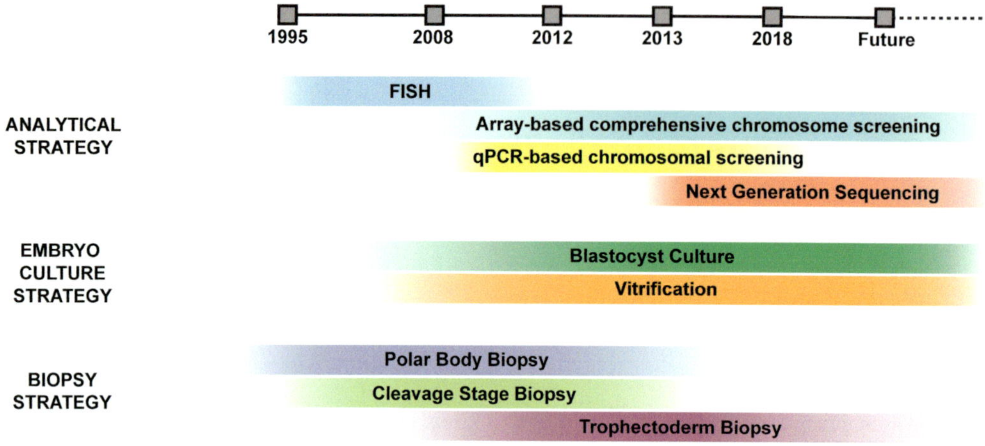

FIGURE 22.1. Overview of different preimplantation genetic testing approaches, their respective objectives, indications, and specific preclinical workflows. *Abbreviations:* PGT-A, preimplantation genetic testing for aneuploidies; PGT-M, preimplantation genetic testing for monogenic disorders; PGT-SR, preimplantation genetic testing for structural rearrangements.

and integrity of the single nuclei fixed onto a glass slide. Nevertheless, FISH rapidly revealed that more than half of all human preimplantation embryos harbored chromosomal abnormalities. Prompted by these findings and the hypothesis that embryo aneuploidy was a key factor affecting the success of assisted reproductive technologies (ART), researchers proposed that identifying and selecting embryos free of chromosomal abnormalities could significantly improve clinical outcomes. This led to the development of PGT-A as a practical tool aimed at enhancing embryo selection. Concurrently, biopsy protocols were successfully replicated and implemented in clinics worldwide, setting the stage for the broader use of PGT in ART.

Novel technologies for genetic testing facilitated the transition from FISH to comprehensive chromosomal analysis. Among these, array comparative genomic hybridization (aCGH) and single nucleotide polymorphism (SNP) arrays have been widely applied on polar bodies, blastomeres, and TE biopsies. Initially, array-based technologies were time-consuming, taking several days to complete. However, with the advent of vitrification, embryos could be efficiently cryopreserved after testing, allowing the transfer of unaffected embryos in a subsequent frozen embryo transfer cycle. With improved culture conditions, embryos were increasingly tested at the blastocyst stage of development, allowing for more cells to be sampled from the TE, increasing accuracy and supporting wider implementation.

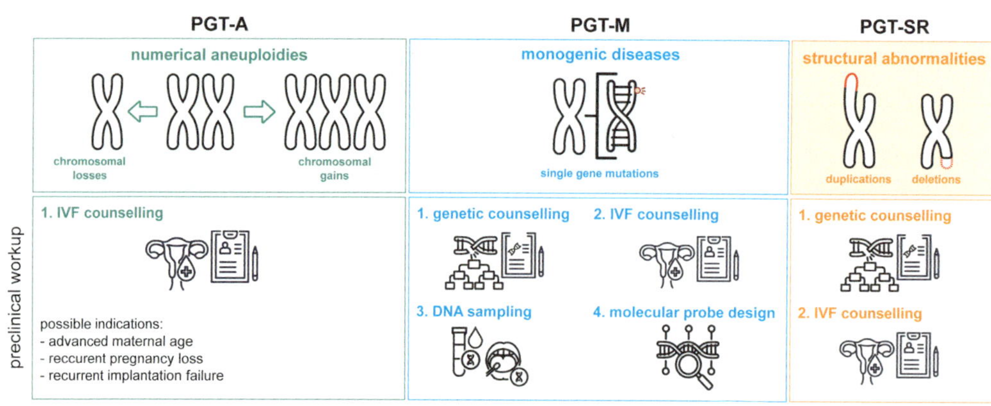

FIGURE 22.2 Historical overview of developments in analytical, embryo culture, and biopsy strategies that have shaped the field of preimplantation genetic testing. *Abbreviations:* qPCR, quantitative polymerase chain reaction.

Today, next generation sequencing (NGS) has gained widespread use for PGT due to its high throughput. The growing commercialization of PGT has expanded access to these technologies through industry-developed kits, protocols, and testing platforms, reducing waiting times and facilitating broader use. Moreover, minimally invasive and non-invasive PGT (niPGT) methods are emerging, though still require careful evaluation. While the evolving landscape of PGT offers the potential to improve efficiency, reduce risks, and optimize outcomes in fertility care, clinicians must remain mindful of the current limitations and thoughtfully integrate these technologies into their practice.

Indications for Preimplantation Genetic Testing

While PGT-A is applied more broadly, PGT-M and PGT-SR are offered to couples with known genetic risks (Table 22.1). These techniques allow for the selection of embryos that are free from genetic or chromosomal abnormalities, ultimately supporting the best possible outcome for the future family. They may also reduce the need for invasive prenatal diagnostics and help avoid difficult decisions of pregnancy termination for therapeutic reasons.

Preimplantation Genetic Testing for Aneuploidies

PGT-A evolved from what was previously known as Preimplantation Genetic Screening, PGS. It tests embryos for aneuploidy, the presence of an abnormal number of chromosomes, with an aim to identify embryos with the highest potential for a successful pregnancy. The clinical implementation of PGT-A revealed that human embryos frequently harbor chromosomal aberrations, a primary determinant of whether they will progress in development. The cytogenetic abnormalities observed in preimplantation embryos are also frequently identified in tissues from spontaneous miscarriages following *in vivo* conceptions. No extensive preclinical workup is typically required for the implementation of PGT-A (Figure 22.1).

Advanced Maternal Age

The success of human reproduction relies heavily on maternal age, with the probability of conception declining steadily after the age of 35. Both the quantity of available oocytes (ovarian reserve) and their quality (oocyte competence) decline with advancing maternal age. These age-related factors ultimately disrupt essential processes of chromosomal alignment and segregation during meiosis, leading to an increase in the frequency of aneuploidies in human oocytes as women age. Gains and losses of entire

TABLE 22.1

Potential Indications for PGT-A, PGT-M and PGT-SR

	PGT-A	PGT-M	PGT-SR
Advanced maternal age	■		
Recurrent pregnancy loss	■		
Recurrent implantation failure	■		
Autosomal dominant or recessive conditions		■	
Late-onset autosomal dominant conditions		■	
X-linked disorders		■	
Cancer predisposition		■	
HLA matching		■	
Risk of hemolytic disease of the fetus and newborn		■	
Carriers of balanced translocation			■
Carriers of inversions			■

chromosomes, trisomies and monosomies, are the most prevalent forms of aneuploidy and significantly impact embryo viability. Aneuploidies ultimately lead to adverse clinical outcomes, including implantation failure, spontaneous miscarriages, and congenital defects. Maternal aneuploidy rates from women under the age of 30 years are estimated to range from 10% to 30%, while for women of advanced maternal age (over the age of 35), aneuploidy rates range from 30% to over 85%. Accordingly, maternal age is among the strongest predictors of ART success. It is also the most common indication for PGT-A, as studies have shown that when euploid embryos are selectively transferred, implantation and pregnancy rates do not significantly differ between younger and older patients, up to the age of 42.

By excluding aneuploid embryos from transfer, PGT-A may help mitigate the age-related decline in fertility, enhancing the likelihood of a successful pregnancy per transfer, and reducing the emotional and financial burden on couples undergoing IVF. Nevertheless, a crucial consideration for women of advanced maternal age is that they may have a limited number of embryos available for testing.

Recurrent Pregnancy Loss

Recurrent pregnancy loss (RPL) was traditionally defined as the loss of three or more consecutive clinical pregnancies. However, updated guidelines from both the American Society for Reproductive Medicine (ASRM) and the European Society for Human Reproduction and Embryology (ESHRE) now broaden the definition to include two or more consecutive or non-consecutive pregnancy losses. With expanded criteria, the reported prevalence of RPL is estimated to affect 2–3% of couples trying to conceive.[1]

RPL has a multifactorial etiology, including parental chromosomal abnormalities, uterine abnormalities, endocrine, and immunological disorders. Yet up to 50% of all RPL cases remain unexplained. Studies have shown that couples with RPL have a higher number of chromosomally abnormal embryos, with rates ranging from 50% to 80%. This association has been further confirmed by research demonstrating an elevated incidence of chromosomal abnormalities in miscarriage tissues from unexplained RPL patients. Therefore, PGT-A has been proposed as a potential approach to reduce the risk of subsequent miscarriages by de-selecting aneuploid embryos. However, conflicting results from various studies have complicated this approach. While some report higher rates of aneuploidy in patients diagnosed with RPL, others show similar rates between RPL and non-RPL patients.

Couples with known chromosomal abnormalities, as well as women with a history of previous aneuploid losses, tend to benefit more clearly from PGT-A in the management of RPL. However, there are limited studies and no established guidelines or recommendations governing the use of PGT-A for couples with unexplained RPL. Research indicates that PGT-A can improve live birth and clinical pregnancy rates, particularly in older women, and suggests that selecting euploid blastocysts for transfer reduces miscarriage risk, even when only a few or poor-quality blastocysts are available. A recent systematic review and meta-analysis demonstrated that patients with unexplained RPL undergoing PGT-A had higher clinical pregnancy rates, lower clinical pregnancy loss rates, and improved live birth rates per transfer compared to those undergoing ART without PGT-A.[1] Nevertheless, the overall efficacy of PGT-A in unexplained RPL cases remains a point of contention. The available data are reported per embryo transfer, leaving some uncertainty about how many women began a cycle but failed to reach the transfer stage, potentially introducing selection bias. Additionally, many studies focus on women with RPL undergoing IVF for other diagnoses, limiting the ability to assess the utility of PGT-A in all RPL patients, particularly those who do not require IVF.

As a result, some suggest that PGT-A should only be recommended after spontaneous conception attempts have been made, and only in cases where fetal aneuploidy has been previously confirmed in miscarriage tissues. The live birth rate after expectant management for patients with RPL is approximately 60–70% depending on maternal age and number of previous losses. Therefore, sufficiently powered randomized controlled trials comparing PGT-A to expectant management are warranted. While awaiting more robust studies, PGT-A may offer benefits to women with a good ovarian reserve, who are likely to produce a sufficient number of embryos for testing, and to women of advanced maternal age who face a higher risk of embryo aneuploidy. By selecting euploid embryos, PGT-A may help reduce miscarriage risks and potentially shorten the time to achieving a live birth. Moreover, the co-occurrence of additional indications for PGT-A, such as known genetic abnormalities, may further enhance its potential benefits for these patients.[1]

Recurrent Implantation Failure

Recurrent implantation failure (RIF) has been historically defined as the failure to achieve a pregnancy after three or more embryo transfers or the cumulative transfer of ten or more high-quality embryos. However, this definition is not standardized, and the multifactorial nature of RIF, encompassing both maternal and embryonic aspects, further complicates diagnosis and treatment. As a result, the true incidence of RIF and the exact role of various implicated factors remain unclear.

Earlier studies estimated that RIF affects approximately 15% of couples undergoing IVF. However, more recent data challenge these figures, indicating that fewer than 5% of women with a normal uterine anatomy fail to achieve pregnancy after transferring three consecutive euploid embryos. These findings were further supported by Gill et al. in their international multicenter study of over 120,000 patients. They observed that after five consecutive euploid embryo transfers, the prevalence of RIF dropped to 2%.[2] They suggest that additional euploid transfers may reduce the prevalence even further, potentially to 0%, questioning the validity of RIF as a diagnosis in the absence of known uterine factors.

These findings are in agreement with a mathematical model based on blastocyst euploidy and implantation rates, which suggest that the likelihood of implantation success largely depends on female age and the probability of obtaining euploid embryos.[3] The authors also stress that the current threshold of embryo transfers used to diagnose RIF may be too rigid and overlook these important factors, particularly since embryo aneuploidy remains the most common cause of implantation failure. Therefore, after a thorough preconception evaluation and exclusion of other potential causes of implantation failure, such as communicating hydrosalpinges, intracavitary pathology, adenomyosis, obesity, or thyroid dysfunction, encouraging patients to proceed with additional euploid embryo transfers may lead to successful outcomes. In cases of unexplained failures, parental karyotyping may be a useful final assessment.[3] Nonetheless, lower live birth rates have been observed in some RIF patients even when euploid blastocysts are transferred, underscoring the need for further research to better define RIF and its underlying causes.

Preimplantation Genetic Testing for Monogenic Disorders

PGT-M, previously referred to as Preimplantation Genetic Diagnosis, PGD, has been primarily used to detect and prevent specific autosomal recessive, autosomal dominant, and X-linked single-gene disorders.[4] While it closely aligns with the scope of conventional prenatal diagnosis, the range of conditions for which PGT-M is applied continues to expand. With advancing technology, best practice guidelines, and external quality assessments, the accuracy of PGT-M has significantly improved, enabling multiple diagnoses from a single sample. The increased accessibility of preconception carrier screening for couples, including those without a family history of genetic disease, has also contributed to the rising number of PGT-M cases. This growth is further supported by the availability of expanded carrier screening panels, reduced costs, and government funding in many countries. PGT-M can now be used to screen embryos for a wide range of genetic disorders, as long as the genetic cause is known. Additional uses include gender selection, HLA typing, identifying hereditary cancers with variable penetrance (such as BRCA1/BRCA2 mutations), and screening for late-onset genetic diseases, all of which have sparked ethical debate.

In the United States, there are currently no formal, nationwide guidelines for determining when to offer or decline PGT-M. Individual physicians, genetic counselors, or PGT laboratories may establish their own internal policies based on ethical considerations and clinical factors. Patients are typically informed of any limitations or policies early in the process. However, in Europe, the approach is more regulated. For instance, ESHRE has issued comprehensive guidelines for the use of PGT-M, including recommendations on patient selection, counseling, and technical procedures.[4, 5] Furthermore, in some countries, such as the United Kingdom or Spain, clinics are required to seek national committee approval for any new genetic conditions being tested, ensuring that only severe conditions with clear genetic causes are considered.

The PGT-M workflow requires careful planning prior to IVF treatment and involves a preclinical phase tailored to the genetic background of each couple (Figure 22.1). The approach allows for a personalized and precise genetic diagnosis that maximizes the chances of selecting healthy embryos.[6]

Couples may become aware of their carrier status and genetic risk through various pathways, such as having an affected child, discovering a family history of a genetic disorder, or undergoing preconception carrier screening. In cases where there is a known risk, genetic counseling is essential both before and after testing to help couples navigate these risks and explore their reproductive options. After thorough genetic counseling, the specific genetic mutation responsible for the condition must be identified, provided that it is located in a region of the genome that can be adequately assessed. Couples should be informed that this process typically requires DNA samples (taken from blood or buccal swabs) from the couple, their parents, family members, and any affected children, if available. This phase can take weeks to months to complete. The DNA samples are analyzed in a specialized genetic laboratory to design unique molecular probes to detect the mutation and its flanking markers in embryos. In cases where the mutation is caused by complex variations, linkage analysis is used to track inheritance across generations. Linkage analysis identifies genetic markers, such as short tandem repeats (STRs) or SNPs, that are inherited alongside the mutation, allowing the identification of embryos carrying the genetic risk. To ensure accuracy, the probes are validated using known genotypes from the couple and their relatives. The protocol can then be applied to embryo biopsies to select healthy embryos. In more complex cases, Karyomapping may also be used, providing a broader genetic overview by mapping multiple genetic markers simultaneously. For further details on the technical aspects of PGT-M workflows, including the validation steps, refer to the ESHRE PGT Consortium good practice recommendations.[4]

Single-Gene Disorders

Single-gene disorders follow distinct inheritance patterns caused by mutations in specific genes. These conditions vary in severity, often leading to a significant reduction in quality of life and, in some cases, mortality, particularly in childhood. While single-gene disorders have been studied extensively, accurately assessing their frequency remains challenging due to underreporting of late-onset conditions and variations in prevalence across different populations. Early estimates placed the incidence of autosomal dominant conditions at 7 per 1000 live births, autosomal recessive conditions at 2.5 per 1000, and X-linked disorders at 0.5 per 1000, accounting for approximately 1% of all live births. Since then, the number of recognized conditions has grown significantly, with advances in DNA analysis revealing that, on average, each individual carries 2.8 recessive gene mutations without exhibiting symptoms. According to the latest ESHRE PGD Consortium data, nearly two-thirds of PGT-M analyses were performed for an autosomal dominant disease (64%), followed by autosomal recessive and X-linked indications, which accounted for 19% and 18%, respectively.[7]

Autosomal dominant disorders can be inherited from an affected parent or arise from a new (*de novo*) mutation in the individual. These conditions require only one mutated copy of the gene for a person to be affected, as the altered gene overrides the normal one. These conditions often run in families, affecting multiple generations. In cases of *de novo* mutations, it is crucial to identify the specific genetic variant prior to PGT-M. The most commonly tested autosomal dominant disorder in PGT-M analyses is Huntington's Disease, accounting for 9% of all tests.[7] Other prominent autosomal dominant conditions tested include hereditary breast–ovarian cancer (associated with BRCA1/BRCA2 mutations), myotonic dystrophy type 1, Marfan syndrome, neurofibromatosis type I, and Charcot-Marie-Tooth disease type 1A.[7]

Autosomal recessive disorders arise from loss-of-function pathogenic variants. They require both parents to pass on the defective allele for the disease to manifest in their offspring. Carriers, who possess a single pathogenic allele, are typically asymptomatic because the second functional allele on the homologous chromosome compensates for the defect. Consequently, children of two carrier parents have a 25% chance of inheriting both pathogenic variants, a 50% chance of being carriers themselves, and a 25% chance of inheriting two functional alleles. In contrast, offspring of affected individuals are obligate carriers of one pathogenic variant. In families with multiple affected generations, these diseases frequently skip one or more generations, as carriers may remain undetected due to their asymptomatic nature. Among the various autosomal recessive disorders, cystic fibrosis is the most frequently tested condition, accounting for approximately 3.7% of all PGT-M analyses, followed by beta-thalassemia.[7]

X-linked disorders are inherited in a manner where healthy carrier mothers pass the pathogenic allele to their male offspring, who are affected due to the absence of a second X chromosome that could compensate for the defective gene. Males with X-linked recessive disorders cannot transmit the condition to their sons; however, their daughters typically become carriers of the disorder, inheriting the affected X chromosome. Duchenne muscular dystrophy and fragile X syndrome are the most commonly evaluated X-linked disorders by PGT-M.[7]

Cancer Predisposition and Late-Onset Diseases

Most PGT-M cases are conducted for severe, life-threatening conditions that manifest during childhood and lack effective treatment. There is general consensus that PGT-M should be available for these situations, as it provides an important opportunity to prevent the transmission of serious genetic diseases. However, approximately a quarter of PGT-M cycles in the United States have been performed for adult-onset conditions.[6] ASRM supports the use of PGT-M in such cases if the condition is severe, and treatments are either ineffective or highly burdensome. For conditions with partial penetrance or where treatments are available, PGT-M can prevent the difficult decision of pregnancy termination by identifying embryos that are free of the mutation before pregnancy. Ethical concerns arise, however, in cases of adult-onset diseases where the risk of developing the condition is uncertain. The growing use of PGT-M for predispositions to cancers such as breast and colon cancer reflects increasing interest in minimizing genetic risks. Non-disclosure and exclusion testing allow patients to avoid knowing their own genetic status while ensuring that at-risk embryos are not selected for transfer. However, these approaches present logistical challenges and demand strict coordination in clinical settings to maintain the integrity of non-disclosure. This strategy is commonly applied for Huntington's disease where patients prefer not to learn their genetic status but wish to ensure their children do not inherit the mutation.

HLA Matching

The use of PGT-M in combination with HLA matching is one of the more controversial applications of PGT. This procedure involves selecting an embryo that is both free of a genetic disorder and HLA-compatible with an affected sibling, enabling the potential use of the embryo as a donor for hematopoietic stem cell transplantation. It is especially beneficial for children suffering from genetic conditions such as β-thalassemia, Fanconi anemia, as well as acquired hematologic disorders. HLA typing on preimplantation embryos is typically carried out using STR markers, which enable highly accurate detection of HLA alleles and recombination events across the HLA region.

Despite its benefits, PGT-M with HLA matching presents significant practical and ethical challenges. One major limitation is the low proportion of embryos that meet both genetic and HLA compatibility requirements. For autosomal recessive conditions, only approximately 18% of embryos fulfill both criteria, substantially reducing the number of blastocysts available for transfer. Furthermore, in cases where umbilical cord blood from an HLA matched sibling provides insufficient stem cells for transplantation, the donor child may need to grow before a bone marrow transplant can be performed. Consequently, time is a crucial factor, as the affected sibling may not survive long enough to benefit from the procedure. Therefore, from an ethical perspective, concerns arise regarding the instrumentalization of the donor child, who is conceived primarily to benefit an existing sibling. These concerns are exacerbated when the procedure is applied in less severe, non-life-threatening conditions. In such instances, the use of HLA matching may be pursued for experimental treatments, such as stem cell therapies, which currently lack established therapeutic efficacy.

Regulations surrounding the use of PGT-M for HLA differ across countries. In the United States, clinics generally have more flexibility in setting their policies, allowing broader access to this technology.

Conversely, European countries, including the United Kingdom, Italy, and France, enforce stricter guidelines, often requiring approval from national committees that evaluate the medical necessity of the procedure. Nonetheless, the demand for HLA matched embryos remains high, particularly in situations where suitable donors are not available within the family or through stem cell banks.

Hemolytic Disease of the Newborn

PGT-M can also be employed to prevent hemolytic disease of the newborn (HDN) by selecting embryos compatible with the maternal blood type, thereby avoiding maternal-fetal blood group incompatibility. HDN, also referred to as erythroblastosis fetalis, occurs when fetal red blood cells carry an antigen, such as RhD or Kell, that the mother lacks, triggering an immune response. This can result in the production of maternal antibodies that attack fetal red blood cells, leading to anemia, or in severe cases, fetal death. Although the incidence of severe RhD alloimmunization has decreased due to the use of prophylactic anti-D immunoglobulin, some women remain at risk of sensitization in future pregnancies. PGT-M can mitigate this risk by selecting Rh-negative embryos in cases where the father is heterozygous for the Rh factor or by ensuring compatibility with other blood group factors like Kell. This reduces the likelihood of HDN and complications such as the need for intrauterine transfusions.

Polygenic and Multifactorial Conditions

Historically, PGT for polygenic and multifactorial conditions has been limited due to the challenges of accurately predicting risks. However, the recent introduction of clinically available PGT for polygenic conditions (PGT-P) has sparked interest. Nevertheless, the application of PGT-P remains controversial and is still evolving. Concerns persist regarding the accuracy of risk prediction and the ethical implications of selecting embryos based on polygenic traits, as the field lacks robust data and a clear consensus on its clinical utility.

Preimplantation Genetic Testing for Structural Rearrangements

PGT-SR is primarily indicated for individuals or couples who are carriers of balanced segmental rearrangements, such as translocations or inversions. These rearrangements do not involve a loss or gain of genetic material, and, therefore, carriers typically present with a normal phenotype. However, during meiosis, these structural rearrangements can result in the formation of unbalanced gametes, which may lead to chromosomal abnormalities in embryos. This increases the risk of infertility, recurrent miscarriages, or congenital abnormalities in offspring. PGT-SR minimizes these risks, potentially reducing the time to achieve a successful pregnancy. Translocations and inversions are the most common types of structural chromosomal rearrangements.

No extensive preclinical workup is typically required for the implementation of PGT-SR (Figure 22.1). Nevertheless, it is important to assess any pathological copy number variations and chromosomal rearrangements in the parental karyotype. These factors need to be considered to confirm that the applied molecular platform has sufficient resolution to detect the specific genomic region involved in the chromosomal rearrangement in embryos.

Inversions

Inversions involve two breaks along the chromosome, followed by the reinsertion of the inverted segment, which changes the linear gene sequence but does not result in a gain or loss of genetic material. As a result, inversions are balanced and do not alter the gene copy number. However, they can disrupt gene function at the inversion breakpoints or affect the expression of nearby genes and regulatory elements. This can lead to varying consequences, such as disrupted gene regulation or coding sequence, although the exact functional impacts of inversions remain poorly understood. Inversions can be further classified as pericentric (involving both chromosomal arms and the centromere) or paracentric (affecting only one arm without involving the centromere). While inversions do not directly cause phenotypic abnormalities, meiotic crossing over within the inverted segment can result in unbalanced gametes. Paracentric inversions often lead to non-viable germ cells due to the presence of either no centromere or two centromeres, while pericentric inversions may result in gametes with deletions or duplications, potentially causing birth defects. The risk of unbalanced gametes is thus dependent on the type as well as the size of the inversion and is proportional to the chance of crossing over occurring within the inverted segment.

Balanced Translocations

Balanced translocations, on the other hand, occur when two chromosomes undergo double-strand breaks and exchange fragments. This leads to a rearrangement of chromosomal segments. The prevalence of balanced translocations in the general population is around 0.2%, but it increases to 0.6% in infertile couples and can be as high as 9.2% in couples experiencing RPL. Many carriers are unaware of their translocation until genetic analysis is conducted after a pregnancy loss or the birth of an affected child.

Carriers of balanced translocations typically have a normal phenotype but are at a higher risk of producing unbalanced gametes, leading to embryos with chromosomal abnormalities. Interestingly, studies have revealed that up to 50% of chromosomally unbalanced embryos obtained from translocation carriers display chaotic cleavage and thus will not develop past the first stages of development. Moreover, it has been suggested that blastocyst formation rates are significantly lower in cases where the female carries the chromosomal translocation. Nevertheless, population selection may be biased, as patients choosing PGT-SR generally have a more severe reproductive history.

Balanced translocations are classified into two main categories: reciprocal translocations, which involve the exchange of segments between two non-homologous chromosomes, and Robertsonian translocations. The frequency of unbalanced gametes varies widely with each translocation carrier. Therefore, assessing the reproductive risks for carriers of reciprocal translocations is particularly challenging, as each case tends to be unique, depending on the chromosomes involved and the breakpoints.

Robertsonian Translocations

Robertsonian translocations occur when two acrocentric chromosomes (13, 14, 15, 21, and 22, in humans) fuse at the centromere. Ultimately, this results in a fusion of long arms and a loss of the short arms of these chromosomes. Comparable to carriers of balanced rearrangements, carriers of Robertsonian translocations generally demonstrate a normal phenotype, they are at risk of producing chromosomally abnormal offspring due to improper segregation of the translocated chromosomes during meiosis. This can result in embryos with trisomies or monosomies.

Robertsonian translocations are more prevalent in individuals with infertility, especially oligospermic men, where incomplete chromosome pairing during meiosis can interfere with spermatogenesis. However, some studies have reported no significant differences in sperm quality between carriers of balanced translocations and individuals with normal karyotypes. Ultimately, it remains challenging to ascertain the influence of translocations on infertility, particularly in the absence of precise experimental tools for gaining clear mechanistic insights and the lack of systematic comparative analyses of Robertsonian carriers. Despite these variations, couples carrying Robertsonian translocations typically produce fewer transferable blastocysts, with rates dropping from 30% in cases of Robertsonian translocations to 20% in reciprocal translocations.

When the indication involves Robertsonian translocations, any molecular technique with sufficient resolution to detect whole chromosome aneuploidies is suitable. In contrast, detecting imbalances caused by reciprocal translocations requires more advanced, high-resolution technologies, such as microarrays or NGS to precisely identify smaller chromosomal imbalances that may not be detectable by conventional methods.

Preimplantation Genetic Testing Techniques

Embryo Biopsy

PGT has been applied at different stages of preimplantation development for sampling polar bodies, blastomeres at the cleavage stage, and TE cells at the blastocyst stage of development, each stage presenting with advantages and limitations (Figure 22.3).

Polar Body Biopsy

As a large proportion of meiotic errors originate from the oocyte, biopsy of the first and second polar body following fertilization provides a feasible option for genetic testing. Several groups have applied this strategy for diagnosing monogenic disorders and translocations and for aneuploidy screening, predominately in cases of advanced maternal age. As embryos are sampled early on, genetic analysis can be performed in time for a fresh embryo transfer. However, this approach only allows the detection of maternal meiotic aberrations. Nevertheless, until recently, this approach was the only PGT platform allowed in some countries, including Italy and Germany.

Cleavage Stage, Blastomere Biopsy

Cleavage stage biopsy encompasses the removal of one or two blastomeres from good quality, day 3 embryos. This approach allows identification of both maternal and paternal chromosomal contributions and, like polar body biopsy, has the advantage of supporting a fresh embryo transfer strategy. Although several groups have strongly criticized this approach due to the potential risk of embryo, others have achieved more optimal results. Nevertheless, with advances in embryo culture and cryopreservation techniques, the current success of PGT has heavily relied on the shift from cleavage to blastocyst stage biopsy.

Blastocyst Stage, Trophectoderm Biopsy

TE biopsy is currently the standard approach for PGT. It is performed at the blastocyst stage, on day 5, day 6, or day 7 of development. As lineage segregation has occurred, biopsy of the extraembryonic

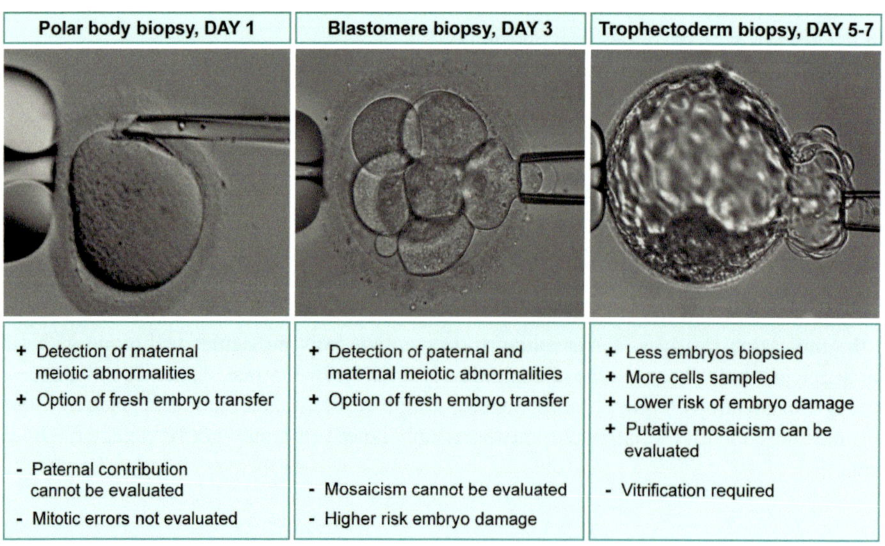

FIGURE 22.3 Different embryo biopsy strategies for PGT. Embryo developmental stage, as well as the advantages and limitations of each approach are described.

TE cells is less likely to affect embryo viability. Moreover, blastocyst culture will inherently result in less embryos being biopsied, while more cells can be tested, reducing the risk of technical artefacts. Embryo biopsies require skilled embryologists and consequently the allocation of additional human resources in IVF laboratories, often associated with an increase in treatment costs. In practice, it is not possible to precisely control the number of cells taken from the TE. Accordingly, removing too many cells increases the risk of impairing embryo viability, while removing too little cells will inherently influence the accuracy of PGT. A robust quality assurance and quality control framework minimizes variability and prevents diagnostic inaccuracies, which could lead to misclassification of embryos. Best practices emphasize optimized sample handling, shipping, and stable long-term storage environments for preserving the quality of the genetic material being tested.[8]

Minimally Invasive and Non-invasive Approaches

In addition to invasive PGT techniques, recent advancements have led to the exploration of minimally invasive and non-invasive PGT (niPGT-A). As of now, niPGT has primarily been applied for PGT-A (niPGT-A). This method analyzes cell-free DNA (cfDNA) found in the spent culture media (SCM) of embryos, which can reflect the chromosomal status of the embryo without the need for an invasive biopsy. Research is ongoing to optimize this approach due to challenges such as lower DNA quantity and potential contamination from non-embryonic cells.

Recent studies have reported the presence of cfDNA in the blastocoel cavity and spent embryo culture media. Less invasive PGT approaches may present several advantages, reducing the cost of extensive micromanipulation, lowering the risk of damaging the embryo, and allowing genetic testing even when blastocyst quality is insufficient for biopsy. While niPGT-A on SCM may present potential benefits, particularly by removing the need for embryo biopsies, its accuracy remains a subject of ongoing investigation. The presence of maternal cumulus cells and amplification artefacts may all account for diagnostic errors. Moreover, the extent to which cfDNA reflects the genotype of all embryonic cells remains to be investigated. Current studies have demonstrated considerable variability in concordance rates between niPGT-A and the gold-standard TE biopsy, ranging between of 33.3% up to 89.1%, and also between niPGT-A and whole blastocysts, ranging from 45.5% to 93.8%. Nevertheless, niPGT-A has been implemented in clinical practice as a ranking tool and may provide additional information for embryo selection. Further refinement of niPGT-A protocols, combined with larger validation studies, will be crucial for its widespread adoption in clinical practice. An alternative approach involves blastocentesis, obtaining cfDNA through the aspiration of blastocoel fluid. Although promising for clinical practice, its application remains difficult, and studies have reported variable accuracy. While we have seen and are likely to experience significant technological progress in embryo sampling approaches, currently, TE biopsy remains the gold standard, providing the most robust and reliable source of embryonic DNA for PGT.

Molecular Diagnostic Techniques

As PGT platforms continue to evolve, it is essential that IVF providers thoroughly understand these technologies to offer the best possible counseling to patients and select the most suitable platform based on specific clinical needs.

Whole Genome Amplification

A major challenge in performing genetic analysis for PGT is the low DNA input available for analysis. A single cell contains approximately 7 picograms of genomic DNA, which is insufficient for most genetic tests presently available. Consequently, the integration of advanced genomic techniques for PGT has fundamentally relied on whole genome amplification (WGA), allowing vast amounts of DNA (>2 μg) to be generated from single cells. Many different WGA protocols have been developed over time, some of which are commercially available. However, different methods of WGA guide downstream applications, each with their benefits and limitations.

Despite the large quantities of DNA produced, it is important to recognize that WGA methods may lead to sampling bias, namely under- or over-representation of the genome at specific loci. None of the currently available WGA methods provide a fully accurate, linear representation of the single- or few-cell genome. The results can vary in terms of allelic dropout (ADO), preferential amplification, genome coverage, and the occurrence of nucleotide copy errors, leading to some degree of inconsistency across different methods. The type and extent of the bias vary with each WGA method and also depend on aspects of the DNA sample itself. Artefacts arising from the cell-cycle phase can also impact the interpretation of results. While computational algorithms can partially mitigate some of the biases introduced by WGA, they cannot completely remove them. More recently, targeted WGA protocols have emerged as an improvement, selectively amplifying specific genomic regions to improve the precision and reduce errors in detecting both aneuploidies and monogenic disease mutations.

Preimplantation Genetic Testing for Aneuploidies

Shallow Whole Genome Next Generation Sequencing

Shallow whole genome NGS is commonly used for PGT-A due to its ability to detect whole chromosome aneuploidies with relatively low genome coverage, typically ranging from 0.1x to 1x. This approach is widely adopted because it offers an efficient and cost-effective method to analyze chromosomal abnormalities by leveraging read-depth data, although it is not suitable for detecting single nucleotide variations or balanced chromosomal rearrangements.

For NGS, most protocols start with WGA. This is followed by library preparation, which includes barcoding and fragmentation of input DNA prior to PCR. The barcoding process allows biopsies to be pooled together in one sequencing run, optimizing cost. Following sequencing, each sample is aligned to the human reference genome, and whole chromosome abnormalities and structural aberrations can be calculated using specific algorithms. The detection of chromosomal abnormalities is based on read depth of the sequencing data for each genomic locus or window. Accordingly, more sequencing reads at a given genomic locus point to a duplication, while less sequencing reads indicate a deletion.

Currently there are two major platforms for NGS, Illumina MiSeq™ and ThermoFisher Ion Proton™. Both platforms utilize benchtop sequencers with fast turnover, targeted for clinical applications, however, employ different sequencing technologies. Illumina MiSeq™ is centered on sequencing by synthesis, while ThermoFisher Ion Proton™ technology uses semiconductor sequencing.

Single Nucleotide Polymorphism Platforms

Today, NGS has gained widespread use in PGT-A due to its high throughput. Nevertheless, both SNP arrays and NGS have significantly enhanced detection capabilities of PGT-A, with the choice of method depending on clinical objectives, cost, availability, and the type of analysis required. In addition, NGS platforms can also sequence SNPs, integrating SNP genotyping with high-throughput sequencing to enhance the resolution of chromosomal abnormalities. This combined approach can yield more precise results.

SNP genotyping offers additional benefits by detecting genome-wide ploidy, parthenogenetic activation, and uniparental heterodisomy. Genome-wide haplotypes and SNP genotypes can also provide information on the origin of a trisomy, which may enhance embryo ranking for transfer. However, to determine inheritance patterns, these tools currently require reference DNA from family members, which may present limitations for its use.

Preimplantation Genetic Testing for Monogenic Disorders

Direct Mutation Analysis

Direct mutation analysis involves PCR-based techniques where specific primers target the mutation of interest. Here, the key strategy is multiplex PCR, which allows simultaneous amplification of multiple loci of interest, including both the mutation and linked markers to reduce the risk of errors such as ADO, where one allele fails to amplify, leading to possible misdiagnosis. By analyzing closely linked STR markers, the accuracy of diagnosis is improved, especially in cases where single mutations are being tested. STR markers are highly specific and differ in the number of repetitions between one allele and another, as well as between individuals. This direct analysis, combined with other mutation-specific detection techniques like quantitative real-time PCR, mini-sequencing, or even Sanger sequencing, helps to precisely identify and confirm the mutation of concern.

Karyomapping

Karyomapping is a comprehensive approach offering a genome-wide analysis of embryos by mapping SNPs across the entire genome. SNPs are the most common form of genomic variation in humans and are responsible for about 90% of human genetic diversity. Karyomapping enables the detection of monogenic disorders through indirect mutation analysis, eliminating the need for patient- or mutation-specific probes.

Karyomapping begins by genotyping both parents and, if possible, a close relative with a known genetic status. SNPs are then analyzed in the parental genomes to create a chromosomal map of the haplotypes they pass on to their offspring. The embryos are subsequently genotyped using SNP arrays. This method provides a high-resolution visualization of the embryonic karyotype, displaying four panels of SNPs for each chromosome. By comparing the embryo SNP data to the parental haplotypes, karyomapping allows the identification of embryos that have inherited the chromosomal segments linked to disease-causing mutations.

SNP genotyping is generally preferred over STRs due to the higher frequency of SNPs in the genome, which makes them more informative in indirect analyses. One of the main advantages of karyomapping is that it serves as a universal platform for diagnosing a wide range of monogenic disorders without the need for mutation-specific tests. It also provides additional advantages such as the ability to concurrently perform PGT-M, PGT-A, and PGT-SR. In cases of meiotic errors, karyomapping can detect trisomies or duplications based on the excess of a parental haplotype, and monosomies or deletions through the absence of a haplotype. However, karyomapping relies on informative SNPs, which limits its ability to detect *de novo* mutations, which are not inherited from the parents. In these cases, direct mutation analysis may still be required.

Next Generation Sequencing

NGS is increasingly being adopted for PGT-M due to its ability to sequence entire genomes or target regions at a high resolution. This method allows for comprehensive screening of monogenic mutations alongside chromosomal aneuploidies in a single workflow. Platforms including OnePGT, GENType, and HaploPGT integrate haplotyping with NGS, allowing for precise detection of disease-associated mutations and surrounding SNPs, while also providing chromosomal copy number analysis. While each of these platforms offers distinct advantages, several limitations have restricted their widespread adoption. These include the need for reference DNA from parents or family members, which may not always be available; high costs due to the extensive sequencing reads and complex bioinformatics analysis required; and the necessity of prior diagnosis using independent technology, which add layers of complexity.

Clinical Value of Preimplantation Genetic Testing

The clinical value of PGT-M and PGT-SR is more clearly established. As these targeted applications offer more direct benefits, particularly for couples at risk of passing on inheritable conditions, the clinical utility of these tests is more straightforward and less controversial compared to PGT-A. What sets PGT-A apart from other diagnostic tests is its predictive nature. Traditional diagnostic tests, such as genetic testing for cystic fibrosis, diagnose an existing condition in a patient, allowing for immediate clinical intervention. In contrast, PGT-A assesses the future reproductive potential of embryos, aiming to streamline the embryo-selection process and improve the efficiency of fertility treatments. While the technology has undoubtedly evolved, the value of PGT-A remains controversial. PGT-A is currently actively marketed as a means for improving clinical outcomes, suggested to increase implantation rates, reduce miscarriages, and decrease the time to pregnancy. However, the evidence to substantiate these claims remains limited. There is a noticeable lack of well-controlled clinical trials to validate its diagnostic accuracy. Ultimately, the rapid evolution of PGT-A technologies highlights the ongoing tension between technological advancement and the need for rigorous analytical validation.

As PGT-A becomes increasingly integrated into clinical practice, significant variability in results between laboratories and clinics has become a pressing concern. This inconsistency complicates embryo transfer decisions and has led to patient counseling practices that are sometimes driven more by opinion rather than by solid, evidence-based conclusions. These discrepancies undermine the reliability of PGT-A, fostering skepticism in the field and ultimately hindering its broader adoption and reducing its perceived clinical value. This ongoing debate reflects the need for a balanced approach that weighs the potential benefits of PGT-A against its limitations and challenges. This will ensure that its intended use and accuracy are closely aligned with clinical outcomes, crucial to avoid overextending the application of PGT-A beyond what current evidence reliably supports.

In the context of PGT-A, uniform whole chromosome abnormalities can be detected with sufficient accuracy, as the TE biopsy is likely to reflect the chromosomal constitution of the embryo. Moreover, such diagnoses are largely predictive of clinical outcomes. In the study by Tiegs and colleagues, embryos were biopsied and transferred without prior knowledge of the genetic results, allowing for a direct comparison of predicted PGT-A diagnoses to actual clinical outcomes.[9] Among the 102 embryos presenting with uniform whole chromosome aneuploidies, 40.2% implanted, 23.5% sustained implantation, however, none progressed to live birth. Therefore, focusing on identifying and excluding embryos with whole chromosome aneuploidies offers a clearer clinical framework for PGT-A.

Findings of Uncertain Clinical Significance: Chromosomal Mosaicism

The introduction of mosaic diagnoses has further complicated our understanding of the clinical utility and the accuracy of PGT-A. Chromosomal mosaicism is biologically defined as the presence of two or more cell lines with different karyotypes within the same embryo. Unlike meiotic errors, which affect all cells uniformly, mosaicism arises during the mitotic divisions that underlie embryogenesis. The presence of mosaicism may thus present inconsistencies across different parts of the embryo, such as between the TE and ICM.

In recent years, diagnoses consistent with chromosomal mosaicism have emerged as a third category of possible embryo ploidy outcomes following PGT-A. A critical factor is that a number of healthy live births have been achieved following the transfer of mosaic blastocysts. In 2015, Greco and colleagues reported the clinical transfer of embryos classified as mosaic for the first time.[10] Previously, mosaic embryos were deemed clinically unsuitable due to inherent reservations about transferring embryos that were suspected to contain some abnormal cells. Since then, several studies have suggested that embryos diagnosed as mosaic can lead to normal live births. The selective elimination of abnormal cells through the competitive growth of normal cells has been proposed as a mechanism by which human mosaic embryos tolerate chromosomal instability. These findings have led to recommendations to transfer mosaic embryos in the absence of a euploid alternative.[11]

Mosaicism is assessed following NGS using chromosome copy number values. If a value falls outside the normal range (typically between 1.8 and 2.2) but does not reach full monosomy or trisomy thresholds (below 1.2 or above 2.8), the embryo is classified as mosaic. However, these intermediate copy number values may be indistinguishable from mosaic results due to technical noise and WGA artifacts. Mosaicism predictions are further complicated by arbitrary intermediate copy number threshold values. For example, some providers classify mosaicism within a 20–80% abnormal cell range (copy number values between 1.2 and 2.8), while others use a narrower range of 30–70% abnormal cells (copy numbers between 1.3 and 2.7). Other factors also lead to variability, including NGS platforms, provider specific guidelines, and bioinformatics algorithms. Such inconsistencies have led to significant variability in interpretations and reporting standards and have ultimately raised concerns about the accuracy of

PGT-A. These discrepancies have also led to varying clinical policies regarding the storage and transfer of mosaic embryos,[11] contributing to further uncertainty in clinical practice. Ensuring high-quality care necessitates greater standardization of PGT-A classification schemes and proprietary algorithms for interpreting mosaic diagnoses. Such standardization will be crucial in establishing evidence-based guidelines for the field.

At present, careful consideration is recommended in cases in which mosaic embryos are considered for transfer. All current guidelines prioritize uniformly normal embryos for transfer, and, therefore, mosaic embryos are only transferred in the absence of this alternative. Recommendations for transferring mosaic embryos have been proposed based on certain parameters of mosaicism, including the percentage of abnormal cells, the size of the abnormality, and the chromosomes involved. However, these recommendations remain largely conceptual and clinical data remain conflicting. It is important to note that current guidelines have been based on retrospective studies that have suggested that mosaic embryos have a reduced reproductive potential compared to normal embryos. In these studies, mosaic embryos were only considered for transfer if no normal embryos were available and thus largely involved poor prognosis patient cohorts, which may ultimately bias conclusions. Prospective studies have now shown similar reproductive outcomes of normal and low-level (<50% abnormal cells) mosaic embryos.[12]

Prevailing concerns regarding the potential risks of mosaicism on development continue to complicate clinical decision-making following PGT-A. Thus, despite recommendations to transfer mosaic embryos, it appears that many patients do not end up using their stored mosaic embryos primarily due to a high-risk perception associated with such diagnoses. Furthermore, recent findings suggest that classifying embryos as mosaic, according to current clinical practice, may come at the expense of euploid diagnoses, potentially leading to the exclusion of viable embryos.[13] Standardizing mosaicism thresholds may help mitigate these inconsistencies. More contemporary platforms for PGT-A that include SNP genotyping may help to distinguish true mosaicism from technical noise, by detecting allele frequency changes in addition to copy number variations.

While there is still little evidence to ascertain which embryos with mosaic results have the best chance of resulting in a successful pregnancy, or the lowest risk for an undesirable outcome, mosaic blastocysts are inevitably being transferred during routine IVF cycles that do not include PGT-A. Importantly, there is currently no evidence of an increased risk of chromosomal mosaicism in children born following ART. If mosaic blastocysts can indeed result in viable pregnancies, excluding them from consideration may unnecessarily compromise treatment outcomes, especially for patients with few or no euploid embryos, such as women of advanced maternal age, a group that commonly undergoes PGT-A. Due to the technical variability among genetic testing laboratories and platforms, it remains essential to exercise caution when interpreting PGT-A results. Clinicians should ask their providers detailed questions about the validation processes for PGT-A results and the quality control measures in place to ensure accuracy. Above all, it is critical to inform patients diligently about the risks, challenges, and limitations of PGT-A, ensuring that decisions are based on transparent, evidence-based information.

Key Points

- PGT platforms continue to evolve offering not only aneuploidy testing but a wider array of genetic testing capabilities.
- It will be essential that IVF providers thoroughly understand these technologies to offer the best possible counseling to patients and select the most suitable platform based on specific clinical needs.

REFERENCES

1. Mumusoglu S et al. Preimplantation genetic testing for aneuploidy in unexplained recurrent pregnancy loss: a systematic review and meta-analysis. *Fertil Steril* 2025;123(1):121–36.

2. Gill P et al. Does recurrent implantation failure exist? Prevalence and outcomes of five consecutive euploid blastocyst transfers in 123 987 patients. *Hum Reprod* 2024;39(5):974–80.
3. Ata B et al. A new definition of recurrent implantation failure on the basis of anticipated blastocyst aneuploidy rates across female age. *Fertil Steril* 2021;116(5):1320–7.
4. ESHRE PGT-M Working Group et al. ESHRE PGT Consortium good practice recommendations for the detection of monogenic disorders. *Hum Reprod Open* 2020;2020(3):hoaa018.
5. ESHRE PGT Consortium Steering Committee, et al. ESHRE PGT Consortium good practice recommendations for the organisation of PGT. *Human Reprod Open* 2020;2020(3):hoaa021.
6. Practice Committee and Genetic Counseling Professional Group, ASRM. Indications and management of preimplantation genetic testing for monogenic conditions: a committee opinion. *Fertil Steril* 2023;120(1):61–71.
7. Spinella F et al. ESHRE PGT Consortium data collection XXI: PGT analyses in 2018. *Human Reprod Open* 2023;2023(2):hoad010.
8. ESHRE PGT Consortium and SIG-Embryology Biopsy Working Group et al. ESHRE PGT Consortium and SIG Embryology good practice recommendations for polar body and embryo biopsy for PGT. *Human Reprod Open* 2020;2020(3):hoaa020.
9. Tiegs AW et al. A multicenter, prospective, blinded, nonselection study evaluating the predictive value of an aneuploid diagnosis using a targeted next-generation sequencing–based preimplantation genetic testing for aneuploidy assay and impact of biopsy. *Fertil Steril* 2021;115(3):627–37.
10. Greco E et al. Healthy babies after intrauterine transfer of mosaic aneuploid blastocysts. *New Engl J Med* 2015;373(21):2089–90.
11. Practice Committees, ASRM and GCPG. Clinical management of mosaic results from preimplantation genetic testing for aneuploidy of blastocysts: a committee opinion. *Fertil Steril* 2023;120(5):973–82.
12. Capalbo A et al. Mosaic human preimplantation embryos and their developmental potential in a prospective, non-selection clinical trial. *Am J Hum Genet* 2021;108(12):2238–47.
13. Popovic M et al. Implicit bias in diagnosing mosaicism amongst preimplantation genetic testing providers: results from a multicenter study of 36 395 blastocysts. *Human Reprod* 2024;39(1):258–74.

23

Challenges in the Laboratory: Fertilization Failure and Poor Blastulation

Marc Torra-Massana and Karina Lattes

Infertility, which is estimated to affect 15% of couples worldwide, results in the impossibility to conceive *in vivo*. In the last years, significant advances in the field of reproductive medicine and assisted reproductive technologies have offered many infertile patients the option to form a family. Nevertheless, success in IVF treatments is far from being guaranteed, as the live birth rate after one cycle remains around 30%. While implantation failure or pregnancy loss are two major contributors to this relatively low rate, there are two additional problems that are frustrating for patients and clinics: fertilization failure and poor blastulation. Both situations are important challenges within the IVF laboratory, leading to the absence of embryos to transfer, and its management is usually difficult from a clinical point of view.

While different factors—–either from the male or the female—have been associated with fertilization and/or blastulation failure, the etiology of both problems is still far from being completely understood. This chapter will provide an overview of fertilization failure and poor blastulation, including the different factors causing or associated with these problems, as well as the different strategies to address them in the laboratory.

Fertilization Failure and Poor Blastulation: Definition and Incidence

In an IVF cycle, total fertilization failure (FF) is defined as the absence of correctly fertilized oocytes (zygotes with two pronuclei and two polar bodies) at 16–19h post-insemination either by ICSI or by conventional IVF. In the laboratory, this can translate to the presence at day 1 of abnormally fertilized oocytes (abnormal number of PN), oocyte degeneration, or, more often, oocyte activation failure (OAF), where the inseminated oocytes remain at metaphase II (MII).

ICSI with ejaculated spermatozoa—the most common insemination technique in fertility clinics from the United States and Europe—results in a mean fertilization rate (FR) of 70–80% per injected MII. In many cases, FF is associated with the insemination of a small number of oocytes: FF occurs in ~17% of cycles with three oocytes or less, and in ~31% of cycles with just one mature oocyte available. However, FF incidence remains at 1–3% even when inseminating a high number of oocytes. Importantly, FF can be repetitive, and it can happen even when morphologically normal sperm and oocytes are used.

Similarly, while not having such a huge impact from a clinical point of view, low or poor fertilization can also lead to the absence of embryos to transfer. Poor fertilization rate occurs when the proportion of oocytes correctly fertilized is considerably lower than the proportion one would expect for a specific insemination technique. For instance, considering that the reported efficiency of ICSI is around 70–80% fertilization rate, a fertilization rate of just 10–20% in an IVF cycle could be considered poor fertilization. However, there is no specific threshold established in the literature to clinically define what is "poor fertilization": 20%, 30%, 33%, or 40% are just some common examples proposed by different authors.

DOI: 10.1201/9781003460275-23

Finally, much less common in an IVF laboratory, zygotic arrest also contributes to the failure of an IVF cycle. In these cases, while the fertilization rate is good, the zygotes fail to undergo the first mitotic division, resulting in embryos arrested at the 1-cell stage.

But even if the fertilization rate is OK and the first mitotic divisions are completed successfully, poor blastulation can happen. Embryonic arrest is a very common phenomenon in IVF, as 50–70% of embryos fail to make it to the blastocyst stage (the embryos do not initiate or complete the compaction and cavitation processes essential for blastocyst formation), and is characterized by downregulation of metabolic activity and cessation of cell division. Nevertheless, poor blastulation can be considered when there is a total absence of viable blastocysts (or an unexpectedly very low number of blastocysts). These cases are usually accompanied by poor embryo quality, usually characterized by high percentages of fragmentation and aberrant cleavage divisions during the first 2–3 days post-insemination.

What Causes FF and Poor Blastulation?

In conventional IVF (c-IVF), where sperm are added to the cumulus oocyte complexes for insemination, successful fertilization is dependent on good motility and the ability of sperm to bind and penetrate the oocyte. Severe defects in sperm motility and morphology are the most common cause of unsuccessful fertilization after c-IVF. In addition, any problem affecting the capacity of sperm to undergo successful capacitation *in vitro* (and subsequent gain of hyperactivated motility) as well as specific alterations affecting the sperm–oocyte interaction (either at the cumulus cells, zona pellucida, or the oolemma) are likely to be a cause of FF.

The situation is completely different when using ICSI. Successful fertilization and the onset of embryo development are more dependent on a specific pattern of intracellular calcium oscillations in the oocyte cytoplasm (triggered by the sperm protein PLCZ1), which promotes oocyte activation. These Ca^{2+} oscillations promote the resumption of meiosis, extrusion of 2nd polar body, cytoskeletal reorganization, and cortical granule exocytosis. Sperm decondensation, formation of the pronuclei, and generation of the first mitotic spindle are also crucial steps to achieve successful fertilization.

The most common etiology of FF after ICSI is by far oocyte activation failure (OAF; the failure to elicit the release from the meiotic block in response to sperm entry in the oocyte), accounting for ~40–80% of non-fertilized oocytes. Cytoplasmic immaturity can explain part of the FF cases: MII oocytes with immature cytoplasm cannot support sperm decondensation, leading to failed fertilization and the formation of aberrant meiotic spindles. Altogether, lack of sperm nucleus decondensation and/or aster formation, defects in the oocyte spindle and cytoskeletal function, the sperm's inability to trigger calcium oscillations, or the inability of the oocyte machinery to respond to its stimuli account for common causes of FF. Deficiencies in key proteins involved in oocyte activation, such as WEE1 and PLCZ1, may explain these problems. For example, abnormal levels and localization of PLCZ1 protein within the sperm head may cause FF. As another example, severe forms of teratozoospermia, such as globozoospermia, characterized by the presence of sperm with round head, lack of acrosome, and non-existing levels of PLCZ1, can lead to OAF after ICSI. Similarly, zygotic arrest seems to be associated with specific morphological features in the zygote, such as uneven pronuclear size, reduced organization of nucleolar precursor bodies, and chromosomal abnormalities.

Regarding preimplantational embryo development, it is largely influenced by inherited maternal/paternal factors. The first divisions and embryonic genome activation (EGA) are largely dependent on stored maternal factors and the participation of multiple genes of maternal origin. Hence, poor oocyte quality is one of the main causes of poor blastulation and, importantly, is highly dependent upon maternal age. Embryonic arrest can be caused by inadequate maternal mRNA content or mutations in relevant genes, and any problem affecting EGA is likely to affect blastulation rate.

Advanced maternal age is associated with a higher incidence of aneuploidies in the embryo. Chromosomal abnormalities represent the major cause of developmental arrest, as most aneuploid embryos arrest their development at the cell or morula stages.

Male infertility also affects embryo preimplantational development. Low fertilization rates and poor embryo development are more common in patients with alterations in sperm condensation, oxidative stress, and/or sperm parameters (such as severe asthenozoospermia, cryptozoospermia, or use of testicular sperm). High levels of sperm DNA fragmentation have also been associated with compromised preimplantational embryo development, especially double-strand DNA breaks. But, overall, the mechanisms behind human embryo developmental arrest remain poorly characterized.

The Important Role of Genetic Alterations Behind FF and Poor Blastulation

Thanks to multiple recent studies using gene sequencing on infertile patients, nowadays we know that genetic alterations can explain a still uncertain but considerable proportion of FF and poor blastulation cases.

Different genetic variants can explain FF after conventional IVF, most associated with asthenozoospermia and affecting genes involved in flagellar assembly and motility regulation in sperm. These include the family of genes encoding dynein axonemal heavy chain proteins (*DNAH1, DNAH2, DNAH6*, etc.), cilia and flagella-associated proteins (*CFAP70, CFAP40*, etc.), *SEPT12, AKAP3*, as well as mutations in *CATSPER* genes (a calcium channel essential for the acquisition of hyperactivated sperm motility during capacitation), as some examples.[1] Moreover, genetic variants affecting the zona pellucida (ZP proteins) or JUNO receptor (in the oocyte) or SPACA6 or IZUMO1 (in the sperm) are potential causes of FF after c-IVF.

So far, more than one hundred genetic variants have been identified in infertile patients as causative of FF after ICSI.[2] Most of the variants causing male-related FF affect the *PLCZ1* gene. These variants are found either in heterozygosis or homozygosis, are independent of the spermiogram results (i.e. can be identified in normozoospermic patients), and mostly affect the enzymatic activity of PLCZ1 protein. During the last decade, phospholipase C zeta (PLCζ/PLCZ1) has emerged as an essential sperm-born factor responsible for oocyte activation. Microinjection of human *PLCZ1* cRNA or recombinant PLCζ protein into human oocytes triggers calcium oscillations and development to the blastocyst stage, while sperm from *PLCZ1* knock-out mice present severe problems in triggering fertilization. Currently, *PLCZ1* is the main genetic marker for the diagnosis of male-related FF, reported to be in about one-third of men that had FF.

However, recently, genetic variants affecting *ACTL9, ACTLA7*, and *DNAH17* genes have also been reported as a cause of FF. These factors are necessary for the normal localization of PLCζ protein. Different mutations in genes like *SPATA16* and *DPY19L2* can cause globozoospermia, and thus male-related OAF after ICSI.

In infertile women, close to 30 genetic variants in *WEE2* gene have been identified.[2] WEE2 is an oocyte-specific MPF inhibitory kinase, an essential factor in the oocyte activation signaling cascade. Ca^{2+} activates CAMKII, which triggers WEE2 phosphorylation, MPF inactivation, and meiosis resumption. Deficiencies in this protein (such as those caused by these variants in homozygosis or compound heterozygosis) cause FF characterized by OAF.

Over 100 genetic variants in *TUBB8*—an essential component of spindle and microtubules within the oocyte—while largely associated with oocyte maturation defects, can also explain a proportion of cases of FF after ICSI. Similarly, genetic variants in *CDC20, PATL2, TRIP13, BTG4*, as well as genes involved in the subcortical maternal complex (SCMC; including *PADI6, NLRP2, TLE6, KHDC3L, NLRP7, NLRP5, OOEP*, or *ZBED3*), have been associated with female-related FF, zygotic arrest, but mainly with poor embryo quality, embryo developmental arrest, and/or poor blastulation.[2, 3] Additional genes have been reported to participate in EGA and early embryo development.[4]

In summary, the spectrum of genes and genetic variants involved in FF and poor blastulation is considerably large and is expected to increase during the following years.

The Importance of a Correct Diagnosis

Considering the high impact of FF and poor blastulation on the patients, it is of utmost relevance to diagnose the problem whenever possible. While an efficient treatment option for these problems is not always available, a diagnostic may help in patient counseling and guide further management.

Currently, assessing PLCζ protein levels or localization has been proposed as a potential diagnostic test for male-related FF. By using immunofluorescence, previous studies reported that the presence of <30% PLCZ1+ sperm may be associated with lower fertilization rates, although this association is still controversial. On the contrary, as previously indicated, *PLCZ1* pathogenic variants are strongly associated with the occurrence of FF. For this reason, sequencing of *PLCZ1* gene has been introduced as a diagnostic tool. Recent studies have demonstrated that genetic alterations in some genes are relatively common among FF patients, not only in *PLCZ1*, but also in genes causing female infertility (such as *WEE2*, *TLE6*, or *TUBB8*). For this reason, targeted gene panels specifically designed to identify mutations related to FF in ART could provide valuable information for genetic counseling of infertility patients. Gene sequencing can be a good diagnostic approach, especially considering that the database of genetic variants associated with FF is increasing every year. Genetic screening as a diagnostic tool is still far from the routine in reproductive health, but it is an affordable technique, can be provided by an external service, and can be performed on a small amount of sample (even single cells). Current research is focused on the creation of diagnostic gene panels for this purpose.

Heterologous ICSI models, using mouse or hamster oocytes, have also been proposed as a diagnostic tool to assess if FF is sperm-related. In the mouse oocyte activation test (MOAT), human sperm is injected into the oocyte to evaluate the oocyte activation (rate of two-cell formation): If 85–100% activation is achieved (MOAT3 group), the sperm potential is adequate; but diminished sperm capacity should be considered for MOAT2 (21–84%) and MOAT1 (0–20%) groups (Figure 23.1). Mouse oocyte calcium analysis (MOCA) is similar, but a Ca^{2+} fluorescent dye and an epifluorescence microscope are used to analyze the Ca^{2+} oscillations pattern after sperm injection. HOCA (human oocyte calcium analysis) is the homologous variant of this test. However, while these methods are accurate in determining sperm activation capacity, they cannot easily be introduced in routine clinical practice because of the need for specific equipment, trained personnel, mouse housing facilities, or the availability of human oocytes for research (strictly regulated or banned in some countries).

As an attempt to improve the diagnostic of poor embryo quality and blastulation, different tests are available to improve the study of male infertility, for example the analysis of sperm DNA condensation, associated with poor embryo quality in some studies. In addition, assessing the levels of sperm DNA fragmentation is gaining relevance as a diagnostic tool in fertility clinics, and can provide a diagnostic and a potential explanation to patients with poor blastulation.[5]

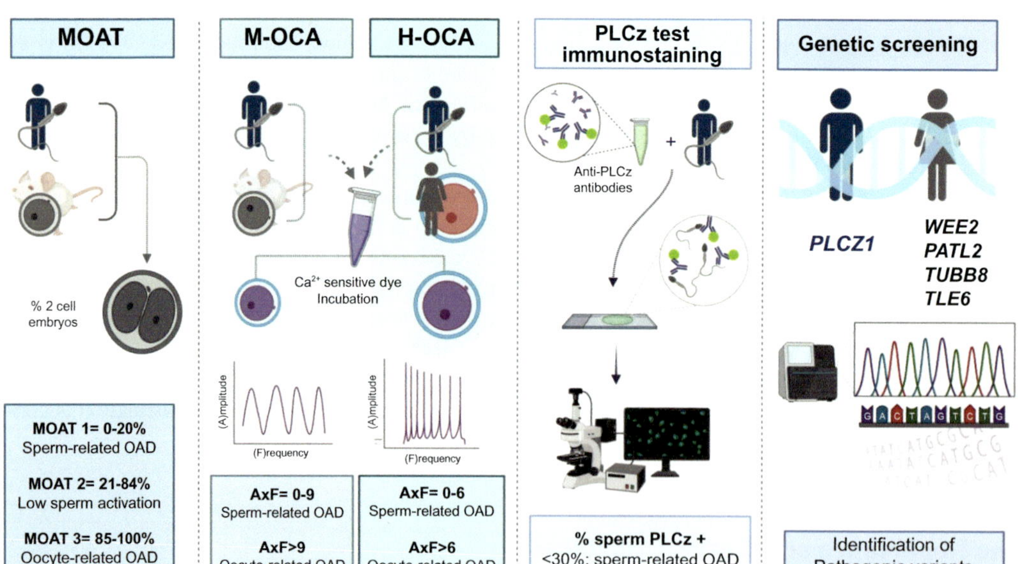

FIGURE 23.1 Summary of the main diagnostic tests for fertilization failure caused by OAD (oocyte activation deficiency)(from ref. 3 with permission).

Despite all the approaches mentioned so far, a clear origin explaining FF or poor blastulation will not be identified in a large proportion of cases, which will be considered as idiopathic infertility.

What to Do in the Clinic? Management of FF and Poor Blastulation

The clinical management of FF is very complex due to the fact that its occurrence is often unexpected and difficult to predict, its molecular pathogenesis is not completely understood (research on the topic suffers from inherent ethical and technical limitations), there is lack of diagnostic tests and clinical options to overcome this problem, and FF has a considerable psychological and economic impact on the patients.

While the routine use of ICSI by many clinics (with the perception that it can reduce the risk of FF) is still controversial, it is still a good option in a subsequent cycle for patients who experienced FF after one or more c-IVF cycles. An unnoticed problem affecting the sperm's ability to bind to the oocyte may explain the original problem.

Another option for FF cases after c-IVF is the use of rescue ICSI (r-ICSI). In this approach, the day after oocyte pick-up and insemination by cIVF, r-ICSI is used for the oocytes showing no signs of fertilization, usually using the previous day's sperm sample. This approach has been reported as especially useful for patients with very low fertilization rates after cIVF (<15%), as with r-ICSI the risk of FF is reduced, around 50% of these cycles have at least one blastocyst, and live birth rates can reach 45%.[6]

However, especially in cases with FF after ICSI, the potential options are reduced. In FF after ICSI, it is relatively common for clinicians and practitioners to offer the patients the option to repeat the cycle without changing much in the treatment. However, it has been reported that FF and poor blastulation can be recurrent, especially when there are unnoticed molecular alterations underlying the problem.

An insufficient or abnormal Ca^{2+} release is a clear cause of low fertilization or total FF after ICSI; assisted oocyte activation (AOA) can be used as a rescue strategy. There are mechanical or electrical AOA strategies, but the most common AOA methodology is chemical AOA, where Ca^{2+} ionophores are used to generate artificial Ca^{2+} oscillations in the oocyte cytoplasm (by increasing membrane Ca^{2+} permeability). Ionomycin or calcymicin (also named A23187) are the two most common ionophores, the former being the most efficient. Ca^{2+} ionophores induce a Ca^{2+} signaling pattern very different from the spikes observed in a physiological situation but enough for the oocyte to complete all events necessary to complete fertilization. AOA using calcium ionophores is a technique especially useful in FF cases after ICSI characterized by OAF, and for patients who carry a pathogenic variant in *PLCZ1* in homozygosis or heterozygosis. While healthy live births have been reported after using this technique, AOA treatment should still be considered an experimental technique and used with caution only to treat couples with clear oocyte activation deficiencies. Some authors also report that injection of *PLCZ1* complementary RNA or PLCZ1 recombinant protein are good options to treat male-related FF, and create more physiologically Ca^{2+} oscillations that are indistinguishable from those occurring during normal fertilization.

On the contrary, it is important to note that conventional AOA (using calcium ionophores) will not work for all cases of FF after ICSI. When the deficiency occurs in molecules acting downstream of the Ca^{2+} signaling, AOA will not be beneficial. For oocyte-related deficiencies, alternative AOA methods which induce MPF inactivation and meiosis resumption can be applied.[3] For example, TPEN [Tetrakis (2-pyridylmethyl)ethylenediamine], CHX (able to inactivate the MPF and promote meiosis resumption) or roscovitine (inhibitor of cyclin-dependent kinases) are reagents proposed for AOA. Similarly, injection of *WEE2*, *TRIP13*, or *CDC20* complementary RNA into the oocyte (for example, in patients carrying a pathogenic genetic variant in these genes) may restore the abnormal protein content and allow correct embryo development.

In addition, specific ovarian stimulation protocols have been investigated for patients with previous cycles with OAF. A modified ovarian stimulation protocol, aiming to reduce oocyte dysmaturity HCG trigger, oocyte retrieval, removal of cumulus cells and ICSI, has been proposed to optimize fertilization rates. Similarly, a dual trigger strategy (adding a GnRH agonist to the hCG) might improve oocyte maturation, fertilization rates, and clinical outcomes in patients with previous poor fertilization compared to standard hCG trigger alone[7], although a recent RCT could not confirm this observation.[8]

Different studies in animal models have highlighted the importance of Ca^{2+} in post-fertilization events, demonstrating that abnormal signaling can affect preimplantational embryo development. For this reason, the use of AOA, either with calcium ionophores or with the use of recombinant PLCZ1 protein, has been proposed also as a method to help patients with poor blastulation. However, according to recent evidence, the use of ionomycin for AOA in patients with recurrent abnormal embryo development (blastulation rate: $\leq 15\%$) does not improve the blastulation rate nor the pregnancy outcomes in subsequent ICSI cycles.[9] These findings have been corroborated by other authors, but there is still controversy on the use of AOA in the treatment of poor embryo development.

During the last few years, the association between high DNA fragmentation levels in sperm and abnormal preimplantational development has gained importance.[10] Hence, sperm selection using microfluidics has been proposed as a good strategy to improve embryo quality and blastulation rate.[11] Nevertheless, other studies fail to demonstrate a clear benefit.

Similarly, to improve sperm selection (and thus improve preimplantational embryo development), the use of modified ICSI protocols has been proposed. This is the case of physiological ICSI (P-ICSI, where sperm are selected based on their ability to bind to hyaluronic acid) and intracytoplasmic morphologically selected sperm injection (IMSI, where sperm are selected under a microscope with high magnification), but as with other techniques, controversy still exists in the literature about their potential to improve blastulation rates in the clinic.

Finally, for patients with suspected alterations in the oocyte cytoplasm, nuclear transfer (NT) represents a general approach with the potential to overcome both FF and poor blastulation. In NT, the cytoplasm of a poor-quality oocyte (containing abnormal proteins required for fertilization and/or embryo development) is replaced by a good-quality cytoplasm from a donated healthy oocyte. In mice, this technique was shown to significantly increase blastocyst formation rates, and similar results have been obtained in humans. This technique is highly complex and is still far from the routine, but further research will elucidate its efficiency in treating infertility.

Important Considerations

Fertilization failure and poor blastulation should be rare circumstances in an IVF laboratory, especially in absence of a clear risk factor. An isolated and unexpected case of FF or poor blastulation is likely to be caused by a molecular or cellular problem affecting the gametes used for insemination. On the contrary, if this occurrence is relatively common or multiple cases of FF occur within a short period, then the problem may be caused by technical problems or suboptimal laboratory or culture conditions. In these cases, strict controls of temperature, pH, and culture media are required, as well as a deep reviewing of all laboratory protocols and equipment (including incubators) to identify potential problems previously unnoticed. The introduction of up-to-date technologies may help optimize the general blastulation rates, and the use of time-lapse incubators and culture media with low lactate concentrations may help in this regard.

Nevertheless, the efficiency of these techniques is far from being guaranteed, and many are still considered experimental. Chemical AOA using calcium ionophores is widely used in patients with previous FF cycles (and even as an attempt to improve embryo development in some cases). However, none of the AOA methods previously detailed have received the CE (*Conformité Européenne*) mark for medical devices, and for most AOA methods, its efficacy and safety have not been demonstrated outside research or diagnostic purposes. Even though AOA is beneficial for patients with sperm-related OAF, most studies and clinics lack a proper diagnosis or fail to discriminate between sperm- or oocyte-related activation failure when using this methodology. Embryologists and clinicians should avoid the indiscriminate use of these techniques and find a balance between attempting to treat these forms of infertility and using treatments that are empirical or not evidence-based.

Another option is gamete donation (either sperm donation, oocyte donation, or double donation), especially if no treatment can solve the problem. However, while gamete donation seems to be justified or is more accepted by the patients for certain types of infertility (i.e. advanced maternal age), patients may

TABLE 23.1

Main Strategies Proposed for the Treatment of FF and Poor Blastulation in the Clinic. The Practitioner Should Note That the Efficiency of Some of These Techniques Is Still Under Debate, Even If Commonly Applied in Fertility Clinics

<table>
<tr><th>FF after cIVF</th><th>FF after ICSI</th><th>Poor blastulation</th></tr>
<tr><td>ICSI</td><td></td><td></td></tr>
<tr><td>r-ICSI</td><td></td><td></td></tr>
<tr><td></td><td colspan="2">Conventional AOA (sperm origin)</td></tr>
<tr><td></td><td>Alternative AOA (oocyte origin)</td><td></td></tr>
<tr><td></td><td>Modified ovarian stimulation protocol</td><td></td></tr>
<tr><td></td><td></td><td>Modified insemination technique (P-ICSI, IMSI)</td></tr>
<tr><td></td><td></td><td>Microfluidics sperm selection</td></tr>
<tr><td></td><td colspan="2">Nuclear transfer (still experimental)</td></tr>
<tr><td colspan="3">Repeating the treatment without major changes</td></tr>
<tr><td colspan="3">Gamete donation (sperm, oocyte, or both)</td></tr>
</table>

be reluctant to change the gamete for FF or poor embryo quality, even if this treatment is the option with higher chances of success.

Finally, independently of the treatment option or clinical management, proper counseling is essential in patients experiencing FF and poor blastulation. IVF centers need to be honest and transparent with the patients and avoid offering false promises or treatments that have not been properly tested (Table 23.1).

Key Points

- During recent years, multiple genetic variants have been described as a cause of FF or abnormal embryo development. Genetic diagnosis of these problems is a practice expected to gain importance in the clinic.
- Rescue ICSI can offer positive results in cases of FF after c-IVF. Use of calcium ionophores for AOA is a good strategy for male-related FF after ICSI, but alternative strategies should be applied in cases of female-related FF.
- Currently, there is a lack of laboratory techniques useful for patients with poor blastulation. Microfluidics sperm sorting or the use of modified insemination techniques have been proposed, but further research is needed to determine their efficiency.
- Gamete donation is, so far, the most efficient approach to treat FF and poor blastulation in the laboratory.

REFERENCES

1. Jiao SY et al. Molecular genetics of infertility: loss-of-function mutations in humans and corresponding knockout/mutated mice. *Hum Reprod Update* 2021;27:154–189.
2. Torra-Massana M et al. Exonic genetic variants associated with unexpected fertilization failure and zygotic arrest after ICSI: a systematic review. *Zygote* 2023;31:316–341.
3. Campos G et al. Total fertilization failure after ICSI: insights into pathophysiology, diagnosis, and management through artificial oocyte activation. *Hum Reprod Update* 2023;29:369–394.
4. Paonessa M et al. Genetic causes of preimplantation embryo developmental failure. *Mol Reprod Dev* 2021;88:338–348.
5. Vallet-Buisan M et al. Contribution of semen to early embryo development: fertilization and beyond. *Hum Reprod Update* 2023;29:395–433.

6. Batha S et al. Day after rescue ICSI: eliminating total fertilization failure after conventional IVF with high live birth rates following cryopreserved blastocyst transfer. *Hum Reprod* 2023;38:1277–1283.
7. Elias RT et al. Combined GnRH-agonist and human chorionic gonadotropin trigger improves ICSI cycle outcomes in patients with history of poor fertilization. *J Assist Reprod Genet* 2017;34:781–788.
8. Zhou C et al. Ovulation triggering with hCG alone, GnRH agonist alone or in combination? A randomized controlled trial in advanced-age women undergoing IVF/ICSI cycles. *Hum Reprod* 2022;37(8):1795–1805.
9. Cardona Barberán A et al. Assisted oocyte activation does not overcome recurrent embryo developmental problems. *Hum Reprod* 2023;38:872–885.
10. Seli E et al. Extent of nuclear DNA damage in ejaculated spermatozoa impacts on blastocyst development after in vitro fertilization. *Fertil Steril. 2004*;82(2):378–83.
11. Godiwala P et al. Embryologic outcomes among patients using a microfluidics chip compared to density gradient centrifugation to process sperm: a paired analysis. *J Assist Reprod Genet* 2022;39:1523–1529.

24

The Future of the IVF Laboratory

Goli Ardestani, Marta Venturas, Denis Vaughan, and Denny Sakkas

Introduction

In the first reported case of *in vitro* fertilization and embryo development in the human, Rock and Menkin [1] made the following description in 1944 about the culture and development of a fertilized embryo: "The eggs were incubated in serum for 22.5 hours, being washed in salt solution before and after incubation, and then exposed to a washed sperm suspension in Locke's solution for two hours at room temperature. They were again washed in Locke's solution and cultured in fresh serum for 45 hours. When examined at the end of the incubation period, one egg was found to be in the two-cell stage; Two blastomeres of fairly uniform size and appearance, and containing granular cytoplasm, were enclosed within a zona pellucida along the border of which were numerous spermatozoa and at least one of them was clearly seen within the zona." Thirty years later, following considerable effort and research, the first IVF birth was described by Steptoe and Edwards in 1978 [2]. Many landmarks occurred in the three decades intervening in these two reports. In the ensuing 46 years since the birth of Louise Brown, some 80 years after the initial studies of Rock and Menkin, dramatic advances in knowledge and technologies have been made in the IVF laboratory, facilitating live birth rates after transfer to surpass the 50% mark in some patient groups and oocyte donors. The crucial laboratory-based advances that have helped these rates to be achieved include ICSI, embryo cryopreservation through vitrification, blastocyst culture, and preimplantation genetic testing. What will the next 10–20 years hold, and how will the IVF laboratory of the future look?

The IVF laboratory, believed to be the cornerstone of successful IVF, will play an increasingly important role in the coming years in improving access to all patients wishing to create a family, increase live birth rates, and most importantly, ensure that the children born from IVF procedures are healthy and not affected by the procedures themselves. The current laboratory workflow comprises of numerous steps (Figure 24.1). This chapter elaborates on the current IVF laboratory workflow and how these steps could be performed in an IVF cycle of the future.

Andrology

Sperm Analysis

One of the first interfaces of the laboratory with IVF patients is the analysis of the semen sample. Remote analysis of a semen sample has already been described in a number of scenarios. This may be as simple as a sample being sent in a solution to a central laboratory from a patient's home or a patient being able to perform an analysis at home by creating a smart phone video that will provide information on sperm quality [3–6]. As will be a consistent theme in the future laboratory, all aspects of the patient's procedure will be accessible through secure access to a patient's individual internet portal. This initial semen analysis could provide the basis for the male's future treatment with their partner.

DOI: 10.1201/9781003460275-24

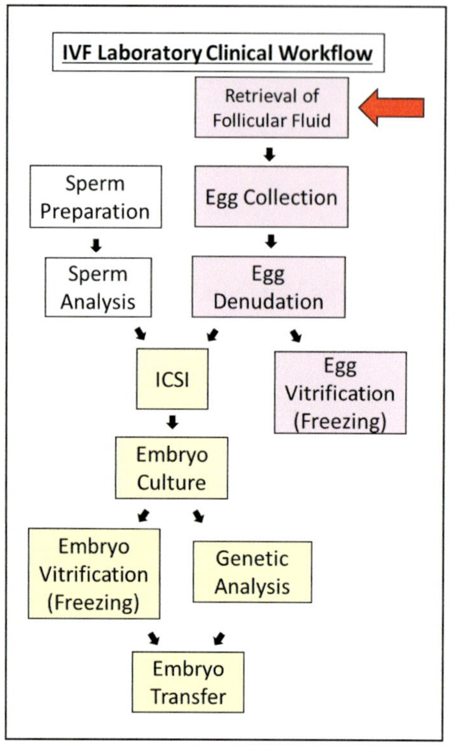

FIGURE 24.1 Major steps in the current IVF laboratory workflow.

The home-based analysis will not only provide analysis of sperm concentration, motility, motility patterns, and morphology but also delve into genetic and methylation patterns of sperm that could streamline and personalize treatment options for patients. Further information on sperm quality, plausibly needed as a marker of child health, will involve molecular analysis of sperm characteristics that should define whether couples will proceed directly to IVF/ICSI or have an equal chance of achieving pregnancy using intrauterine insemination. Specific methylation and microRNA profiles of sperm characteristics could be examined to ascertain whether the semen profile of the male will negatively impact success rates. Indeed, there is emerging data suggesting that the predictive power of DNA methylation and RNA signatures in sperm likely exceeds that which can be found with traditional assessments of male infertility [7, 8]. The group of Carrell and colleagues have already shown that the unique nature of the sperm epigenome and the patterns found in mature sperm that appear to reflect perturbations in spermatogenesis may ultimately have an effect on pregnancy outcomes [7–10]. More recently, Inherent Biosciences Path Fertility has shown that specific methylation profiles can not only be indicative of whether a patient should avoid insemination, even with normal semen parameters, but also of whether they are likely to have sperm in their biopsy if they were assessed as azoospermic [11]. mRNAs in the semen have been shown to have epigenetic properties whereby specific adult traits may be inheritable, such as anxiety [12]. Sperm may also be frozen in younger men to avoid inheritable traits that have been linked to older fathers [13].

It is therefore highly likely that semen analysis will provide predictive insight that can be exploited as a diagnostic tool for both infertility treatment and even health. The future andrology laboratory will be equipped with greater molecular diagnostic capabilities in the context of male infertility. Much of the testing will be done at the patients' homes and analysis likely provided remotely via secure connections [4].

Sperm Preparation and Selection

Sperm preparation will also be performed in a manner that will be aimed at identifying populations or single sperm that have limited or no risk of passing on paternal traits that could affect fertilization, embryo development, pregnancy, and the health of the offspring. Human epidemiological studies have suggested a relationship between advanced paternal age at conception and adverse neurodevelopmental outcomes in offspring, including an increased risk for psychiatric conditions such as autism and schizophrenia [9]. In one study, over 40 million documented live births were examined by the Centers for Disease Control and Prevention and the National Center for Health Statistics database between 2007 and 2016 in the USA [14, 15]. The study investigated the impact of advanced paternal age on maternal and perinatal outcomes and found a higher paternal age was associated with an increased risk of premature birth, low birth weight, and low Apgar score. Although currently clear evidence is not available that sperm selection technologies provide dramatic improvement in improving pregnancy rates, a common theme in such studies has been reduction in miscarriage rates [16–18].

How will sperm be prepared and selected in the future? The most promising methodology will likely involve selection via a microfluidic platform for IVF/ICSI cases [19]. These platforms have already entered into a testing phase in many IVF laboratories. For example, in the early 2000s, Takayama and Smith used two parallel laminar flow channels where non-motile spermatozoa and debris would flow along their initial streamlines and exit one outlet, whereas motile spermatozoa had an opportunity to swim into a parallel stream and exit a separate outlet. They found that both motility (98%) and morphology (22%) improved significantly [20, 21].

Relying solely on the motility characteristics and size to sort sperm by microfluidics will most likely be surpassed by further innovations to these systems. Artificial intelligence has also been investigated as a technology to provide rapid sperm selection capabilities. The team of Chavez-Badiola have developed AI that relates characteristics of sperm to fertilization, blastocyst and pregnancy outcomes, allowing quick identification of sperm so that they can be picked by embryologists performing ICSI [22–24].

The IVF Laboratory Processes

It is envisaged that all aspects of clinical embryology over the coming decades, including the retrieval, ICSI, embryo culture, and cryopreservation, will become automated. Such advances may be achieved through microrobotics and microfluidic systems, which are already being adapted into many processes of IVF [25–27].

Egg Collection and Processing

The first step in an IVF procedure is to collect oocytes. There have been no automated and continuous processing systems that can reduce the dependence on well-trained embryologists to obtain ICSI-ready oocytes from patients; however, using mouse models, a microfluidic device to denude oocytes from the surrounding cumulus-corona cell mass was reported [28, 29]. Oocytes that were denuded by the device showed comparable fertilization and developmental competence compared with mechanical pipetting. The same microfluidic device has also been shown to provide an automated way of identifying human cumulus-oocyte complexes from follicular fluid and denuding oocytes that would be ready for either ICSI or vitrification (unpublished data). Similarly, this has also been performed using robotics by a company called Conceivable Life Sciences [30].

Intracytoplasmic Sperm Injection (ICSI) and Routine Insemination

The advent of ICSI [31] revolutionized the treatment of the infertile male. Its adaptation in the IVF laboratory has surpassed its traditionally intended role, and it is now applied to nearly 70% of cases worldwide [32]. In many clinics it is used in 100% of cases. The automation of this skill has been attempted by various groups in recent years [33]. In particular, the group of Sun in Toronto has used a robotic system to track sperm and inject them with variable success [34]. The first automated ICSI pregnancies have been reported [35]. Microfluidic cradles that hold the oocyte in place have also been developed to facilitate and improve ICSI; some initial results show improvement in embryo development using these systems [36].

Although the use of ICSI has been adopted on a more regular basis, the use of microfluidics may allow more improved access of sperm to oocytes in smaller chambers, similar to that seen in the oviduct or fallopian tube. In fact, microfluidics may better mimic oocyte–sperm interactions in drastically reduced volumes (mimicking those present in the female tract), allowing for fertilization rates to be achieved with minimal numbers of surrounding spermatozoa, eliminating the wider use of ICSI. Han et al. [37] developed a microwell array used to capture and hold individual oocytes during the flow-through process of oocyte and sperm loading, medium substitution, and debris cleaning. Different microwell depths were compared by computational modeling and flow washing experiments for their effectiveness in oocyte trapping and debris removal. Fertilization was achieved in the microfluidic devices with similar fertilization rates to controls. The use of shorter exposure and low sperm numbers for insemination has long been argued to improve embryo quality [38], and the use of these systems may translate to improvements in not only process but outcomes.

Embryo Culture

Our ability to culture preimplantation embryos has improved dramatically over the last 40 years. Incubators, culture media, and culture environment have significantly improved and can now facilitate development of the fertilized oocyte to the blastocyst stage in all laboratories [39–42]. Although many aspects of embryo culture have improved, the actual hardware we culture embryos in has not changed. Standard culture conditions still call for embryos to be grown in a Petri dish using relatively large media volumes, when compared to embryo size, under oil. The major change in embryo culture in the past 10 years has been in the utilization of time-lapse systems, which has allowed clinics to assess embryos in a continuous temperature and gas phase without environmental perturbations. A number of studies have now shown that the time-lapse systems surpass the older standard incubators [43, 44], indicating that one benefit may definitely be a non-disturbed environment.

One of the unperceived advantages that coincide with time-lapse incubation is the use of specifically designed culture wells that can better create microenvironments around the embryo. These wells are characterized by lower incubation volumes per embryo, and by their columnar design in which embryos reside in the base of a small column of medium. These changes to dish design alone have been shown to improve embryo development, compared to that seen in a conventional Petri dish in drops of medium under oil [45].

The concept of a non-disturbed environment for culture lends itself well to microfluidic culture systems. Various microfluidic platforms have already been tested experimentally for embryo culture [46]. Some of the original studies reported by Heo et al. [47–49] cultured mouse embryos in a microfluidic system and found that blastocyst development was significantly enhanced in development to the hatching stage and in the average number of cells per blastocyst. Importantly, dynamic microfluidic culture (in which embryos moved) significantly improved embryo implantation and ongoing pregnancy rates over static culture to levels approaching that of in utero derived preimplantation embryos [48]. Unfortunately, although many systems have been developed that allow microfluidic embryo culture to be performed, their adaptation has yet to be realized. However, this could change in the future as the microfluidic platforms also allow two major adjunct improvements to embryo culture. First, they allow the manipulation of the media so that it can better suit the dynamic nature of preimplantation embryo development [41]. The adoption of single step culture media, although perceived to be equivalent to sequential, does not cater to the embryos' real metabolic needs. Microfluidics will allow these metabolic needs to be synchronized more closely to embryo stages [50–52]. For example, we envisage a future where embryos are monitored individually, and as they progress in development, they are exposed to changing gradients of nutrients to maximize the physiology of each stage [46, 51, 53]. This could be performed for multiple factors including carbohydrates, amino acids, vitamins, growth factors, cytokines, and macromolecules [45]. More importantly, interactive culture systems could be developed whereby embryo culture may finally be able to mimic that of an in vivo environment. In a study by Ferraz et al. [54], bovine embryos were cultured in a microfluidic chamber in addition to oviductal feeder cells. The authors concluded that cultured embryos were able to show in vivo characteristics as culture using "oviduct-on-a-chip" yielded 50% of zygotes with no discernible difference in gene expression pattern to in vivo zygotes. They postulated that their results highlight the importance of a more in vivo-like environment when studying pathways related to normal fertilization and zygote formation *in vitro*, and they suggested that future studies should focus on the relevance of this improved environment for further (epi)genetic reprogramming events in developing embryos.

A second benefit of microfluidic platforms is the ability to perform in-line diagnostics of embryos as they are growing. This concept was proven by Urbanski et al. [55], who showed that a microfluidic device could be employed in which media samples are loaded or integrated into microfluidic culture systems for in-line, real-time metabolic evaluation. Similar systems integrating microfluidics and diagnostics have been developed by the group of Horta [56] with an optofluidic device capable of obtaining high-resolution 3D images of the NAD(P)H autofluorescence of live mouse embryos using a light-sheet on-a-chip device.

Embryo Cryopreservation

Since the first report of a frozen IVF pregnancy in 1983 by Trounson and Mohr [57], embryo cryopreservation has become a major part of any IVF cycle. Although embryo freezing was able to provide limited successes, the advent of vitrification has revolutionized freezing of eggs and embryos [58, 59] to the extent that frozen embryo transfers are now surpassing fresh transfers as an option for embryo transfer. In the future, it is plausible that the current benefits seen in the transfer of vitrified embryos will translate to all cycles being completed by a frozen embryo transfer. In addition, change in clinical practice may provide a better luteal support and improve live birth outcomes [60].

The challenges to improving freezing protocols are both related to time- and outcome-efficiency. Automated vitrification systems are already under development which are aimed at improving laboratory efficiency [58, 61–67]. A further improvement will be the ability to provide greater control over the cryopreservation process. For example, Pyne et al. [63] have described a digital microfluidic device that automates sample preparation for mammalian embryo vitrification. The automated operation allowed gametes or embryos to pass through a cryoprotectant concentration gradient, which is distinct from current practice where they are passed through several steps of solutions. This in itself may improve outcomes. Further refinements have now been adopted clinically in shortening the times for both vitrification and warming with excellent clinical results [68].

Egg and Embryo Analysis

The development of precise methods for assessing oocyte and embryo quality has long remained a critical goal in ART. Forty years after the first IVF procedures were performed, morphological assessment remains the primary method of evaluation, despite its well-known limitations [69, 70]. Morphological features per se, however, have no clear connection to the underlying biochemical factors that are essential for viability, such as metabolic function and genetic integrity [71]. However, using time-lapse to quantitate the timing of key events such as initiation of cavitation to full blastocoel expansion could well be linked to metabolic activity over a defined period [69]. Current technology for embryo assessment is largely based on biopsy of the trophectoderm followed by genetic analysis. This, however, has raised a number of concerns not only because the procedure is invasive and requires removal of cells from the embryo but also as it is only representative of part of the embryo. We consider that in the future, these tests will be superseded by non-invasive testing that will give a more holistic evaluation of the entire embryo, that will provide information about genetic, metabolic, and transcriptional activity; thereby not only reflecting the ploidy and viability of the embryo, but providing important information regarding the health of the embryo itself [70, 72, 73].

Metabolic

The metabolic state of an embryo is not only predictive of viability (defined as the ability to implant) but is also reflective of the actual health of the embryo (as defined by the development of the resultant fetus). To date, assessment of metabolic function has relied heavily on specialized miniaturized procedures, available to only a few laboratories worldwide. Non-invasive embryo assessment of the embryo's metabolic state can now be performed indirectly through a number of novel imaging platforms that can obtain information about the metabolic functions of the embryo. Raman spectroscopy, Fourier transform infrared spectroscopy (FTIR), or fluorescence-lifetime imaging microscopy (FLIM) and hyperspectral analysis can all be used to provide additional spectroscopic data on embryos, and they thus have the potential to produce superior clinical tools for embryo assessment [74]. One methodology that has recently provided interesting data on mouse eggs and embryos is FLIM [74]. Interestingly, experiments on human blastocysts have shown that FLIM parameters exhibit strong differentiation between various parameters including inner cell mass and trophectoderm and day of development [75] as well as ploidy status [76]. FLIM analysis of blastocysts was recently tested in a pilot trial to understand if metabolic signatures existed that could identify viable versus non-viable embryos but failed to improve outcomes when compared to blastocyst morphology alone [77].

Genetic

Non-invasive/Semi-invasive PGT

Currently the most reliable embryo analysis technology is PGT-A using trophectodermal biopsies. This technology consistently provides greater than 50% live birth rates when an euploid embryo is found for transfer [78]. Unfortunately, the technique requires significant laboratory resources, including the actual trophectoderm biopsy itself and the addition of cryopreservation of all blastocysts prior to analysis. Recently, however, the advent of non-invasive PGT-A may circumvent much of the need for biopsying embryos. Promising non-invasive methods to genetically analyze the embryo include blastocoelic fluid [79–81] and/or media assessment [82–84] and the use of advanced microscopy techniques [76, 85]. In several years, the need to biopsy an embryo will most likely be unnecessary. Recent publications have shown that >95% concordance rates can be achieved using non-invasive PGT methods to examine the culture media of embryos [86].

Artificial Intelligence

Through the introduction of time-lapse microscopy, we are now in the unique position of collecting more data than a clinical embryology laboratory can utilize. With embryos being imaged every 10 minutes, during a 4-to-5-day culture period, over 700 pictures (each with several focal planes) are amassed, therefore making the total number of images available for consideration into the thousands. With the ability to annotate embryo development and the application of algorithms to model the significance of discrete events, we can now utilize the potential of time-lapse to a greater extent than first imagined [71, 87]. However, even the most sophisticated algorithms to date use only a small percent of the available information. Artificial Intelligence (AI) is a means to maximize the potential of time-lapse microscopy in clinical IVF [88]. Rather than taking a sample of images into consideration, AI can utilize every image at every focal plane in order to learn what time-dependent features are associated with a successful transfer outcome, such as fetal heart rate [89]. Furthermore, AI will be of value in integrating the growing amount of clinical data collected per embryo, allowing patient parameters also to be combined into decision-making with the images acquired throughout development [90, 91]. Although many retrospective analyses have shown promise with AI for embryo selection, a number of randomized clinical trials have failed to show any benefit when compared to the standard selection of blastocysts using morphology alone [92, 93]. In particular, the Illingworth et al. study [92] was unable to demonstrate the non-inferiority of deep learning for clinical pregnancy rate when compared to standard morphology and a predefined prioritization scheme. This brings into question how AI will produce benefits above that of morphology [94].

A final benefit of AI in combination with microfluidics will be added safety for tracking patients' gametes and embryos, allowing all the data to be assimilated into electronic medical records which would include witnessing systems. This will allow patients' gametes and embryos to be tracked more efficiently with the ultimate aim of eliminating any errors in the laboratory.

Conclusion

The initial laboratory conditions responsible for the creation of Louise Brown have changed significantly over the intervening decades. We predict that more changes will be forthcoming through innovation in automation, microrobotics, microfluidics, all combined with AI. Hence, the laboratory of tomorrow is more likely to be an integral component in "Personalized Medicine" in order to better diagnose and treat couples. Clinical profiles will be fundamental in choosing how a patient's gametes and embryos are monitored individually as they progress in development. Culture and selection could be performed in a microfluidic device allowing greater efficiency, safety, and overall efficacy in the laboratory. Gamete and embryo data created, via imaging and media sampling for metabolites and DNA, will be integrated into algorithms that could also incorporate the couple's own clinical profile. This will allow a truly personalized approach in handling the gametes and embryos of each patient in the laboratory. Importantly, such an approach will enable the laboratory to maximize each couple's chance of achieving a healthy singleton live birth. It should also provide a rapid and meaningful diagnosis in the advent of a failed cycle, thereby facilitating the patient to be treated efficiently in future treatment cycles, or even to provide closure in the event of extremely poor prognosis. Ultimately, however, the approaches considered will improve laboratory efficiencies and reduce time to pregnancy.

Key Points

- Remote, home-based sperm analysis will become standard, assessing not just basic parameters (motility, morphology), but also advanced genetic and epigenetic markers.
- AI and microfluidics will enable precise, non-invasive sperm selection to minimize hereditary risks and improve reproductive success rates.
- Critical IVF steps (e.g., egg collection, ICSI, embryo culture, and cryopreservation) are being automated using robotics and microfluidics.
- Embryo diagnostics will be revolutionized with integrated metabolic and genetic monitoring using technologies like FLIM, Raman spectroscopy, and in-line microfluidic sensors.
- Non-invasive PGT-A via spent culture media or blastocoelic fluid shows high concordance with traditional biopsies, reducing the need for invasive embryo testing.
- AI will be increasingly used to analyze time-lapse imaging data, integrating thousands of developmental images and patient data for embryo selection. It will also be used to enhance laboratory safety and traceability, reducing human error by integrating witnessing systems into EMRs.

REFERENCES

1. Rock J, Menkin MF. In vitro fertilization and cleavage of human ovarian eggs. *Science* 1944;100: 105–107.
2. Steptoe PC, Edwards RG. Birth after the reimplantation of a human embryo. *Lancet* 1978;2:366.
3. Gonzalez D et al. Clinical update on home testing for male fertility. *World J Mens Health* 2021;39:615–625.
4. Kanakasabapathy MK et al. An automated smartphone-based diagnostic assay for point-of-care semen analysis. *Sci Transl Med* 2017;9. https://doi.org/10.1126/scitranslmed.aai7863

5. Kim KS et al. Ability and accuracy of the smartphone-based O;VIEW-M(R) sperm test: useful tool in the era of Covid-19. *PLoS One* 2022;17: e0269894.
6. Park MJ et al. Accuracy comparison study of new smartphone-based semen analyzer versus laboratory sperm quality analyzer. *Investig Clin Urol* 2021;62:672–680.
7. Jenkins TG et al. Sperm epigenetics in the study of male fertility, offspring health, and potential clinical applications. *Syst Biol Reprod Med* 2017;63:69–76.
8. Jenkins TG, Carrell DT. The paternal epigenome and embryogenesis: poising mechanisms for development. *Asian J Androl* 2011;13:76–80.
9. Jenkins TG et al. Age-associated sperm DNA methylation alterations: possible implications in offspring disease susceptibility. *PLoS Genet* 2014;10:e1004458.
10. Jenkins TG et al. Sperm epigenetics and aging. *Transl Androl Urol* 2018;7:S328-S335.
11. Miller RH et al. Epigenetic determinants of reproductive potential augment the predictive ability of the semen analysis. *F S Sci* 2023;4:279–285.
12. Dickson DA et al. Reduced levels of miRNAs 449 and 34 in sperm of mice and men exposed to early life stress. *Transl Psychiatry* 2018;8:101.
13. Eisenberg ML. Can a father be too old? *Fertil Steril* 2022;118:999–1000.
14. Khandwala YS et al. The age of fathers in the USA is rising: an analysis of 168 867 480 births from 1972 to 2015. *Hum Reprod* 2017;32:2110–2116.
15. Gil M et al. Sperm selection using magnetic activated cell sorting (MACS) in assisted reproduction: a systematic review and meta-analysis. *J Assist Reprod Genet* 2013;30:479–485.
16. Niederberger C. Re: the age of fathers in the USA is rising: an analysis of 168 867 480 births from 1972 to 2015. *J Urol* 2018;199:1099.
17. Kirkman-Brown J et al. *Sperm Selection for Assisted Reproduction by Prior Hyaluronan Binding: The HABSelect RCT.* National Institute for Health Research, Evaluation, Trials and Studies Coordinating Centre, 2019.
18. West R et al. Sperm selection with hyaluronic acid improved live birth outcomes among older couples and was connected to sperm DNA quality, potentially affecting all treatment outcomes. *Hum Reprod* 2022;37:1106–1125.
19. Vaughan DA, Sakkas D. Sperm selection methods in the 21st century. *Biol Reprod* 2019;101:1076–1082.
20. Schuster TG et al. Isolation of motile spermatozoa from semen samples using microfluidics. *Reprod Biomed Online* 2003;7:75–81.
21. Suh RS et al. IVF within microfluidic channels requires lower total numbers and lower concentrations of sperm. *Hum Reprod* 2006;21:477–483.
22. Mendizabal-Ruiz G et al. Artificial intelligence in human reproduction. *Arch Med Res* 2024;55:103131.
23. Mendizabal-Ruiz G et al. Computer software (SiD) assisted real-time single sperm selection associated with fertilization and blastocyst formation. *Reprod Biomed Online* 2022;45:703–711.
24. Montjean D et al. Automated Single-Sperm Selection Software (SiD) during ICSI: a prospective sibling oocyte evaluation. *Med Sci (Basel)* 2024;12.
25. Campbell A et al. In vitro fertilization and andrology laboratory in 2030: expert visions. *Fertil Steril* 2021;116:4–12.
26. Meseguer M et al. Full in vitro fertilization laboratory mechanization: toward robotic assisted reproduction? *Fertil Steril* 2012;97:1277–1286.
27. Simon C et al. In vitro fertilization and andrology laboratories in 2030. *Fertil Steril* 2021;116:2–3.
28. Weng L et al. On-chip oocyte denudation from cumulus-oocyte complexes for assisted reproductive therapy. *Lab Chip* 2018;18:892–3902.
29. Zhai R et al. Automated denudation of oocytes. *Micromachines (Basel)* 2022;13.
30. Conceivable Life Sciences [internet]: www.conceivable.life.
31. Palermo G et al. Pregnancies after intracytoplasmic injection of single spermatozoon into an oocyte. *Lancet* 1992;340: 17–18.
32. Kupka MS et al. International committee for monitoring assisted reproductive technology world report: assisted reproductive technology, 2015 and 2016. *Fertil Steril* 2024;122:875–893.
33. Thompson JG et al. A brief history of technical developments in intracytoplasmic sperm injection (ICSI). Dedicated to the memory of J.M. Cummins. *Reprod Fertil Dev* 2024;36.
34. Sun Y et al. High-speed automated robotic microinjection. *Fertil Steril* 2009;92:S147.

35. Costa-Borges N et al. First babies conceived with automated intracytoplasmic sperm injection. *Reprod Biomed Online* 2023;47:103237.
36. McLennan HJ et al. A micro-fabricated device (microICSI) improves porcine blastocyst development and procedural efficiency for both porcine intracytoplasmic sperm injection and human microinjection. *J Assist Reprod Genet* 2024;41:297–309.
37. Han C et al. Integration of single oocyte trapping, in vitro fertilization and embryo culture in a microwell-structured microfluidic device. *Lab Chip* 2010;10:2848–2854.
38. Kattera S, Chen C. Short coincubation of gametes in in vitro fertilization improves implantation and pregnancy rates: a prospective, randomized, controlled study. *Fertil Steril* 2003;80:1017–1021.
39. Bavister BD. Culture of preimplantation embryos: facts and artifacts. *Hum Reprod Update* 1995;1:91–148.
40. Gardner DK, Lane M. Culture of viable human blastocysts in defined sequential serum-free media. *Hum Reprod* 1998;13 Suppl 3:148–159; discussion 160.
41. Gardner DK, Lane M. Culture of viable mammalian embryos. In Cibelli J, Lanza R, Campbell K and West MD (eds) *Principles of Cloning*. Academic Press, San Diego, 2014;63–84.
42. Gardner DK et al. Physiology and culture of the human blastocyst. *J Reprod Immunol* 2002;55:85–100.
43. Armstrong S et al. Time-lapse systems for embryo incubation and assessment in assisted reproduction. *Cochrane Database Syst Rev* 2018;5: CD011320.
44. Pribenszky C et al. Time-lapse culture with morphokinetic embryo selection improves pregnancy and live birth chances and reduces early pregnancy loss: a meta-analysis. *Reprod Biomed Online* 2017;35:511–520.
45. Gardner D, Kelley RL. Impact of the IVF laboratory environment on human preimplantation embryo phenotype. *J Dev Orig Health Dis* 2019;8:418–435.
46. Francés-Herrero E et al. Bioengineering trends in female reproduction: a systematic review. *Hum Reprod Update* 2022;28:798–837.
47. Heo YS et al. Characterization and resolution of evaporation-mediated osmolality shifts that constrain microfluidic cell culture in poly(dimethylsiloxane) devices. *Anal Chem* 2007;79:1126–1134.
48. Heo YS et al. Dynamic microfunnel culture enhances mouse embryo development and pregnancy rates. *Hum Reprod* 2010;25:613–622.
49. Heo YS et al. Real time culture and analysis of embryo metabolism using a microfluidic device with deformation based actuation. *Lab Chip* 2012;12:2240–2246.
50. Kushnir VA et al. The future of IVF: the new normal in human reproduction. *Reprod Sci* 2022;29:849–856.
51. Smith GD, Takayama S. Application of microfluidic technologies to human assisted reproduction. *Mol Hum Reprod* 2017;23:257–268.
52. Swain JE et al. Thinking big by thinking small: application of microfluidic technology to improve ART. *Lab Chip* 2013;13:1213–1224.
53. Gardner DK. 'The way to improve ART outcomes is to introduce more technologies in the laboratory'. *Reprod Biomed Online* 2022;44: 389–392.
54. Ferraz M et al. An oviduct-on-a-chip provides an enhanced in vitro environment for zygote genome reprogramming. *Nat Commun* 2018;9:4934.
55. Urbanski JP et al. Noninvasive metabolic profiling using microfluidics for analysis of single preimplantation embryos. *Anal Chem* 2008;80:6500–6507.
56. Vargas-Ordaz E et al. Novel application of metabolic imaging of early embryos using a light-sheet on-a-chip device: a proof-of-concept study. *Hum Reprod* 2025;40/1:41–55.
57. Trounson A, Mohr L. Human pregnancy following cryopreservation, thawing and transfer of an eight-cell embryo. *Nature* 1983;305:707–709.
58. Lane M et al. Vitrification of mouse and human blastocysts using a novel cryoloop container-less technique. *Fertil Steril* 1999;72:1073–1078.
59. Rienzi L et al. Oocyte, embryo and blastocyst cryopreservation in ART: systematic review and meta-analysis comparing slow-freezing versus vitrification to produce evidence for the development of global guidance. *Hum Reprod Update* 2017;23:139–155.
60. Drakopoulos P et al. The future of luteal phase support in ART and the role of dydrogesterone. *Front Reprod Health* 2020;2:618838.
61. Feng H et al. A microfluidic hanging droplet as a programmable platform for mammalian egg vitrification. *Lab Chip* 2024;24:5225–5237.

62. Miao S et al. A robotic system with embedded open microfluidic chip for automatic embryo vitrification. *IEEE Trans Biomed Eng* 2022;69:3562–3571.
63. Pyne DG et al. Digital microfluidic processing of mammalian embryos for vitrification. *PLoS One* 2014;9: e108128.
64. Shen J et al. Oocytes vitrification using automated equipment based on microfluidic chip. *Ann Biomed Eng* 2024.
65. Tirgar P et al. Toward embryo cryopreservation-on-a-chip: a standalone microfluidic platform for gradual loading of cryoprotectants to minimize cryoinjuries. *Biomicrofluidics* 2021;15:034104.
66. Wang S et al. A compact, high-throughput semi-automated embryo vitrification system based on hydrogel. *Reprod Biomed Online* 2024;48:103769.
67. Zhu Y et al. Automation in vitrification and thawing of mouse oocytes and embryos. *Front Cell Dev Biol* 2023;11:1330684.
68. Liebermann J et al. Fast and furious: pregnancy outcome with one-step rehydration in the warming protocol for human blastocysts. *Reprod Biomed Online* 2024;48:103731.
69. Gardner DK, Balaban B. Assessment of human embryo development using morphological criteria in an era of time-lapse, algorithms and 'OMICS': is looking good still important? *Mol Hum Reprod* 2016;22:704–718.
70. Sakkas D, Gardner DK. Embryo selection through the analysis of morphology and physiology. In Gardner DK et al. (eds) *Textbook of Assisted Reproduction Techniques*. CRC Press, Boca Raton, 2023:161–175.
71. Gardner DK et al. Diagnosis of human preimplantation embryo viability. *Hum Reprod Update* 2015;21:727–747.
72. Ferrick L et al. Metabolic activity of human blastocysts correlates with their morphokinetics, morphological grade, KIDScore and artificial intelligence ranking. *Hum Reprod* 2020;35:2004–2016.
73. Sakkas D, Gardner DK. Noninvasive methods to assess embryo quality. *Curr Opin Obstet Gynecol* 2005;17:283–288.
74. Sanchez T et al. Will noninvasive methods surpass invasive for assessing gametes and embryos? *Fertil Steril* 2017;108:730–737.
75. Venturas M et al. Metabolic state of human blastocysts measured by fluorescence lifetime imaging microscopy. *Hum Reprod* 2022;37:411–427.
76. Shah JS et al. Fluorescence lifetime imaging microscopy (FLIM) detects differences in metabolic signatures between euploid and aneuploid human blastocysts. *Hum Reprod* 2022;37:400–410.
77. Sakkas D. The 'golden fleece of embryology' eludes us once again: a recent RCT using artificial intelligence reveals again that blastocyst morphology remains the standard to beat. *Hum Reprod* 2024.
78. Munné S et al. Preimplantation genetic testing for aneuploidy versus morphology as selection criteria for single frozen-thawed embryo transfer in good-prognosis patients: a multicenter randomized clinical trial. *Fertil Steril* 2019;112:1071–1079.e1077.
79. Gianaroli L et al. Failure to detect DNA in blastocoel fluid is associated with a higher live birth rate in both PGT-A and conventional IVF/ICSI cycles. *Hum Reprod* 2023;38:1268–1276.
80. Kuznyetsov V et al. Minimally invasive cell-free human embryo aneuploidy testing (miPGT-A) utilizing combined spent embryo culture medium and blastocoel fluid–towards development of a clinical assay. *Sci Rep* 2020;10:7244.
81. Zhang Y et al. Molecular analysis of DNA in blastocoele fluid using next-generation sequencing. *J Assist Reprod Genet* 2016;33:637–645.
82. Rubio C et al. Noninvasive preimplantation genetic testing for aneuploidy in spent culture medium as a substitute for trophectoderm biopsy. *Fertil Steril* 2021;115:841–849.
83. Shamonki M et al. Proof of concept: preimplantation genetic screening without embryo biopsy through analysis of cell-free DNA in spent embryo culture media. *Fertil Steril* 2016;106:1312–1318.
84. Xu J et al. Noninvasive chromosome screening of human embryos by genome sequencing of embryo culture medium for in vitro fertilization. *Proc Natl Acad Sci USA* 2016;113:11907–11912.
85. Tan TCY et al. Non-invasive, label-free optical analysis to detect aneuploidy within the inner cell mass of the preimplantation embryo. *Hum Reprod* 2021;37:14–29.

86. Ardestani G et al. Culture time to optimize embryo cell-free DNA analysis for frozen-thawed blastocysts undergoing noninvasive preimplantation genetic testing for aneuploidy. *Fertil Steril* 2024;122:465–473.
87. Giménez C et al. Time-lapse imaging: morphokinetic analysis of in vitro fertilization outcomes. *Fertil Steril* 2023;120:218–227.
88. Khosravi P et al. Deep learning enables robust assessment and selection of human blastocysts after in vitro fertilization. *NPJ Digit Med* 2019;2:21.
89. Tran D et al. Deep learning as a predictive tool for fetal heart pregnancy following time-lapse incubation and blastocyst transfer. *Hum Reprod* 2019;34:1011–1018.
90. Letterie G. Moonshot. Long shot. Or sure shot. What needs to happen to realize the full potential of AI in the fertility sector? *Hum Reprod* 2024;39:1863–1868.
91. Youngster M et al. Optimizing workload balance using artificial intelligence. *Fertil Steril* 2024;122:178–180.
92. Illingworth PJ et al. Deep learning versus manual morphology-based embryo selection in IVF: a randomized, double-blind noninferiority trial. *Nature Medicine* 2024.
93. Kieslinger DC et al. Clinical outcomes of uninterrupted embryo culture with or without time-lapse-based embryo selection versus interrupted standard culture (SelecTIMO): a three-armed, multicentre, double-blind, randomised controlled trial. *Lancet* 2023;401:1438–1446.
94. Sakkas D et al. Metabolic imaging of human embryos is predictive of ploidy status but is not associated with clinical pregnancy outcomes: a pilot trial. *Hum Reprod* 2024;39:516–525.

25

Oncofertility: Fertility Preservation for Patients Undergoing Gonadotoxic Treatment

Denis Vaughan and Pietro Bortoletto

Based on estimates of new cancer cases in 2024, approximately 84,000 cases will be diagnosed among adolescents and young adults (AYAs, ages 15–39). This represents 4.2% of all new cancer cases at any age. Breast and thyroid cancers represent the most common malignancies diagnosed in this age group (15% for each), followed by testis cancer (8%) and melanoma of the skin (1). Using statistical models for analysis, rates of new cancer cases of any site among AYAs have been stable each year over 2012–2021, the last 10 years of available data. Death rates have been falling on average 0.9% each year over 2013–2022, owing to improved cancer surveillance and treatment regimens. More than 85% of AYAs will survive five years or more after being diagnosed with cancer. Future fertility is an issue of concern for many young patients diagnosed with cancer. Previous studies have estimated that about one-third of young women desire future children at the time of breast cancer diagnosis, and half have some degree of concern about infertility following treatment. Addressing this concern ahead of cancer treatment can decrease future regret concerning fertility.

In the United States, cancer is the leading cause of death by disease after infancy among children. The most common types of cancer diagnosed in 2016–2020 among children and adolescents were leukemias, malignant brain, and other central nervous system (CNS) tumors, lymphomas, epithelial neoplasms and melanomas, soft tissue tumors, malignant germ cell tumors, and bone tumors. Cancer survival rates have improved dramatically among children and adolescents. In the mid-1970s, 58% of children (ages 0 to 14 years) and 68% of adolescents (ages 15 to 19 years) diagnosed with cancer survived at least five years. In 2013–2019, five-year survival was 83.2% for children younger than 1 year, 87.8% for children ages 1–4 years, 85.7% for children ages 5–9 years, 85.5% for children ages 10–14 years, and 87.3% for adolescents ages 15–19 years (2). As of January 1, 2020, approximately 495,739 survivors of childhood and adolescent cancer (diagnosed at ages 0 to 19 years) were estimated to be alive in the United States.

Effects of Chemotherapy and Radiation on Female Fertility

Many treatments that have improved survival among both adults and children diagnosed with cancer are gonadotoxic, especially those that employ high doses of alkylating agents and pelvic radiation therapy. The impact on ovarian reserve is related to the accelerated depletion of the primordial germ cell pool resulting from these therapies.

Oogenesis is a process that begins in utero, approximately three weeks after conception, when the primordial germ cells derived from the endodermal yolk sac initiate their migration to the developing ovaries. These cells then undergo an inexorable differentiation to become primary oocytes, which at the time of birth are arrested in the prophase of the first meiotic division. At this time, there is no further differentiation of the germ cells, but a continuous apoptotic loss that depletes the supply from 1–2 million at birth to 300,000–500,000 at the time of puberty. Through ovulation and continued atresia of the

 DOI: 10.1201/9781003460275-25

non-dominant follicles, the ovarian reserve is eventually depleted with an accelerated loss of oocytes occurring at the age of 37 years up until the time of the menopause.

Alkylating agents (such as cyclophosphamide, ifosfamide, nitrosoureas, chlorambucil, melphalan, and busulfan), which are not cell-cycle specific, confer their deleterious effect on the vast supply of primordial germ cells and carry the highest risk of ovarian failure. Anti-metabolites (such as methotrexate, bleomycin, 5-fluorouracil, actinomycin-D, mercaptopurine, vincristine) impact the cells (granulosa and oocyte) of the metabolically active ovarian follicles and are lower risk for gonadal dysfunction, while cisplatin appears to carry intermediate risk between the anti-metabolites and alkylating agents (3). Women over the age of 40 years have a 90% chance of amenorrhea subsequent to multiagent chemotherapy, whereas the potential for premature ovarian failure in younger patients varies between 20–90% (4).

The tolerance of the ovary and uterus to radiation exposure is dependent on several factors including the age of the patient, ovarian reserve, the volume of irradiated tissue, the total dose of radiation, the risk of scatter, and the fractionation schedule. When applied conventionally, radiation doses of 24 Gy will result in ovarian failure. If the pelvis is included in the radiation field of an adult patient, the dose will typically exceed this level (5). Doses of radiation between 14 and 30 Gy result in uterine dysfunction, increasing the risk of obstetric complications in future pregnancies.

Unfortunately, one of the challenges in shielding the ovaries from direct or indirect radiation from pelvic radiation is that the ovaries are both small in size and mobile in terms of their positioning. This makes it challenging, but not impossible, for dose planning to protect the ovaries fully. For a given dose of radiotherapy at a known chronological age, oncologists can predict the size of the surviving fraction of oocytes and, therefore, the age at which ovarian failure can be expected for a patient. These projections will serve the patient well, as patients and physicians contemplate the timing and utility of fertility preservation strategies.

The greatest risk for developing premature ovarian failure occurs in the setting of the intensive multiagent chemotherapy and total body irradiation that is required for both adults and children who undergo bone marrow stem cell transplantation (BMSCT) for treatment of their malignancies. The doses required cause immediate ovarian failure in nearly all cases. Chemotherapy treatments, most including cyclophosphamide, and BMSCT are also utilized in the treatment of benign and chronic diseases such as sickle-cell anemia, thalassemia, aplastic anemia, lupus, and autoimmune thrombocytopenia. Additional benign indications for fertility preservation technologies include recurrent ovarian endometriosis, ovarian cysts, and the need for prophylactic oophorectomy in women affected by BRCA1 and 2.

Fertility Preservation Guidelines

In March 2005, the Practice Committee of the American Society for Reproductive Medicine (ASRM) first published their guidelines for the preservation of fertility in cancer patients, and it has been reaffirmed and updated several times since, most recently in 2019 (6).

The guidelines emphasize the importance of rapid access to care and the benefits of a multidisciplinary approach involving oncologists, reproductive endocrinologists and urologists, and reproductive surgeons. In addition, fertility preservation programs should have prompt access to mental health professionals and genetic counselors.

For females, the guidelines stress that embryo cryopreservation and mature oocyte cryopreservation should be considered first-line treatment for fertility preservation among post-pubertal females.

Since the 2019 update to the ASRM guidelines, ovarian tissue cryopreservation is no longer deemed experimental. Ovarian tissue banking is the only method to preserve fertility for prepubertal girls since ovarian stimulation and IVF are not options.

The authors of the guidelines point out that the use of gonadotropin-releasing hormone (GnRH) antagonist for ovarian protection during chemotherapy remains controversial with mixed data to support its use. They do, however, point out the beneficial effect in preventing heavy bleeding in patients with thrombocytopenia.

The authors of the ASRM Ethics Committee Report express that concerns about the welfare of the potential offspring *should not* be cause for denying cancer patients assistance in reproducing. When raised in a loving and nurturing environment, children should be given the opportunity to thrive, despite the misfortune of an early death of one parent.

These recommendations parallel those initially published by the American Society of Clinical Oncology (ASCO) in 2006, last updated in 2018, and is concordant with ASRM in designating sperm, oocyte, and embryo cryopreservation as standard practice (7). They also acknowledge the conflicting data to support GnRHa and other means of ovarian suppression and that the field of ovarian tissue cryopreservation is advancing quickly and may become standard therapy in the future. The authors recommended that oncologists should consider the options for fertility preservation expediently, so as to facilitate discussions with reproductive specialists and advocacy groups that support these treatments. Established methods, in addition to embryo, oocyte, and sperm cryopreservation, include gonadal shielding and ovarian transposition in cases involving exposure of the pelvis to radiation therapies. Encouragingly, the ASCO guidelines confirm that there appears to be no increased risk of disease recurrence associated with the use of the established treatments, even in tumors that might be hormonally sensitive, i.e., breast cancer. There is also no evidence of an increased risk of congenital abnormalities in the progeny of patients who have attempted to preserve their fertility, except in those cases that involve hereditary genetic syndromes.

Male Fertility Preservation

On the male side, cryopreservation of ejaculated sperm remains the gold standard in post-pubertal males. Penile vibratory stimulation or electroejaculation may be used in those men with neurologic injuries or other factors negatively impacting the ejaculatory reflex. Cryopreservation of surgically extracted sperm is a viable alternative strategy in males who cannot ejaculate or have azoospermia/severe oligospermia.

In prepubertal males, testicular tissue cryopreservation is the only method to preserve future fertility. Animal research demonstrates the feasibility and safety of next generation reproductive technologies using frozen and thawed testicular tissues (15). No human live births have been reported using those technologies; this should be considered experimental and done as part of a clinical trial.

Non-surgical Fertility Preservation Techniques

Embryo Cryopreservation

Embryo cryopreservation, routinely performed in patients undergoing IVF, affords the patient an optimal chance to preserve fertility, with excellent live birth rates depending on the age of the patient at the time of oocyte retrieval. However, this approach requires a source of sperm, which many young, unpartnered patients do not have access to. Additionally, the treatment cannot be offered to prepubertal patients who have an undeveloped reproductive endocrine axis or to adolescents who can neither provide consent nor use donor sperm.

Due to our enhanced understanding of the female hypothalamic-pituitary-gonadal axis and the ability to use sophisticated ovarian stimulation protocols, the timing and implementation of fertility preservation techniques can be done expediently. Traditional approaches required the initiation of fertility preservation treatment in the early follicular phase of the patient's menstrual cycle, adding time constraints that conferred unacceptable delays with respect to beginning chemotherapy or radiation treatments. The novel "cycle-independent" or "random-start" approach to ovarian stimulation for the purpose of oocyte retrieval and eventual embryo and/or oocyte cryopreservation can complete the process within two to three weeks of the patient's presentation to the reproductive endocrinologist. Protocols for ovarian stimulation that include agents such as Letrozole (aromatase inhibitor) and Tamoxifen (selective estrogen receptor modulator) in conjunction with gonadotropins appear to yield high-quality embryos and counteract the theoretical negative impact of high estradiol levels. When implemented in close collaboration with the patient's oncology team, these protocols can be completed for breast cancer patients during the four-to-six-week interval that typically occurs between the patient's surgery and the initiation of chemotherapy. Outcomes regarding oocyte yields and fertilization rates, comparing the traditionally timed technique of ovarian stimulation vs. the "cycle-independent" approach, show similar results.

Oocyte Cryopreservation

Similar to embryo cryopreservation, oocyte cryopreservation results in elevated serum estradiol levels and requires a mature reproductive axis, the use of gonadotropins for ovarian stimulation, and small, clinically insignificant delays in initiation of cancer treatment. However, there is no need for a male partner or donor sperm, and issues related to the creation of surplus embryos are avoided. The use of cryoprotectants that limit osmolarity changes, rapid freezing techniques known as vitrification, and fertilization with ICSI have increased success of subsequent oocyte thaw cycles. Randomized controlled trials of fresh vs. vitrified/warmed oocytes indicate that implantation and clinical pregnancy rates are similar (8, 9).

Along with the reassuring outcome data, the cryopreservation of oocytes offers more flexibility in future and full ownership of gametes. Previous studies have demonstrated that cancer survivors are 77% more likely to get divorced or separated.

In Vitro Maturation

As an alternative, *in vitro* maturation (IVM) of oocytes retrieved from unstimulated ovaries is an option for fertility preservation for young women that would not require the participation of a male partner or delays in cancer treatments. In the IVM and freezing of these oocytes, like oocyte and ovarian tissue cryopreservation, efficiency is lower than mature oocyte cryopreservation. This technology has been used in conjunction with ovarian tissue cryopreservation, allowing the aspiration of antral follicles prior to the cryobanking of ovarian tissue that has been surgically retrieved. However, its application is limited to specialized centers.

Surgical Fertility Preservation Techniques

For female patients facing gonadotoxic chemotherapy or pelvic radiation, several surgical interventions exist to help preserve future fertility beyond oocyte and embryo cryopreservation. While some are out of the scope of practice of REIs, such as radical trachelectomy, others such as ovarian transposition and ovarian tissue cryopreservation remain in the scope of REI.

Oophoropexy and ovarian transposition, which limit gonadotoxicity induced by radiation exposure, are established surgical techniques offered to women who are undergoing radiation therapy for cancers involving the pelvis, such as cervical cancer, colon cancer, or metastatic Hodgkin lymphoma. As mentioned, uterine exposure to pelvic/abdominal radiation may require the use of gestational carriers in future pregnancies to eliminate the risk of obstetric complications related to these treatments. In one recent meta-analysis of 892 women undergoing ovarian transposition followed by brachytherapy, 94% had preserved ovarian function after radiotherapy, but this number fell to 65% in those who underwent external beam radiation therapy with or without brachytherapy. Following gonadotoxic treatment, the ovaries are typically left in the transposed position for ovarian stimulation and retrieval as migration back to the radiated area is associated with increased rates of ovarian failure.

Ovarian Tissue Cryopreservation

Perhaps the most promising surgical tool for fertility preservation is ovarian tissue cryopreservation and transplantation. As of 2019, it is estimated that over 130 live births have occurred from the transplantation of cryopreserved ovarian tissue. The procedure involves laparoscopic excision of strips of ovarian cortex that are processed and then cryopreserved. The thawed tissue can then be implanted orthotopically, into a remaining ovary or other areas within the pelvis such as ovarian fossa or broad ligaments, or heterotopically. Heterotopic transplantation is typically performed in the retroperitoneum within the pelvis or abdominal wall, with the obvious advantage of ease of access for eventual ovarian stimulation or in cases of severe pelvic adhesions or disease that precludes orthotopic transplantation. One of the concerns with heterotopic transplantation has been graft viability with regard to tissue tension, temperature, and blood supply, amongst others.

Concerns with the transplantation of cryopreserved-thawed ovarian tissue focus on the risk of disease recurrence emanating from the exposure of cancer survivors to diseased tissue that harbor malignant cells. Fortunately, the ovary is not considered to be a typical metastatic site for blood-borne malignancies. In an Israeli study in 2008, 58 patients with hematologic malignancies, including non-Hodgkin lymphoma, acute leukemia, myelodysplastic syndrome, chronic myeloid leukemia (CML), and Hodgkin lymphoma, were evaluated for storage of ovarian tissue for fertility preservation. Two of the subjects were excluded from the study due to preoperative imaging confirming the presence of macroscopic ovarian metastases. Of the remaining patients, post-thawing tissue analysis confirmed the presence of minimal residual disease in only one patient, retrieved from a patient with CML.

Testicular Tissue Cryopreservation

For male patients, particularly prepubertal boys, testicular tissue cryopreservation is a promising surgical fertility preservation option. Testicular tissue cryopreservation (TTC) is an investigational fertility preservation strategy for prepubertal patients at risk of gonadotoxicity from chemotherapy, radiation, or other medical conditions. As spermatogonial stem cells (SSCs) are present in the testes before puberty but do not produce mature sperm, cryopreservation of testicular tissue aims to preserve these cells for future autotransplantation or *in vitro* maturation. Feasibility studies have demonstrated successful tissue retrieval, cryostorage, and maintenance of SSC viability, with reports of spermatogenesis in animal models following transplantation (10). Parental acceptance of TTC is increasing, particularly in high-risk pediatric populations, despite its experimental nature and the absence of reported live births. As research advances in SSC expansion and transplantation techniques, TTC holds promise for future clinical application in restoring fertility in prepubertal males exposed to gonadotoxic treatments.

Conclusion

Cancer treatments, despite their gonadotoxicity, have allowed survivors to focus on an enhanced quality of life, including the ability to have a biologic child. Both established and experimental therapies can now be utilized to allow these women to overcome the infertility that may result from their chemotherapy and radiation therapies. Continued research into the surgical and non-surgical approaches to fertility preservation is warranted.

Key Points

- Approximately 84,000 new cancer cases will be diagnosed among adolescents and young adults (AYAs) in 2024, with breast and thyroid cancers being the most common malignancies in this group. Given that more than 85% of AYAs will survive at least five years, addressing fertility concerns before treatment can significantly reduce future regret among cancer survivors.
- High-dose alkylating agents and pelvic radiation therapy pose the greatest risk to ovarian reserve, with women over 40 years old facing a 90% likelihood of amenorrhea after multiagent chemotherapy. Ovarian tissue cryopreservation, now considered a standard-of-care rather than experimental, is the only viable fertility preservation option for prepubertal girls.
- For males, sperm cryopreservation remains the gold standard for post-pubertal patients, while testicular tissue cryopreservation is an investigational option for prepubertal boys. Emerging

research on spermatogonial stem cell transplantation and *in vitro* maturation holds promise for future fertility restoration, but clinical application remains experimental.

REFERENCES

1. SEER, Cancer among Adolescents and Young Adults (Ayas) - Cancer Stat Facts [internet]: https://seer.cancer.gov/statfacts/html/aya.html (accessed Oct 2024).
2. Siegel RL et al. Cancer Statistics, 2021. *CA Cancer J Clin.* 2021;71(1):7–33. doi: 10.3322/caac.21654. Erratum in: *CA Cancer J Clin.* 2021;71(4):359.
3. Bokemeyer C et al. Long-term gonadal toxicity after therapy for Hodgkin's and non-Hodgkin's lymphoma. *Ann Hematol.* 1994;68(3):105–110.
4. Lobo RA. Potential options for preservation of fertility in women. *N Engl J Med.* 2005;353(1):64–73.
5. Critchley HO, Wallace WH. Impact of cancer treatment on uterine function. *J Natl Cancer Inst Monogr.* 2005;(34):64–68.
6. Practice Committee, ASRM. Fertility preservation in patients undergoing gonadotoxic therapy or gonadectomy: a committee opinion. *Fertil Steril.* 2019;112(6):1022–1033.
7. Oktay K et al. Fertility preservation in patients with cancer: ASCO clinical practice guideline update summary. *J Oncol Pract.* 2018;14(6):381–385.
8. Grifo JA, Noyes N. Delivery rate using cryopreserved oocytes is comparable to conventional in vitro fertilization using fresh oocytes: potential fertility preservation for female cancer patients. *Fertil Steril.* 2010;93(2):391–396.
9. Rienzi L et al. Embryo development of fresh 'versus' vitrified metaphase II oocytes after ICSI: a prospective randomized sibling-oocyte study. *Hum Reprod.* 2010;25(1):66–73.
10. Goossens E et al. Fertility preservation in boys: recent developments and new insights. *Human Reprod Open.* 2013;28(5):897–907.

26

Egg Freezing

Samuel A. Pauli, Kerri L. Luzzo, and Karishma Patel

Oocyte cryopreservation has grown in popularity for both medical and elective reasons. The laboratory technique to freeze oocytes has improved such that we have confidence that eggs that have been frozen have a high probability of surviving the thaw, can be fertilized and result in a pregnancy. This chapter provides an overview of the application of this technology.

Oocyte Cryopreservation Technology

Cryopreservation, a process in which tissues are cooled to sub-zero temperatures thereby placing the cell in an arrested biologic state, allows women to freeze oocytes at a particular reproductive age to preserve for potential future use. This rapidly developing technology has progressed over the last couple of decades with improvements in cooling techniques and alterations in cryoprotectants. These changes led to the first human birth from cryopreserved oocytes in 1986. Challenges with initial methods of oocyte cryopreservation included cellular damage related to oocyte plasma membrane stability, osmotic damage, changes in salt concentrations, cellular ice formation, and meiotic spindle sensitivity to dehydration and rehydration. The two methods of cryopreservation, slow freezing and vitrification, use different concentrations of cryoprotectants and differing rates of cooling and warming. Vitrification, the most current method of cryopreservation, utilizes high concentrations of cryoprotectant and rapid cooling and warming resulting in a solid glass-like cell that is free of ice crystals. A Cochrane review in 2014 suggested higher clinical pregnancy rates with oocyte vitrification versus slow freezing (RR 3.86, 95% CI 1.63–9.11, p=0.002) (1). A 2013 meta-analysis of 10 studies and 2265 oocyte cryopreservation cycles with slow freeze and vitrification revealed lower oocyte survival and fertilization rates as well as lower implantation and live birth rates with slow freezing (2).

Indications for Oocyte Cryopreservation

While embryo cryopreservation is a well-established, reliable technology, it requires a partner or donor sperm and is not suitable for all patients. In 2012, the American Society for Reproductive Medicine (ASRM) removed the experimental label from oocyte cryopreservation (3). Oocyte cryopreservation has various indications including preserving fertility in women facing gonadotoxic treatment with chemotherapy or radiation, minimizing the formation of excess embryos due to religious/legal concerns, or in the setting of *in vitro* fertilization (IVF) where sperm in unobtainable.

For women undergoing gonadotoxic therapy, the potential negative outcomes include irregular menses, premature ovarian failure, or infertility. The American Society of Clinical Oncology (ASCO) recommends that health care providers address fertility preservation prior to cancer treatment, to discuss the possibility of infertility and fertility preservation options and/or refer to reproductive specialists. Information regarding oocyte cryopreservation for cancer patients specifically is addressed in another chapter in this handbook. As more women delay childbearing for social reasons, elective oocyte

 DOI: 10.1201/9781003460275-26

cryopreservation, now referred to as planned oocyte cryopreservation, is increasing as a method to potentially preserve reproductive potential. Notably, there was an 880% increase in oocyte cryopreservation cycles in the United States between 2010 and 2016 for both medical and planned reasons, and recent SART data from 2016–2019 shows a continued increase of 89% (4).

In addition, planned oocyte cryopreservation includes providing fertility preservation and reproductive care to transgender persons. Oocyte cryopreservation offers trans men the opportunity to preserve their fertility without committing to a male partner or sperm donor at the time of cryopreservation. The effect of long-term testosterone therapy on ovarian function and egg quality is unclear, with some reports that trans men can still experience pregnancy while on testosterone and regain fertility after discontinuing it (5). Although it is recommended that transgender individuals receive counseling regarding the potential loss of fertility and future reproductive options before initiating gender affirming hormone therapy, there are ultimately no guidelines on actual fertility risks of gender affirming hormone treatment, which fertility preservation options are appropriate, and what point in the medical intervention process that fertility preservation should occur.

Oocyte Cryopreservation Outcomes

Early experience with oocyte cryopreservation reported pregnancy rates between 8–33% due to slow freezing technology, but studies examining outcomes in the era of vitrification show that frozen oocytes have a similar potential to fresh oocytes. A retrospective cohort study from 2016 examined oocyte vitrification outcomes for indications including elective fertility preservation, limiting excess embryo creation, or cases in which a sperm sample was not obtainable on the day of oocyte retrieval. Comparing fresh oocyte versus vitrified oocytes, they found similar fertilization rates, higher implantation and pregnancy rates for vitrified versus fresh oocyte cycles but no differences in live birth rates between fresh and frozen cycles. The overall per oocyte live birth rate, or efficiency, which is important with regards to number of oocytes to freeze and proper patient counseling, of 6.4% was dependent on maternal age (6). The ASRM practice guidelines on mature oocyte cryopreservation summarizes four randomized, controlled trials showing similar implantation and clinical pregnancy rates when comparing fresh to vitrified warmed oocytes that were cryopreserved (3).

More recently, literature has focused not only on the outcomes of oocyte cryopreservation for planned or medical indications but also trends in how many patients return to use frozen oocytes. A retrospective study in 2018 looked at over 8000 medically indicated and planned oocyte cryopreservation cycles. Patients undergoing planned oocyte cryopreservation were older, underwent more treatment cycles, and had fewer oocytes retrieved and vitrified per cycle. In addition, the utilization rate was higher for planned oocyte cryopreservation at 12.5% compared to 7.4% for medically indicated oocyte cryopreservation. The thaw survival rates of vitrified oocytes were similar in both groups, and overall there was no difference in clinical or ongoing pregnancy rates (7). Another study that specifically looked at planned oocyte cryopreservation found that of 921 patients, 7.4% returned to use their oocytes. The cumulative live birth rate per patient who initiated thawing–warming was 32.4% in this group (8). Utilization rates of frozen oocytes remain low, thus it is difficult to make meaningful conclusions on differences in reproductive outcomes. Overall, however, the literature suggests that fresh and frozen oocytes are similar with respect to fertilization and pregnancy rates.

Neonatal Outcomes After Oocyte Cryopreservation

The data thus far suggests that oocyte cryopreservation does not increase perinatal/neonatal risk. A 2013 observational study and comparative analysis of obstetric and neonatal outcomes from pregnancies achieved with fresh and/or cryopreserved oocytes showed no differences in fetal or perinatal complications or congenital anomalies (9). A large retrospective cohort study examining obstetric and perinatal outcomes between fresh and vitrified oocytes showed no differences in obstetrical complications such as pregnancy-induced hypertension, premature rupture of membranes, cesarean delivery, diabetes, or preterm delivery. Adverse neonatal outcomes including low birth weight, birth defects, and NICU admission were also similar between fresh and vitrified oocytes (10). Overall, the ASRM recommends that patients should be counseled that neonatal outcomes appear similar after using their own previously cryopreserved oocytes compared with outcomes after the use of fresh oocytes (11).

Planned Oocyte Cryopreservation

In the United States, the only age demographic seeing an increased rise in the rate of pregnancies are in women ages 35–39 and 40 and older, highlighting a trend of delayed childbearing for reproductive-age women. Most women face infertility not from cancer or systemic disease, but rather from the passage of time and age-related fertility decline. Today, multiple social and demographic pressures conspire to encourage women to delay and defer childbearing including education and career aspirations, later marriage, no partner, economic barriers, media images of late-in-life celebrity motherhood, and a host of other factors. Given these reasons, women may wish to postpone childbearing for social reasons. Supporting this notion is the decreasing average age of those undergoing oocyte cryopreservation for any indication, from 36.7 years in 2010 to 34.7 years in 2016 (4).

Given the progressive loss of oocyte quantify and quality with aging, the use of oocyte cryopreservation can be used as a strategy by women to defer childbearing to maintain reproductive autonomy. The ASRM endorsed oocyte cryopreservation for medically indicated fertility preservation but initially did not endorse it directly for oocyte cryopreservation for the sole purpose of reproductive aging (3). Since then, there has been increased data suggesting that oocyte cryopreservation is both effective and safe when used for elective deferring of childbearing. Given these reassuring findings, the ASRM, in 2023, deemed planned oocyte cryopreservation ethically permissible (12). The discussion raised concerns about the inherent risks of single and multiple ovarian stimulation(s) and retrieval(s), absence of long-term outcomes, and inequitable access. It was concluded, however, that planned oocyte cryopreservation increases flexibility with life circumstances and increases options to have genetically-related offspring at a time when natural fertility would be in decline. Regardless, planned oocyte cryopreservation appears favorable to patients; a survey study of 338 patients who underwent initial consultation for planned oocyte cryopreservation showed that 47.3% of patients had not undergone preservation. Of those patients, 50% experienced moderate-to-severe regret with their decision compared to respondents who had undergone at least one cycle of planned oocyte cryopreservation (13).

Patient selection, counseling, and informed consent for oocyte cryopreservation is paramount when counseling women on future reproductive choices. The ASRM acknowledges that the available data support improved outcomes for women who undergo planned oocyte cryopreservation at a younger age, but there are insufficient data to pinpoint an optimal age (11). Ideally, women should be 38 years old or younger given age-related declines in fertility and increased risk of chromosomal aneuploidy. Evaluation typically starts with an assessment of ovarian reserve to determine if a patient will be a good candidate for oocyte preservation and to give a realistic assessment of the number of oocytes to be retrieved. It is important to stress that there is no guarantee of future success of oocyte cryopreservation, and, therefore, the technology should not be used to encourage women to delay childbearing. Rather, it should be used as a tool for women who wish to electively freeze their eggs as part of their longer-term reproductive goals.

Quantity of Oocytes Cryopreserved

Patients may commonly ask how many frozen eggs are considered enough to ensure future reproductive potential. Of course, oocyte efficiency decreases with increasing age, but there are limited data to specify the optimal number of oocytes needed with planned OC. Some authors have used retrospective

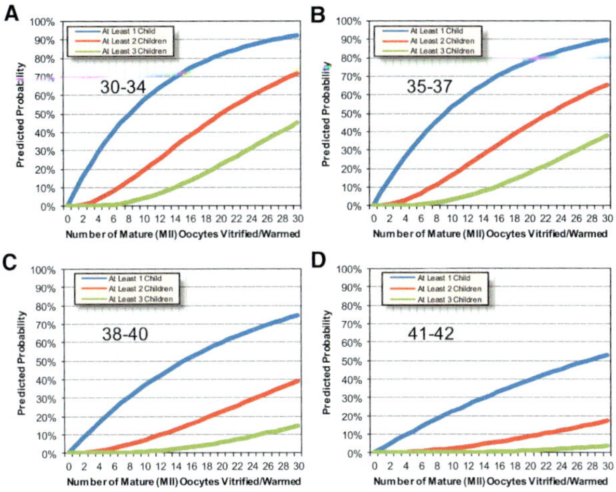

FIGURE 26.1 Predicted probabilities of having at least one, two, and three live-born children according to the number of mature oocytes cryopreserved for elective fertility preservation, according to age at oocyte retrieval and the associated oocyte to live-born child efficiency estimates: (A) 30–34 years, 8.2% efficiency; (B) 35–37 years, 7.3% efficiency; (C) 38–40 years, 4.5% efficiency; (D) 41–42 years, 2.5% efficiency. (From ref 6 with permission.)

data and statistical modeling to create counseling tools on ideal number of oocytes cryopreserved to achieve a live birth.

A model by Doyle and colleagues in 2016 used outcomes from both fresh and frozen IVF cycles to estimate the oocyte-to-child efficiency for each retrieved oocyte after stratification by age group. They estimated that to achieve a 70% chance of one live birth, women aged 30–34 need 14 mature oocytes, women aged 35–37 need 15 mature oocytes, and women aged 38–40 need 26. Their visual counseling tool is illustrated in Figure 26.1 (6). Also in 2016, Cobo and colleagues retrospectively reviewed outcomes of 137 women who returned to use vitrified oocytes that were either cryopreserved electively due to age or for a non-cancer medical condition. Kaplan–Meier curves were created to estimate the live birth rate per oocyte used for women ≤35 and ≥36. They found that women ≤35 who used 10 mature oocytes had a 60.5% likelihood of live birth, while women ≥36 y who used the same number of oocytes had a 29.7% likelihood of live birth (14).

Notably, a 2022 study published data for the largest cohort of patients that underwent specifically planned oocyte cryopreservation (15). This study included oocyte utilization data on 543 patients over a 15-year study period. The median time between the first cryopreservation and thaw was 4.2 years, and

Age at the first cryopreservation	0–9 M2s thawed	10–14 M2s thawed	15–19 M2s thawed	≥20 M2s thawed
All ages (n = 467)	24% (43/176)	45%[a] (54/120)	44%[a] (38/87)	58%[a] (49/84)
<38 y (n = 187)	36% (16/45)	54% (32/59)	41% (16/39)	70%[b] (31/44)
38–40 y (n = 219)	23% (23/100)	37%[a] (18/49)	49%[a] (19/39)	48%[a] (15/31)
≥41 y (n = 61)	13%[c] (4/31)	33% (4/12)	33% (3/9)	33%[c] (3/9)

FIGURE 26.2 Final live birth rate per patient by age at the first cryopreservation and number of M2s thawed (15).

61% underwent one or more transfers. The live birth rate per transfer was 55% for euploid embryos and 31% for non-biopsied embryos, which is similar to age-matched IVF outcomes. Their data also supported the notion that age at the time of cryopreservation and the number of M2 oocytes thawed were predictive of live birth rate. A >50% live birth rate was achieved for patients aged <38 years old and for patients who thawed ≥20 M2 oocytes. Data from the study, illustrated in Figure 26.2, can also be used as a counseling tool.

Ultimately, after review of the literature, the ASRM notes that currently there is insufficient evidence to counsel women of various ages on the absolute number of oocytes necessary to achieve a reasonable probability of a live birth after planned OC (11).

Key Points

- With the development of vitrification, oocyte cryopreservation has become a more efficient process allowing women to freeze oocytes at a particular reproductive age.
- Indications for oocyte cryopreservation include preserving fertility in women undergoing gonadotoxic treatment (ex. chemotherapy/radiation), minimizing the formation of excess embryos, preserving oocytes when sperm is unobtainable during IVF, and preserving fertility in transgender men prior to gender affirming hormone therapy. Given the recent trend to delay childbearing, planned (elective) oocyte cryopreservation is increasing as a method to preserve reproductive potential and autonomy.
- Although the utilization rate of cryopreserved oocytes remains low, several studies have shown similar fertilization rates and pregnancy rates when comparing the use of fresh oocytes to the use of warmed oocytes that were previously cryopreserved via vitrification.
- There is currently insufficient data to pinpoint an optimal age to proceed with planned oocyte cryopreservation. Patients should be counseled on age-related decline in fertility and increased risk of chromosomal aneuploidy.
- There is currently insufficient data to pinpoint an optimal number of oocytes to cryopreserve to achieve a reasonable probability of a live birth. Patient counseling can be guided by published retrospective data that outlines the oocyte-to-child efficiency stratified by age.

REFERENCES:

1. Glujovsky D et al. Vitrification versus slow freezing for women undergoing oocyte cryopreservation. *Cochrane Database Syst Rev* 2014(9):CD010047.
2. Pelin Cil A et al. Age-specific probability of live birth with oocyte cryopreservation: an individual patient data meta-analysis. *Fertil Steril* 2013;100:492–499.
3. Practice Committees, ASRM. Mature oocyte cryopreservation: a guideline. *Fertil Steril* 2013;99:37–43.
4. Johnston M et al. A major increase in oocyte cryopreservation cycles in the USA, Australia and New Zealand since 2010 is highlighted by younger women but a need for standardized data collection. *Hum Reprod* 2021;36(3):624–635.
5. Tishelman AC et al. Health care provider perceptions of fertility preservation barriers and challenges with transgender patients and families: qualitative responses to an international survey. *J Assist Reprod Genet* 2019;36(3):579–588.
6. Doyle JO et al. Successful elective and medically indicated oocyte vitrification and warming for autologous in vitro fertilization, with predicted birth probabilities for fertility preservation according to number of cryopreserved oocytes and age at retrieval. *Fertil Steril* 2016;105:459–466.
7. Cobo A et al. Elective and Onco-fertility preservation: factors related to IVF outcomes. *Hum Reprod* 2018;33(12):2222–2231.
8. Leung AQ et al. Clinical outcomes and utilization from over a decade of planned oocyte cryopreservation. *Reprod Biomed Online* 2021;43(4):671–679.

9. Setti PE et al. Comparative analysis of fetal and neonatal outcomes of pregnancies from fresh and cryo-preserved/thawed oocytes in the same group of patients. *Fertil Steril* 2013;100:396–401.
10. Cobo A et al. Obstetric and perinatal outcomes of babies born from vitrified oocytes. *Fertil Steril* 2014;102:1006–1015.
11. Practice Committees, ASRM. Evidence-based outcomes after oocyte cryopreservation for donor oocyte in vitro fertilization and planned oocyte cryopreservation: a guideline. *Fertil Steril* 2021;116:36–47.
12. ASRM Ethics Committee Documents. Planned oocyte cryopreservation to preserve future reproductive potential: an ethics committee opinion. *Fertil Steril* 2024;121:604–612.
13. Korkidakis A et al. Decision-making in women considering planned oocyte cryopreservation: decision satisfaction or regret? *Reprod Biomed Online* 2024;103944.
14. Cobo A et al. Oocyte vitrification as an efficient option for elective fertility preservation. *Fertil Steril.* 2016;105(3):755–64.
15. Cascante SD et al. Fifteen years of autologous oocyte thaw outcomes from a large university-based fertility center. *Fertil Steril.* 2022;118(1):158–166.

27

Tools for Effective Nursing in the Care of the Infertile Patient

Sharon Edwards

Introduction

Reproductive Endocrinology and Infertility (REI) or Assisted Reproductive Technology (ART) nursing is a relatively new field that began in the 1970s with hospital-based infertility clinics where nurses were considered the doctor's "assistant." The field has expanded considerably from those days into a complex and unique specialty requiring a vast amount of knowledge, empathy, understanding, and patience. The REI nurse is the crucial link between the patient and the physician as an advocate, giving support and helping to navigate the complicated system the patient has just entered. On any given day, the REI nurse may discuss the areas of reproductive anatomy, lab procedures, genetics, insurance, law, and ethics. The REI nurse is also the "glue" that holds the rest of the team together by being a liaison for medical staff, embryology, endocrinology, clinical and surgical procedures, financial services, and mental health practitioners. Since REI nurses are such an integral part of the patient's journey, they must be well trained and understand their role has a far-reaching impact on each patient they encounter. There truly is an "art" to ART nursing.

Acquiring a Knowledge Base

What brings someone to REI nursing? For some it is a personal experience, either themself, a family member, or friend. Experiencing the emotional struggle and stress of infertility has a profound effect on many nurses and leads to a desire to help others. For many it represents a change from the typical hospital-based practice on a floor or critical care unit, allowing a better life/work balance in a field that is constantly changing and growing. For most it is having a background in women's health nursing and the interest and challenge of a specialty practice. Whatever the reason or past experience, REI is an innovative field that requires intensive training and learning from a variety of sources. It takes about six months to understand all the mechanics of infertility and up to a year to feel competent and knowledgeable as an REI nurse. This is not a static specialty; REI is an ever-changing field requiring nurses to keep abreast of new clinical protocols, medications, laboratory innovations, and genetic testing regimens, to name a few related topics.

Sources of Education

- There is no uniform standardization or universal curriculum of teaching nurses that are unaccustomed to REI. Clinics often rely on their current nursing staff to train those inexperienced in the field, and in-depth training may be lacking. Fortunately, there are resources for a

DOI: 10.1201/9781003460275-27

nurse unfamiliar with the infertility field to access—the American Society for Reproductive Medicine (ASRM) has dozens of modules for both new and seasoned nurses, from basic infertility to embryology for the nursing professional [1]. The nursing arm of ASRM, the Nurses' Professional Group (NPG), has developed a certificate course acknowledging nursing excellence in the field, which is the gold standard for REI nursing [2]. Several pharmaceutical companies have PhDs who provide one-on-one nurse training in the clinic setting on basic infertility and a variety of specialty subjects. In addition, there are annual conferences that offer courses on many topics needed to acquire a solid knowledge base for infertility.

- On-the-job training is an important and crucial aspect of nursing education as it deals with day-to-day, real-life situations that are important to develop a "feel" for what the patient experiences. Seasoned REI nurses can mentor the in-training nurse on the nuts and bolts of the specialty, offering experience and wisdom in a practical application. The best training method is to have a comprehensive orientation schedule over the course of two to three months, with specific elements that gradually progress the inexperienced nurse from observation to fielding calls, with a seasoned nurse as a mentor. An effective tool during this training period is "role playing." The seasoned mentor nurse "pretends" to be a patient, asking questions in different ways. Doing this ensures the unseasoned nurse understands the content and is not just memorizing what was taught and is a known effective teaching method. A checklist to "sign off" the newly-trained nurse as having been exposed to and understands all the necessary elements rounds out the educational experience. With so much information to learn, the use of checklists and digital notebooks (OneNote, for example) to keep information easily organized and accessible are great tools. At the end of the day, nurses learn best by "doing," sitting at the computer themselves learning and alongside their mentor, not sitting by passively only observing or reading protocols.

What the REI Nurse Needs to Know

- Infertility 101: This comprises the "basics" of infertility, explaining to the patient the male and female reproductive anatomy, the menstrual cycle, endocrine hormones, and how they interact.
- The infertility evaluation: Many diagnostic tests are needed to evaluate the cause of infertility, and it is the REI nurse's responsibility to explain and schedule these tests, which could include a fallopian tube and cavity study (hysterosalpingogram [HSG]), saline sonohysterogram (SIS) with Hysterosalpingo-Contrast Sonography (HyCoSy), office hysteroscopy, endocrine hormone assay (cycle day 3 testing, which can include follicle stimulating hormone, anti-Müllerian hormone, and estradiol levels), ultrasound (basal antral follicle count), or semen analysis for male patients.
- Abnormalities and what they mean: Sometimes abnormalities can interfere with cycle timing, so understanding and explaining how this impacts a patient is important. Things such as fibroids or polyps can negatively impact implantation to carry a fetus to term. Other factors such as polycystic ovary syndrome (PCOS), premature ovarian insufficiency (POI), endometriosis, to name a few, can impact egg release and embryo implantation. The REI nurse must be able to assist with an explanation on courses of treatment to resolve these issues.
- Treatment options: The variety of options can be overwhelming for a patient to grasp, and the decision-making process stressful. Understanding the many protocols, medications, and regimens is a key ingredient for successful REI nurse–patient interactions. Patients often do not understand everything being said in the follow-up visit with their physician and look to the nurse to explain what has just been discussed. They may be nervous or don't want to appear unknowledgeable and, therefore, don't ask questions of their physician. At the other end of the spectrum, patients now have access to more information online than ever before and are trying to sift through what's relevant and what's not. Because of the strong bond formed with their nurse, patients feel safe and cared for and look to their nurse to go through the treatment options again to come to an informed decision. It is, therefore, imperative that an REI nurse be

adept at explaining treatment options. These options can include timed intercourse, IUI with Clomid/Letrozole, IUI with gonadotropins, natural cycles, IVF cycles, natural insemination versus ICSI, PGTa/SR/M, as well as third-party reproduction. In the end, the REI nurse is the one who takes the information given to a patient, breaks it down step-by-step in a way that can be understood, and implements it in a way that the patient doesn't feel so overwhelmed. This can be accomplished in a variety of ways to fortify the verbal communication that has already taken place, such as written materials or handouts pertinent to each cycle, treatment, or test, and this is often the most effective communication. This underscores and validates what the nurse has explained and gives patients a reference to refer to as and when needed. The materials can be generic templates tailored to each patient, and can be sent by email, posted in an electronic patient portal, or a paper handout to the patient depending on the resources of the center. Quite an impressive amount of knowledge to master!

Elements for Effective REI Nursing

Once REI nurses have learned the medical and scientific basis of their craft, they must follow through on the other necessary elements needed as part of the care team. Communication and attention to detail are critical components of effective nursing for both the patient and other members of the team. As the primary liaison for the patient, the REI nurse must have good documentation practices, detailed notes for all team members to easily access, communicate with all parties, and be articulate in those communications.

The landscape has changed post-Covid to shift how we communicate with patients, and now more than ever it is important to build connections via the way we communicate as so much is now done digitally. Finding a middle ground between personalized/individualized communication and the expectations of the digital age has brought added challenges.

- Attention to detail: This is imperative due to the multifactorial aspect of the patient's care. As the "go to" member of the team, the REI nurse is the "quarterback" for the team and must be meticulous in detailing all aspects of treatment. Decisions are made that must be coordinated, from the physician to the embryologist to the financial counselor to the appointment scheduler; all are fed through the REI nurse. Attention to every detail must be noted and acted on, whether it be to the team or to the patient. Treatment plans are modified, patients change their minds, and many things happen daily requiring the quarterback to monitor and ensure these details are attended to and implemented.
- Communication and documentation: Nurses learn early on in their education, "if it wasn't documented, it wasn't done." Every interaction with the patient must be clearly and concisely written. It is the REI nurse's obligation to ensure that the next health care team member who accesses the patient chart is aware of all that has transpired and that all interactions with the patient are documented. It is also imperative that the nurse is clear and concise with the patient, whether it be in person, by phone, or by email. Patients hang on to every word expressed, give great value to what is said, and great value to anything said that may be expressed differently or perceived as contradictory. For this reason, every interaction must be documented in objective terms with precise language to prevent misinterpretation and provide clarity to both patient and team members.

Timely and effective communication can be accomplished through a variety of means; infertility nurses may field 50–80 calls a day. Email, texting, and an EMR patient portal are a few of the ways nurses communicate in the modern paradigm. Patients are anxious and stressed, and if they are unable to speak to their nurse live, they expect a return call quickly. A policy should be in place that all calls are returned by the end of that day, regardless of whether there is a solution or not. While all issues may not be resolved, the patient will understand that their issue is being addressed and reassured their concerns are taken seriously. The patient experience involves not only good medical care but good customer service care as well.

Informed Consent

While informed consent is ultimately the responsibility of the physician, the process begins with a discussion of the proposed treatment plan with the physician and ultimately involves multiple staff across departmental lines. After the initial discussion, the nursing team provides educational materials and consent forms for the patient to review. The pandemic brought a shift in the way signed consents were obtained. Patients and partners typically signed paper consent forms when they were in the office after their consultation for treatment. However, with the adoption of telehealth and drastically decreased number of patients in the office, many clinics had to quickly convert to electronic consent forms. It is imperative to have a form of authentication for identification. This can be done with SMS authentication and geolocation.

When the patient and partner (if applicable) are ready to move forward, they either meet with the nurse to review and sign the consents or they receive/sign the consents electronically and review with the nurse via telehealth or phone. If any issues arise from the wording of the consent or it appears the patient requires clarification of the treatment plan that the nurse has already addressed, the nurse will arrange for the patient to meet again with the physician. Informed consent is a shared responsibility that the REI nurse contributes to in a meaningful way, and the patient looks to his or her nurse as a guide through understanding the elements.

Triage

The nurse plays an important role in the triage of medical and emotional issues that need to be addressed during treatment and brought to the attention of the physician. For example, ectopic pregnancies can be more common in the infertile population who undergo IVF treatment. A patient who calls with a menses that is lighter than usual, has bleeding at an anticipated time of the menstrual cycles, has abnormal rising hCG titers, or complains of pain should be considered at risk of having an ectopic pregnancy. Ovarian hyperstimulation syndrome (OHSS) complicates any fertility treatment but is more common in the patient undergoing IVF and being triggered with hCG. Symptoms can occur any time from the time of the egg retrieval through the pregnancy test. Initial symptoms include abdominal distention and pain. Symptoms of more advanced OHSS include SOB, N/V, and severe pain—–these patients need to be brought in for evaluation expeditiously. These are just a few examples of why REI nurses must have a thorough understanding of complications and be aware of the signs and symptoms of many concerns presented by patients. Since the nurse is in frequent contact with the patient, the nurse is the person fielding these important calls—if not properly triaged, these patients can be at risk for serious consequences.

Patient Education

Patient education begins the moment a patient walks into the clinic and it lasts through the entire journey. REI nurses daily encounter patients who need accurate and compassionate information about the process of infertility treatment. There are many ways to provide the necessary information, and a formal patient education program should be in place to teach patients not only the details of their treatment plan but to guide patients through all the steps along the way.

The nurse guides the patient through many medical and non-medical aspects, such as financial implications, insurance benefits, appointment setting, consenting, as well as medications and treatment. A comprehensive system is set up to teach and instruct patients with each new phase of the process encountered, and there are two main elements of a good patient education program:

- Instruction by the primary nurse each time the patient meets with the physician.

- A formal education consultation with an experienced nurse each time the patient has a treatment she/he hasn't done before (such as the first time a patient does IUI or IVF).

When the patient has a consult with the physician, there is usually a "next step" that the primary nurse helps to explain; comprehensive testing after the initial consult, the results of that testing after the follow-up consult, discussion about progress once treatment begins, to name a few. This is ongoing throughout the patient's experience. The second, and very important patient education interaction, is when a first-time regimen is ordered, such as an IUI or IVF cycle. There are several ways clinics set up education forums: large group teaching sessions, one-on-one in-person sessions, and on-line programs. Large group sessions are difficult to teach as they involve multiple treatment plans and medications and are not individualized to the patient. They tend to be ineffective and often create more questions than they answer. One-on-one in-person sessions are individualized and effective, but terribly inefficient and not practical for the primary nurse to do as each session is an hour-long process. The most efficient and beneficial method is to do an online program that involves computer-based information, real-time medication video, and a follow-up phone consultation with the nurse educator. This allows the patient to review the literature and instructions at home at a time of their choosing. It is less stressful as the patient can do this over a period of time and review the information as many times as needed. The key part of this type of program is the follow-up phone call by the nurse to make sure the patient has read the material and understands it; a short "quiz" can take place during the conversation. If the nurse feels the patient does not fully understand the treatment plan or what is involved, the patient is brought into the clinic to go over it in person. This method has a high patient satisfaction index and respects the patient's time as well as being more manageable by the clinic. However, not all clinics have the necessary staffing to do this and will incorporate other methods of comprehensive teaching that is handled through a third party. This includes detailed patient modules on various aspects of treatment as well as step-by-step injection training and has quizzes along the way to ensure patient understanding. There is a modest cost to this, and many clinics use this method as an adjunct to complete the necessary patient education.

Being a Patient Advocate

REI nurses are in a unique position to help guide the patient experience, since patients identify their nurse as their most important contact and see or speak to their nurse more often than they do with their physician. The inability to conceive or maintain a pregnancy often creates a crisis for women and their partners and they look to their nurse for care, compassion, and help. Many patients put on their best faces in front of the physician but confide in the nurse how they are truly feeling, and it is a special role that nurses take on to reduce the patient's anxiety and validate their feelings. Nurses guide patients through the grief of failed treatment, provide empathy after a loss, and allow the patient to feel safe in expressing their loss of control. Nurses are more in tune with the emotional aspects of what the patient experiences and often will recognize anxiety and depression in patients they work with. When this happens, it is crucial that the nurse speak to the physician and formulate a plan of care that includes a mental health professional—most patients will deny they have an issue, but prolonged depression will affect all aspects of the patient's life and must be addressed. A clinic should have access to or a list of qualified professionals who are experienced in patients undergoing infertility. The ideal would be to have a social worker or psychologist on site to meet with patients or intervene if there is an urgent need.

Conclusion

The scope of REI nursing practice continues to expand as cutting-edge developments in science, treatment protocol, medication, and laboratory procedures evolve, along with the ever-changing political landscape and norms of society. The scientific, emotional, legal, and changing patient population provides an exciting environment with many opportunities for a nurse to grow. Every day we learn something from our patients and from each other, and this makes our field amazing. Strong, qualified nurses will always be needed to provide a foundation for the patient struggling with infertility; they are a critical link when a patient is successful and an empathic friend when the patient isn't. The role is complex, but the rewards are many and it is a privilege to be a part of the journey.

Key Points

- The nursing arm of ASRM, the Nurses' Professional Group (NPG), has developed a certificate course acknowledging nursing excellence in the field, which is the gold standard for REI nursing.
- Every interaction with the patient must be clearly and concisely written. It is the REI nurse's obligation to ensure that the next health care team member who accesses the patient chart is aware of all that has transpired and that all interactions with the patient are documented.
- REI nurses are in a unique position to help guide the patient experience since patients identify their nurse as their most important contact and see or speak to their nurse more often than their physician.

REFERENCES

1. Academy, ASRM [internet]: /www.asrm.org/asrm-academy/.
2. Nurses Professional Group, ASRM [internet]: www.npg-asrm.org/programs/nursecertificatecourse?ssopc=1

28

The Role of the Infertility Counselor

Jeanie Ungerleider and Lynn Nichols

Infertility is a medical condition that can affect every part of an individual's or couple's life. It can challenge the ways in which people feel about themselves, their relationships with their partner, family, and friends. It often can distract them in their work and general outlook on life. Few situations are as stressful and overwhelming, which is why infertility is considered a life crisis.

When going through infertility, a person can feel that the process is totally beyond their control. Most people assume that if they work hard enough, they will achieve their goal to become parents. These feelings can get amplified by the disappointment of repeated failed treatments. Their uncertainty about whether they will ever conceive and have a healthy baby can increase one's level of anxiety. They also see their peers who are pregnant with their first, second, or third child, while they are struggling with infertility, feeling increasingly resentful, angry, and isolated from the people whom they usually turn to for support.

Infertility is a crisis of identity where one questions their sense of self and self-worth. Over time, women may express feeling inadequate, depressed, and anxious about their failed cycles, which can stir up a sense of helplessness and hopelessness. For men struggling with male factor problems, this can be devastating and challenging to their sense of masculinity, potency, and identity.

Many factors contribute to the different ways in which people cope with stress. This includes personality differences, family history, and life experiences, which shape how people experience and handle this life crisis. Moreover, women and men may demonstrate very different ways of coping with the diagnosis and treatment process. Women often feel anxious about the limits of their biological clocks. There is the heightened awareness of the urgency of time and a painful reminder each month when there is not a pregnancy. Women tend to blame themselves or their partner for not starting sooner to conceive and are burdened with guilt and regrets about the delay. When a woman has had a prior pregnancy termination, they may experience their infertility as a punishment for having had an abortion.

Women often want to discuss feelings and concerns about the infertility with their partner, which can dominate the conversation when they are together. Generally speaking, men may tend to respond with optimism, assuring their partner of a positive outcome, not wanting to add to their partner's distress, thereby limiting or avoiding the conversation, which can contribute to a growing sense of disconnect and isolation from each other. This can affect the couple's sexual relationship; no longer is their lovemaking pleasurable and intimate. Sometimes a couple is in conflict about moving forward with the infertility treatment.

The Role of the Counselor in an Infertility Practice

Most major infertility practices have licensed independent clinical social workers (LICSWs) or psychologists available who specialize in infertility counseling. Many of these clinicians are members of the American Society for Reproductive Medicine (ASRM) and the Mental Health Professional Group of ASRM that offer practice guidelines and guidance for the mental health professionals. The role of the counselor is multifaceted and ever-changing depending on the expressed needs of the individual or

DOI: 10.1201/9781003460275-28

couple and their level of distress. Sometimes they consult with members of the health care team, offer supportive counseling, a patient advocate, or more broadly, a psychotherapist. Furthermore, the infertility counselor can make referrals to resources in the community and be a liaison to other mental health professionals, such as psychopharmacologists and psychotherapists, on behalf of the health care team. The roles of the infertility counselor can shift with the individual or couple over time and reflect this complex process and their changing needs. If an individual or couple are having a difficult time going through the medical process, seeing a counselor one-on-one can help address specific issues and provide the support and strategies needed for coping.

Counseling is helpful for those who are having difficulty making informed treatment decisions or choosing treatment options. It is also useful for those who have experienced a miscarriage and are grieving this loss and need acute bereavement counseling that can help build emotional resilience. When appropriate, the counselor can make a referral to a bereavement support group or suggest other resources.

Counseling is also recommended for people who are facing the end of medical treatment and are having difficulty making this decision or wishing to discuss other options and alternatives, such as the use of donor egg or donor sperm, donor embryo, gestational care arrangement, adoption, or child-free living. Some of these issues are covered later in this chapter.

In making a clinical assessment of the individual's or couple's needs, the counselor can determine the most appropriate treatment modality. This can be in the form of individual counseling, couples counseling, a support group, a mind/body program, or a combination of these options. In individual and couples counseling, the counselor can help sort out feelings of how their infertility has impacted them and their partner as well as help them deal with family and friends. Couples learn ways to strengthen their relationship and develop skills to navigate the emotional roller coaster of infertility.

If a patient presents with a complicated trauma history and other heightened stress, the counselor can effectively help to facilitate the woman's care with her health care team and intervene, when necessary, in a particular area of concern in order to assist her going forward with treatment.

The Role of the Infertility Counselor in Assisted Conception

Newer ways of having a family with the use of donor egg, donor sperm, egg freezing, gestational carrier arrangement, and embryo donation have become increasingly successful ways for individuals and couples to have a child. These choices for family building raise unique social, emotional, and ethical issues. As part of most IVF programs, it is considered invaluable for people to meet with a counselor to discuss these complex issues.

Donor Egg or Donor Sperm Consultation

When the use of a third party in the reproductive process (donor egg or donor sperm) is recommended to infertile individuals and couples, new sets of concerns and feelings arise. These include feelings about the medical condition that necessitated the use of a donor. Additionally, the loss of the genetic tie to the prospective mother or father and its meaning may become central. Practical issues such as disclosure must also be addressed. While the decision to tell the child about its genetic origins is a personal one, it is an issue that should be explored with the couple before treatment begins. Those coming into infertility clinics with the hopes of creating their own child have often gone through, and continue to go through, a multitude of emotional experiences from positive anticipation to frustration, disappointment, and continued loss. Here, the counselor can continue to assist couples to manage the emotional roller coaster associated with infertility treatment.

The topics covered in the psychoeducational consultation of third-party reproduction may include transitioning from a traditional form of treatment to the use of a third party; the feelings involved in making this decision; choosing an anonymous or known donor and the benefits and challenges associated with either choice; issues of disclosure, including when and how to tell the child, the notion of privacy versus secrecy, and how to discuss disclosure with family and friends; transitioning to parenthood and parenting at an older age, if applicable; and the possibility of treatment failure and alternatives for future planning.

The counselor as a member of the medical team participates in the screening of the anonymous and known egg donor. While the donor undergoes a thorough medical screening, it is the responsibility of the counselor to conduct a psychosocial evaluation. The purpose of this portion of the donor screening is to have an understanding of the donor's current life situation as well as assess her personal and family psychiatric history. It is also to determine whether or not she is aware of and prepared to meet the responsibilities and demands present in an egg donation cycle. The counselor follows the ASRM general guidelines for the psychological assessment of oocyte donors and recipients to help determine if a donor is an appropriate candidate. It is also the responsibility of the counselor to inform the donor about the potential emotional benefits and risks associated with egg donation and help her determine if the decision to serve as a donor is well thought out and in her best interest, thus helping her make a psychologically informed consent.

In instances where a known donor is considered, it is important for the infertility counselor to explore and discuss with the recipients and donor together their feelings about the relationship and future expectations between all parties, including the future child. It is essential that everyone involved meet at the time of the medical screening and be in agreement with decisions that have the potential to affect a future family.

Gestational Carrier Arrangement Consultation

The use of gestational carrier arrangement is rarely the first choice for family building in assisted conception. More often, people come to this after exhausting other options, such as intrauterine insemination (IUI) and IVF. Medical conditions on the part of the woman, such as the loss of or impaired uterus, can also determine the use of gestational carrier arrangement in some cases. The most common gestational carrier arrangement these days is for the intended or prospective mother or an egg donor to provide the egg and the intended or prospective father or sperm donor to provide the sperm. The resulting embryo is transferred to the gestational carrier, who does not have a genetic connection to the embryo.

The role of the professional counselor in gestational carrier arrangement consultation is to determine what is best for all the participants involved, including the existing children, and to foresee the range of psychological issues that occur in third-party reproduction and pregnancy and address these to the individualized, psychosocial situations of the participants. The standard practice is for the counselor to have the first consultation with the intended parents to discuss the psychological issues related to gestational carrier arrangement and to assist them in assessing their readiness to take part in a gestational carrier arrangement. This consultation is followed by one evaluative consultation with the prospective gestational carrier and her husband or partner to assess their psychological readiness to participate in a gestational carrier arrangement. Lastly, a joint consultation is provided to the intended parents and gestational carrier and husband or partner together to discuss and assess their readiness to take part in a gestational carrier arrangement with one another. This joint meeting is an important opportunity to define everyone's mutual expectations with regard to the nature of their relationship during the medical process, pregnancy, and after the delivery, as well as to discuss their agreement on potential decision-making ahead, such as twin pregnancy, selective reduction, or circumstances for the termination of a pregnancy.

The counselor also either provides or makes arrangement for standardized psychological testing of the prospective gestational carrier (GC) as part of the screening process. This typically includes a personality test, such as the Minnesota Multiphasic Personality Inventory-2 (MMPI-2) or the Personality Assessment Inventory (PAI), to access the GC's capacity to cope with stress and the quality of her interpersonal relationships.

The evaluation of the carrier by the counselor is an in-depth process and also involves evaluation of her husband or partner as well. Many factors go into the selection of an appropriate gestational carrier, including understanding her motivation or underlying reason to be a gestational carrier for someone. It is important that she has had positive experiences with previous pregnancies and is raising a child of her own. It is critical to assess her psychosocial history and current life situation as well as her psychological history and emotional well-being. It is also important for the gestational carrier to have an adequate support system, in particular, her husband or partner, who supports her wish to be a gestational carrier and helps her and her children during a pregnancy, especially should she require bed rest or hospitalized bed rest. She must be at peace about the relinquishment of the child to the intended parents. The goal is for the prospective gestational carrier to leave the program whole and unharmed and feel satisfied with the process and her relationship with the intended parents.

It is important for all participants involved to have legal, medical, and psychological consultations. Once the medical process is underway, ongoing psychological counseling for the intended parents on an as-needed basis as well as follow-up with their gestational carrier can be an option offered in an effort to help facilitate the gestational carrier process and support their relationship during the pregnancy and afterward. If participants are well matched and invested in the psychological preparedness and considerations, the experience can be mutually fulfilling and satisfying. Additionally, it is a wonderful opportunity to create a positive legacy for the forthcoming child. In addition to heterosexual individuals and couples, most clinics work with gay and lesbian individuals and couples, transgender, and queer patients who look to the donor process or gestational care arrangement as a way of becoming parents.

Preimplantation Genetic Diagnosis for Gender Selection Consultation

Preimplantation genetic diagnosis or PGD is a technology used in conjunction with IVF to test for healthy embryos prior to transfer to the woman's uterus. One indication for performing PGD is when the couple is at risk for having a child with an inherited genetic disorder (i.e., cystic fibrosis, Tay–Sachs disease). A single cell is removed from each embryo and can be tested for the specific genetic disorders. Only embryos free of genetic abnormalities are selected for implantation. Prior to the advent of PGD, testing for genetic disorders was limited and could only be done during the first trimester of pregnancy. The woman would have to endure the stress of waiting for the results. If carrying a genetically abnormal fetus, she would be faced with the psychological trauma associated with decision-making around pregnancy termination. PGD now offers individuals the opportunity to determine healthy embryos prior to transfer, which also reduces much emotional distress with pregnancy.

PGD can also be performed to determine the chromosomal makeup of the embryo including an assessment of the sex chromosomes. There are now some IVF centers that offer PGD to determine the gender of the embryo. Gender selection can be used to eliminate those embryos of a certain gender with a transmittable genetic disorder. Some prospective parent(s) may have a strong gender preference and may request the use of PGD for gender selection. Still others may choose PGD for family balancing, for example, if the couple already has a child or children of one gender and expresses the desire to have another child of the opposite gender. In this situation, all the embryos would be tested to determine their gender, and then the healthy embryos of the preferred sex would be transferred to the woman's uterus.

Sex selection raises various psychosocial, ethical, and controversial issues, such as if a couple has not yet had a child, should they be allowed to select the sex of their offspring? Just because the technology exists, should it be used in this way? Some IVF centers only offer sex selection for family balancing.

It is important for counseling to be available to individuals and couples who are considering PGD for gender selection to allow them to think through the unique psychosocial and ethical questions that are inherent in this technology. For example, if a person wants to have a female child and they undergo IVF with PGD and there are no healthy female embryos, would they transfer the healthy male embryos instead? If they decide not to transfer the healthy male embryos, then what would be the disposition plan for these newly created embryos? The possible options would be to consider freezing the embryos and postpone making any decisions, donating them for medical research, or donating the embryos to another couple or individual. They could also choose to discard the embryos. Thorough discussion of each of these choices needs to be carefully explored before commencing the IVF cycle. If there is a difference of opinion between the couple, they may need assistance in reaching a decision that they can both agree upon.

Embryo Donation Consultation

When a couple or individual have created embryos through IVF and successfully completed their family building, they may have extra embryos that they no longer intend to use. There are a number of options they have for making a dispositional plan. They could decide to continue to keep them frozen, paying a yearly storage charge until they are ready to make a final decision. With the success of IVF, there are now more than 600,000 extra frozen embryos stored in laboratories across the United States. Some people decide to donate their embryos to the clinic laboratory for training embryologists, some decide to discard them, some choose to donate their embryos to another person(s) or an agency that matches donors with recipients. Some embryo donors and recipients find each other online. There are varying degrees of contact the two families will have with each other as well as the nature of the relationship with future offspring. These discussions are finalized in a contract drawn up by a lawyer specializing in reproductive law. Becoming a recipient of donated embryos can be another way for single women or same sex couples to create their families. In the last few years embryo donation has become more common. Some people want to avoid transmitting a genetic disease to their offspring. In some instances, recipients may favor embryo donation instead of only one partner having a genetic link to the child. For some recipients, the cost is another major factor in their decision to use donated embryos. It is considerably less than paying for an IVF cycle with donor gametes. Becoming a recipient of embryo donation takes considerably less time than going through an adoption process. Finally, it gives the prospective mother the opportunity to experience pregnancy and bond with her baby from the beginning.

Sometimes when an infertile couple finally achieves a successful pregnancy and birth, they may initially consider donating their extra embryos to another couple or individual struggling to conceive. However, once they have become parents and completed their family, they sometimes feel different about donating their unused embryos to another person. Some parents begin to think about the fact that their frozen embryos would become full genetic siblings to their children. Anticipating these complex psychological, ethical, and legal issues raises a host of emotions, questions, and thoughts to carefully consider.

Counseling for embryo donors and recipients is extremely helpful in thinking through the psychosocial, ethical, and legal issues unique to embryo donation. The Practice Committee of the ASRM and the Practice Committee of the Society for Assisted Reproductive Technology (SART) provide guidelines for gamete and embryo donation. The complex and often charged emotions that embryo donation raises need to be thoroughly explored and understood. It is useful for both embryo donors and recipients to thoroughly understand the implications of their decision and the nature of the relationship they would want to have with the family and offspring of their embryo donation so they can make a psychological informed consent. Some of the issues to consider are as follows: Will they choose a known donor/known recipient situation? What kind of relationship would the donor family have with the recipient family? What would be the expectations of the relationship with the child who was created through embryo donation? Would the recipient's children and donor's children know about each other? And if so, when and how do they explain this unique situation to their children? In an anonymous embryo donation, the donors and recipients independently decide how much information to share about each other's family and if they would want the option to have contact with the child at 18 years or older.

Parents choosing to donate their extra embryos to an infertile couple or individual often feel tremendous empathy and identification with those who are struggling to conceive. Donating can be an opportunity to help another family in a powerful way and at the same time be compatible with the donating couple's values, religious, and spiritual beliefs. For some it can be an ethical and moral solution for their embryos.

Conclusion

While no one can predict or guarantee the outcome of the infertility treatments, the counselor can help make the process as supportive and helpful as possible. The individual or couple generally value the team approach, expressing appreciation for their health care providers' attention to their medical, physical, emotional, and psychosocial well-being.

In the future, there will be even further advances in assisted reproductive technologies and genetic testing. These new developments may open up more complex ethical, emotional, and psychosocial issues. With the increased success of the assisted reproductive technologies, including third-party reproduction, these new ways to create a family give a renewed sense of hope for patients beginning this journey. There can be several people involved in creating a child. They can include the ovum donor, sperm donor, gestational carrier, intended parents, and recipients of embryo donation. These complex ways of starting the process necessitate careful understanding of the issues involved and exploration of their implications for the individual, couple, and future child. The infertility counselor's role is ever expanding as people make use of these new pathways to parenthood.

Key Point

- Counseling is imperative during the difficult journey of assisted reproduction treatment.

29

Fertility Care for the LGBTQIA+ Community

Samuel Pang and Nina Resetkova

Introduction

For many years, children have been raised in families where their parents are lesbian, gay, bisexual, transgender, queer, intersex, asexual, and more (LGBTQIA+; see Table 29.1 for definitions). Studies have found that children of lesbian or gay parents are not different than children of heterosexual parents in terms of their emotional development or relationships with others (1). Historically, many of these children were conceived and born from heterosexual relationships, after which one parent (or in some cases both parents) "come out" as LGBTQIA+. More recently, LGBTQIA+ people are "coming out" in their youth so that they are less likely to have children from prior heterosexual relationships. Therefore, they are building their families by having children as LGBTQIA+ people. Some choose adoption, but many lesbian couples use donor sperm to conceive. Some use donor sperm from friends, acquaintances, or family members of their partners, but the majority use donor sperm from a commercial sperm bank. For lesbian couples in which one (or both) has infertility, many are able to conceive with assisted reproductive technologies (ART). Historically, gay male couples have built their families through adoption or co-parenting arrangements with lesbian friends, but some have used surrogacy to have children. More recently, transgender people have also been able to use ART to have genetically-related children (2).

Following the U.S. Supreme Court *Obergefell vs. Hodges* decision, which legalized same-sex marriage in the U.S., same-sex couples are marrying in increasing numbers (3–5). Same-sex couples who marry are increasingly seeking to build families, which has resulted in increased demand for ART services (6). The percentage of people who identify as LGBTQIA+ is also growing. Data from the Williams Institute and Gallup poll corroborate that >5% of U.S. adults identify as LGBTQIA+, with higher rates in the 18–24-year old population, suggesting that this proportion may increase over time (6, 7).

LGBTQIA+ individuals frequently experience discrimination or disparities in their health care. The Ethics Committees of the American Society for Reproductive Medicine (ASRM) and the American Congress of Obstetricians and Gynecologists (ACOG) have opined that ethical arguments supporting denial of access to fertility services on the basis of marital status, sexual orientation, or gender identity cannot be justified (8, 9). Healthcare providers need to be informed regarding ART options available to LGBTQIA+ people so that they may counsel their patients appropriately.

Psychosocial Counseling

Psychosocial counseling associated with the use of ART services is not unique to LGBTQIA+ patients. All couples who plan to conceive with donor gametes (sperm or eggs) or a surrogate need to have psychoeducational counseling to discuss concerns and feelings which arise when family-building involves the assistance of a third party. For the parent who is not contributing genetic material, there is the lack of a genetic connection to the child(ren) conceived with donor gametes. There are also practical issues,

DOI: 10.1201/9781003460275-29

TABLE 29.1

Glossary

Sexual orientation:	A person's sexual, physical, romantic, and/or emotional attraction to a particular sex (male or female)
Heterosexuality:	Sexual, physical, romantic, and/or emotional attraction between persons of the opposite sex or gender
Homosexuality:	Sexual, physical, romantic, and/or emotional attraction between persons of the same sex or gender
Gay:	Describes a man whose enduring sexual, physical, romantic and/or emotional attraction is to other men
Lesbian:	Describes a woman whose enduring sexual, physical, romantic, and/or emotional attraction is to other women
Bisexual:	An individual who is sexually, physically, romantically, and/or emotionally attracted to both genders, although not necessarily to the same degree
Gender identity:	A person's internal perception of their gender
Transgender:	An individual who identifies with a gender different than what society expects based on the sex the individual was assigned at birth. Transgender individuals can be heterosexual, lesbian, gay, or bisexual in their sexual orientation
Cisgender:	An individual who identifies with the gender that society expects based on the sex the individual was assigned at birth. Cisgender individuals can be heterosexual, lesbian, gay, or bisexual in their sexual orientation

such as the challenges of choosing the appropriate gamete donor, the differences between known and recruited donors, the option of selecting donors who are open to contact with offspring in the future, and when and how to discuss with the child(ren) conceived with donor gametes the circumstances of their conception. When surrogacy is part of the treatment plan, group counseling involving all parties is mandatory to ensure that everyone is in agreement regarding the expectations of their relationship during and beyond the surrogacy process. For LGBTQIA+ couples, who may experience situations or remarks that are inappropriate or hurtful, it is important to discuss feelings and responses to sociocultural challenges for these families who are marginalized and discriminated against in subtle ways. Counseling with a professional counselor is done prior to proceeding with treatment.

Donor Sperm

Donors who donate sperm to a commercial sperm bank have all been tested for a standard list of infectious diseases mandated by the Food and Drug Administration (FDA), which has published regulations regarding donation of human tissues (10). These regulations mandate testing of all non-identified donors for these infectious diseases which may potentially be transmitted in semen, prior to collecting semen specimens intended for donation. Sperm specimens are frozen and quarantined for a period of six months, after which the donor is retested for the same list of infectious diseases. If all the repeat tests for infectious diseases results are negative, the quarantined frozen sperm specimens may then be released by the sperm bank for donation. If any test for infectious diseases is positive, the quarantined sperm specimens may not be released for donation and must be discarded.

Sperm donated to a commercial sperm bank have usually been washed with special cell culture media fluids and concentrated into a small volume prior to cryopreservation. These vials are designated for intrauterine insemination (IUI) and are ready for immediate use upon thaw. If the vial of donor sperm obtained from a commercial sperm bank is labelled "ICI," it is intended for intra-cervical or intravaginal insemination and needs to be washed with special culture media fluids in the laboratory and concentrated into a small volume prior to IUI.

Occasionally, some lesbian couples choose to use sperm from a known (or directed) donor, typically a family member of the partner who is not conceiving, or friend or acquaintance. Family-building with sperm from a known donor has significant psychosocial and legal ramifications; therefore, psychosocial and legal counseling, as well as legal contracts, are mandatory. The counseling and legal contracts address the questions of who owns the donor sperm specimens and controls their use, parental rights and obligations of the intended parents (IPs), as well as the lack of parental rights and obligations of the donor. If a lesbian couple wishes to use sperm from a known donor, the most efficient process for the designated donor is to bank his sperm at a commercial sperm bank and specifically designate the banked sperm specimens for use by the recipient-intended parents. Some fertility clinics may also offer this service. There are FDA regulations specifically governing use of sperm from a known/directed donor if the insemination is being performed by a clinician in a medical facility, which are similar to the regulations governing use of sperm from donors recruited by a commercial sperm bank (10). After initial testing for potentially transmissible infectious diseases, sperm specimens are frozen and quarantined for a period of three to six months, after which the donor is retested for the same list of infectious diseases. If all the repeat tests results are negative for these infectious diseases, the frozen sperm specimens may then be released by the sperm bank for use by the recipient IPs. If any test for infectious diseases is positive, the recipient IPs must be counseled regarding the potential risk of infection with the infectious disease, following which they may choose to use the frozen donor sperm specimens for insemination, but would have to sign a waiver acknowledging that they have been counseled regarding the risk of potential infection from use of these donor sperm specimens.

Options for Lesbian Couples

1. **Insemination with Donor Sperm**

Donor sperm insemination is the least invasive procedure and is the primary method of conception for lesbians who do not have fertility issues. One option is intra-vaginal insemination at home, timed with urinary ovulation predictor kits (OPK). Alternatively, insemination performed by a clinician in a medical facility is typically IUI, in which donor sperm are placed directly inside the uterus on the day that the patient is determined to be ovulating. IUI serves to deliver the maximum number of sperm to the fallopian tubes where fertilization of the oocyte takes place.

IUI may be done with or without the use of fertility medications. Most lesbians who do not have fertility issues may do donor sperm IUI without the use of fertility medications. However, those who have ovulatory dysfunction may benefit from the use of fertility medications such as letrozole, clomiphene, or injectable gonadotropins. There is an increased risk of multiple gestations in pregnancies resulting from the use of fertility medications.

2. **IVF with Donor Sperm**

Some lesbians are unable to conceive with donor sperm IUI because they have an infertility-related diagnosis such as endometriosis, pelvic adhesive disease, advanced reproductive age, or unexplained infertility. The success rate of IUI treatment is also significantly influenced by age, thus more patients will have unsuccessful outcomes after the completion of several IUIs with advancing age. These patients may benefit from treatment with *in vitro* fertilization (IVF). Optimal outcomes from IUI are achieved within the first four treatment cycles, after which point proceeding with IVF should be considered (11).

3. **IVF with Partner's Oocytes**

A lesbian who is unsuccessful in conceiving with her own eggs due to primary ovarian insufficiency (premature ovarian failure), diminished ovarian reserve, advanced reproductive age, or other infertility diagnosis may potentially conceive with IVF using oocytes provided by her partner. This process has variously been referred to as Reciprocal IVF, Partner Assisted Reproduction (PAR), Co-IVF, Shared Motherhood IVF, and ROPA (Reception of Oocytes from the Partner).

4. **Reciprocal IVF**

Some lesbian couples who have never attempted conception with donor sperm insemination and do not have infertility may choose to have children with IVF using the eggs from one partner, inseminated with donor sperm, and have the resultant embryo(s) transferred into the uterus of the other partner, who then gestates the pregnancy and gives birth. This enables both partners in the relationship to be directly and physically involved in having their child(ren) and is an appealing concept for many lesbian couples. After the birth of their first child, they may choose to repeat the reciprocal IVF process, but reverse roles so that the partner who gestated the pregnancy for their first reciprocal IVF cycle then provides oocytes for their second reciprocal IVF cycle, and the partner who provided oocytes for their first reciprocal IVF cycle then gestates the pregnancy.

Some couples choose to use reciprocal IVF if one of them has no intentions of ever being pregnant, so this is an option to have a genetically-related child without carrying a pregnancy. After they have a child successfully with reciprocal IVF, the partner who gestated the pregnancy may then return to conceive a genetically-related child with donor sperm insemination so they each have genetically-related child(ren).

5. **IVF with Donor Eggs**

Some lesbian couples may need to use donor eggs from a third party due to the absence of ovaries or the inability of both partners to produce viable oocytes. In this situation, their egg donor may either be a known or directed donor (family member, friend, or acquaintance), or an egg donor recruited by an approved egg donor agency or frozen donor eggs from a frozen donor egg bank. (See section on Egg Donor Agencies and Anonymous Donors in chapter titled "Donor oocyte use in IVF.")

6. **IVF with Gestational Surrogacy**

In rare situations, some lesbian couples may need to use a gestational surrogate due to the absence of a uterus, or the absence of a normally functional uterus in both partners, or the presence of other medical impediments to a healthy pregnancy. In this situation, embryos may be created with oocytes provided by either of the two partners, inseminated with donor sperm, and the resulting embryo(s) transferred into the uterus of a gestational surrogate. (See section on Gestational Carrier in chapter titled "Donor oocyte use in IVF.")

Options for Gay Male Couples

Historically, gay men who desired genetically-related children have had children through co-parenting arrangements with close friends (often lesbian friends) or through traditional surrogacy. In traditional surrogacy, sperm of the intended father(s) are inseminated into the surrogate. At birth, the baby conceived in this manner is given up by the traditional surrogate for adoption by the IPs. Traditional surrogacy has significant pitfalls due to historical cases in which the traditional surrogate changed her mind and decided to keep the baby after birth. These cases have led to litigation in which the IPs have sued for custody of their baby. In these cases, the courts have historically ruled in favor of the traditional surrogate who then retains custody of the baby. Nowadays, traditional surrogacy is rarely, if ever, done.

With the advent of IVF, the option of gestational surrogacy became possible. A gestational surrogate has no genetic relationship with the fetus that she carries. Gay male couples have been using IVF with donor eggs and gestational surrogacy to build their families since the late 1990s. Oocytes donated by an egg donor may be inseminated with sperm provided by one or both of the intended fathers, and a resulting embryo is transferred into the uterus of the gestational surrogate. In 1998, the Reproductive Science Center of New England (now a part of Boston IVF) was the first IVF center in New England, and one of the first IVF programs in the U.S. and in the world, to treat a gay male couple with donor eggs and gestational surrogacy.

There are significant psychosocial and legal ramifications to having a child through gestational surrogacy, so psychosocial and legal counseling of all parties involved are mandatory, as are legal contracts. Surrogacy is prohibited by law in some states, surrogacy laws vary from state to state, and some states have no laws specifically addressing surrogacy, so it is critical to have legal counseling regarding the implications of the state in which the surrogate delivers the baby.

The roles of egg donor and gestational surrogate may be filled by female relatives or friends, or by women who provide these services through a fee-based agreement facilitated by an agency.

Egg Donors

Ideally, donors recruited by egg donor agencies are healthy young women who are between the ages of 21–29 years, although women who are up to the age of 32 years may be acceptable as recruited egg donors. However, known egg donors (family members or close friends of the IPs) may be women in their mid- to late-thirties and may be acceptable as egg donors if they are healthy and have good ovarian reserve.

Donors recruited and matched through an egg donor agency are typically compensated for their time, effort, inconvenience, time off from work, and the pain of undergoing a surgical egg retrieval procedure under anesthesia. They are not considered to be "selling" their eggs and are compensated a fixed amount (that is agreed upon) per donation cycle, regardless of the number of eggs retrieved. They are compensated even if no oocyte is retrieved, assuming that the failure to retrieve oocytes is not a result of reckless non-compliance on the part of the donor. A legal contract is mandatory between the egg donor and the IPs, who must be represented by separate attorneys.

Donor egg cycles can be coordinated with the woman who is carrying the pregnancy such that fresh embryo(s) is(are) transferred, and any untransferred embryos are cryopreserved for potential future use. More commonly, the cohort of embryos is cryopreserved, allowing for selection of the best embryo from the cohort for thaw and subsequent transfer. This pathway also permits time for genetic testing results to become available, if elected by the IPs. More recently, the ability to successfully cryopreserve unfertilized human oocytes has resulted in the development of frozen donor egg banks, which has become an alternative source of donor oocytes for those needing to use donor eggs to conceive. Women who are recruited for frozen donor egg banks are extensively evaluated in the same way that all egg donors are evaluated. These donors are stimulated with gonadotropins and undergo transvaginal oocyte retrieval, following which all the mature oocytes are cryopreserved. Their detailed profile is then posted on the list of available donors on the website of the frozen donor egg bank. IPs who need donor eggs may choose to use frozen donor eggs instead of searching for a donor through an egg donor agency. The live birth success rates from frozen donor egg treatment cycles are comparable to those from fresh donor egg treatment cycles. The frozen donor egg option eliminates the need to search for an appropriate donor through an egg donor agency, waiting for evaluation of the potential donor, and coordination of treatment dates. The overall cost of using frozen donor oocytes is also significantly lower than the cost of using donor oocytes from a donor recruited and matched through an egg donor agency and may result in significant overall cost savings for a male couple who choose this option. The main advantage of a fresh donor egg treatment cycle is the higher probability of having excess untransferred embryos cryopreserved for potential future use. Since frozen donor egg treatment cycles are typically allotted 6–8 frozen eggs per treatment cycle, they usually yield 1–2 usable embryos. The likelihood of having surplus embryos available to achieve two successful surrogacy journeys is reduced with this option, thus many couples wishing for two children will choose a fresh donor cycle.

Gestational Surrogates

Gestational surrogates (or gestational carriers) may be known to the intended parent IP(s) (such as a female relative or friend) or may be recruited and matched through a surrogacy agency. Regardless of whether a surrogate is known or recruited through an agency, psychosocial and legal counseling for all parties involved, and a legal contract between the surrogate and IPs are mandatory. Legal counseling must be provided by an attorney (or law firm) who specializes in reproductive law.

Once the prospective surrogate has been selected and matched, she undergoes an extensive evaluation, including psychological testing, medical testing, and screening for potentially infectious diseases that may inadvertently infect the fetus during pregnancy or childbirth. After comprehensive evaluation, the treatment pathway is selected. Although more rarely used given the advent of improved cryopreservation techniques, it is possible to synchronize the surrogate's cycle with that of the egg donor. Synchronization of the two women's cycles is typically accomplished with a combination of oral contraceptive pills and a gonadotropin-releasing hormone agonist such as leuprolide acetate. If frozen-thawed embryos or frozen donor oocytes are being used, synchronization with the egg donor's cycle is unnecessary. The surrogate's endometrial development is programmed with estradiol and progesterone, such that the window of implantation is optimal when the embryo is ready for transfer.

Screening embryos for aneuploidy using Preimplantation Genetic Testing for Aneuploidy (PGT-A) has become more popular in Third-Party Reproduction (see chapter titled "Preimplantation Genetic Testing"). The current technology for PGT-A is very accurate, and the cost of the technology is very reasonable considering the total cost of having a baby with donor eggs and gestational surrogacy. Many IPs, especially those who are using a donor recruited and matched through an egg donor agency, opt for PGT-A testing on their embryos, which are then cryopreserved for future FET into their gestational surrogate. The advantage of doing PGT-A for aneuploidy is the lower risk of first trimester spontaneous abortion or pregnancy with a fetus affected with aneuploidy such as Trisomy 21 (Down syndrome). When the IPs have euploid embryos (as determined by PGT-A) that are cryopreserved and suitable for transfer, their gestational surrogate is then brought in for the FET. This strategy results in more efficient utilization of their gestational surrogate's time. It also decreases the risk of their gestational surrogate experiencing a spontaneous abortion due to aneuploidy or the unfortunate situation of pregnancy with an aneuploid fetus, where the IPs are faced with the dilemma of considering a termination of pregnancy. PGT-A testing has also permitted for a more consistent utilization of single embryo transfer, thus reducing the risks involved with multiple gestations.

Options for Transgender People

The desire to become a parent is compelling for many people, regardless of sexual orientation or gender identity. Transgender individuals who want to have genetically-related children need to plan ahead, as some of the hormonal and surgical procedures employed in their transition to their affirmed gender identity may render them incapable of having genetically-related children post-transition. Reproductive options for transgender individuals depend on where in the transition process they are and whether they are ready to have children immediately or in the future.

Fertility Preservation

Most transgender individuals are not ready to have children prior to or at the time of their transition, so they choose to undergo fertility preservation procedures. While the ability to cryopreserve sperm has been available for decades, effective and reliable cryopreservation of unfertilized human oocytes was not consistently available until the 2010s. There is good evidence that fertilization and pregnancy rates are similar to IVF with fresh oocytes when previously vitrified oocytes from young women are thawed for use in IVF. Although data are limited, no increase in chromosomal abnormalities, birth defects, and developmental deficits have been reported in the offspring born from cryopreserved oocytes when compared to pregnancies from conventional IVF and the general population. Therefore, the ASRM declared in 2012 that vitrification of mature oocytes should no longer be considered experimental (12). Oocyte cryopreservation technology is currently being used for frozen donor egg banks, as well as for the purpose of fertility preservation in young women who have been diagnosed with cancer or women who are freezing oocytes for delayed childbearing. This same technology is also used for the purpose of fertility preservation in transgender men.

1. Fertility Preservation for Transgender Men

Transgender men may cryopreserve their oocytes for potential future use. This can be done prior to initiation of testosterone therapy, which suppresses ovulation. However, transgender men who have initiated testosterone therapy may also undergo oocyte cryopreservation if they are willing to discontinue testosterone therapy for a short period of time in order to undergo oocyte cryopreservation procedures, after which they may resume testosterone therapy after their oocytes have been successfully cryopreserved. The process for oocyte cryopreservation for transgender men is virtually identical to the process that is used for egg donors who are donating oocytes for a frozen donor egg bank. Controlled ovarian stimulation is achieved with daily gonadotropin injections for an average of 10 to 12 days, after which transvaginal oocyte retrieval is performed under anesthesia. Depending on how many oocytes are desired, more than one oocyte cryopreservation cycle may be done. Outcomes of this treatment are correlated with age and appear to be comparable to the cisgender population, even for the subgroup of trans men who have had prior testosterone exposure (13). There have also been case reports of transgender men undergoing oocyte stimulation while on testosterone with good results; however, there are no randomized trials comparing outcomes of fertility preservation with or without cessation of testosterone (14–16).

2. Fertility Preservation for Transgender Women

Transgender women may cryopreserve their sperm for potential future use. Ideally, this should be done prior to initiation of estrogen therapy, which suppresses spermatogenesis. There is data to show that long-term use of estrogens or anti-androgens reduces sperm production (17–19). Some transfeminine individuals may not have recovery of sperm production after cessation of gender affirming hormones, while some may need surgical procedures to retrieve sperm from the testicular tissue. Sperm banking can be done conveniently at any commercial sperm bank. Banking of multiple specimens is recommended.

Reproductive Options for Transgender Individuals Who Are Ready to Have Children

Transgender individuals who have planned ahead and have cryopreserved their gametes (either sperm or eggs) may return to use their cryopreserved gametes to have children when they are ready to do so.

1. **Use of Cryopreserved Oocytes in Transgender Men**

When transgender men are ready to use their cryopreserved oocytes to have children, the frozen oocytes may be thawed for IVF. Intracytoplasmic sperm injection (ICSI) is recommended when IVF is being done with previously vitrified oocytes which have been thawed, as the fertilization rate with conventional drop insemination may be very low with previously vitrified oocytes.

Depending on the relationship status of the transgender man, his previously vitrified oocytes may be thawed for insemination with donor sperm or sperm from his cisgender male partner. Depending on his relationship status, the resulting embryo(s) may be transferred into the uterus of his cisgender female partner or a gestational surrogate. If he has not had a hysterectomy, he may choose to gestate the pregnancy himself, in which case the embryo(s) would be transferred into his own uterus. It is also reasonable to consider initiating treatment with IUI prior to thawing the previously frozen oocytes.

2. **Use of Cryopreserved Sperm in Transgender Women**

When transgender women are ready to use their cryopreserved sperm to have children, their frozen sperm may be thawed for either IUI or IVF, depending on the quantity and quality of the frozen sperm, as well as their partnership status.

If the transgender woman is partnered with a cisgender woman, her frozen sperm may be thawed for either IUI or IVF in her cisgender female partner. If the transgender woman is partnered with a cisgender man or another transgender woman, her frozen sperm may be thawed for IVF with donor oocytes and the resulting embryo(s) transferred into a gestational surrogate.

If the transgender woman is partnered with a transgender man, her frozen sperm may be thawed for IVF with oocytes previously cryopreserved by her partner or with donor oocytes, and the resulting embryo(s) may be transferred into a gestational surrogate or into the uterus of her partner if he has not had a hysterectomy and chooses to gestate the pregnancy himself.

Reproductive Options for Transgender Individuals Who Have Not Cryopreserved Their Gametes

Transgender individuals who have not cryopreserved their gametes may have the opportunity to have genetically-related children if they have not undergone any surgical procedures during the course of their transition which render them permanently sterile.

1. **Reproductive Options for Transgender Men**

Transgender men who transitioned prior to the availability of oocyte cryopreservation or who have not previously cryopreserved their oocytes can have genetically-related children if they have not had bilateral oophorectomy and are willing to discontinue testosterone therapy temporarily. Their options for procreation depend on their relationship status and whether they have had a hysterectomy. A transgender man who is partnered with a cisgender woman may do reciprocal IVF in which he provides oocytes that are inseminated with donor sperm, and the resulting embryo(s) is(are) transferred into the uterus of his partner.

A transgender man who has not had bilateral oophorectomy or hysterectomy may choose to conceive himself with sperm from his cisgender male partner or with donor sperm insemination. Alternatively, he may do IVF with sperm from his cisgender male partner, or sperm from his transgender female partner who previously cryopreserved her sperm, or with donor sperm. The resulting embryos may be transferred into a gestational surrogate, or into his own uterus if he chooses to carry the pregnancy himself, or into the uterus of his transgender male partner who may choose to carry the pregnancy (reciprocal IVF).

2. **Reproductive Options for Transgender Women**

Transgender women who transitioned without having previously banked their sperm may or may not be able to have genetically-related children, depending on whether they have had bilateral orchiectomy or whether spermatogenesis is still present if they have not had bilateral orchiectomy. In general, estrogen therapy suppresses spermatogenesis to the point of azoospermia, but spermatogenesis may or may not recover if estrogen therapy is discontinued. According to published studies, sperm recovery may take anywhere between 3–27 months after stopping gender affirming therapies, and for some, surgical procedures will be needed to recover sperm (19). If there is sperm present in the ejaculate but in low counts (oligozoospermia), these may be used in an IVF cycle with ICSI. If the transgender woman is partnered with a cisgender woman, her female partner may undergo an IVF cycle in which the oocytes are inseminated with sperm provided by the transgender woman and the resulting embryo(s) transferred into the uterus of her female partner.

If the transgender woman is partnered with a transgender man, her sperm may be used to inseminate donor oocytes or oocytes previously cryopreserved by her partner, and the resulting embryo(s) transferred into the uterus of a gestational surrogate to gestate the pregnancy, or into the uterus of her partner if he has not had a hysterectomy and chooses to carry the pregnancy himself. If the transgender woman is partnered with a cisgender man or another transgender woman, sperm from either one or both of them may be used to inseminate donor oocytes and the resulting embryo(s) transferred into the uterus of a gestational surrogate.

Conclusion

The same ART which are used to treat heterosexual couples with infertility has been used very successfully to assist members of the LGBTQIA+ community to have genetically-related children. In addition to being informed about the treatment options that may be offered to LGBTQIA+ people, it is also very important that medical providers (and their office staff) who treat LGBTQIA+ people be culturally competent and sensitive to their needs.

Key Points

- Historically, there has been little published on LGBTQIA+ fertility care to inform patients and providers. More research is emerging, allowing for evidence-based approaches to the provision of care.
- Lesbian patients have several options with donor sperm, including insemination, IVF, reciprocal IVF, and the use of donor oocytes. A fertility workup is recommended prior to initiating treatment to rule out causes of infertility and optimize the chances of treatment success.
- Transgender patients have options to preserve their fertility prior to initiating gender affirming hormones or having definitive gender affirming surgery. The effect of long-term testosterone use on fertility for transmasculine persons is not known, whereas data indicates that long-term use of estrogens for transfeminine persons may negatively impact sperm parameters.
- Male-male couples require the use of donor oocytes and a gestational carrier to have a genetically-related child. There is a complex screening process required in third-party reproduction to ensure the safety of oocyte donors, gestational carriers, and intended parents.

REFERENCES

1. Wainright JL et al. Psychosocial adjustment, school outcomes, and romantic relationships of adolescents with same-sex parents. *Child Dev* 2004;75(6):1886–1898.
2. James-Abra S et al. Trans people's experiences with assisted reproduction services: a qualitative study. *Hum Reprod* 2015;30:1365–1374.
3. Flores A. Examining variation in surveying attitudes on same-sex marriage: a meta-analysis. *Public Opin Q* 2015;2:580–593.
4. Gates GJ, Brown TNT. *Marriage and Same-Sex Couples After Obergefell* [internet]. The Williams Institute, UCLA School of Law 2015: https://williamsinstitute.law.ucla.edu/wp-content/uploads/Marriage-Post-Obergefell-Nov-2015.pdf.
5. Gates GJ. Marriage and family: LGBT individuals and same-sex couples. *Future Child* 2015;2:67–87.
6. Flores AR, Conron KJ. Adult LGBT population in the United States [internet], 2023: https://williamsinstitute.law.ucla.edu/wp-content/uploads/LGBT-Adult-US-Pop-Dec-2023.pdf
7. Jones JM. U.S. LGBT Identification Steady at 7.2% [internet], 2023: https://news.gallup.com/poll/470708/lgbt-identification-steady.aspx
8. Ethics Committee, ASRM. Access to fertility treatment irrespective of marital status, sexual orientation, or gender identity: an Ethics Committee opinion. *Fertil Steril.* 2021;116(2):326–330.
9. Ethics Committee, ASRM. Access to fertility services by transgender and nonbinary persons: an Ethics Committee opinion. *Fertil Steril.* 2021;115(4):874–878.

10. Food and Drug Administration. Eligibility determination for donors of human cells, tissues and cellular and tissue-based products, final rule. *Fed Regist.* 2004;69(101):29785–29834.
11. Heyward QD et al. Reproductive outcomes following insemination in same-sex female couples, unpartnered female patients, and heterosexual couples. *Fertil Steril.* 2024:S0015-0282(24)01948-4.
12. Practice Committees, ASRM and SART. Mature oocyte cryopreservation: a guideline. *Fertil Steril.* 2013;99:37–43.
13. Leung A et al. Assisted reproductive technology outcomes in female-to-male transgender patients compared with cisgender patients: a new frontier in reproductive medicine. *Fertil Steril.* 2019;112(5):858–865.
14. Gale J et al. Oocyte cryopreservation in a transgender man on long-term testosterone therapy: a case report. *F S Rep.* 2021;2(2):249–251
15. Stark BA, Mok-Lin E. Fertility preservation in transgender men without discontinuation of testosterone. *F S Rep.* 2022;3(2):153–156
16. White J et al. Oocyte cryopreservation and reciprocal in vitro fertilization in a transgender man on long term testosterone gender-affirming hormone therapy: a case report. *F S Rep.* 2023;5(1):111–113.
17. Rodriguez-Wallberg KA et al. Sperm quality in transgender women before or after gender affirming hormone therapy-A prospective cohort study. *Andrology.* 2021;9(6):1773–1780.
18. Jiang DD et al. Effects of estrogen on spermatogenesis in transgender women. *Urology.* 2019;132:117–122.
19. de Nie I et al. Successful restoration of spermatogenesis following gender-affirming hormone therapy in transgender women. *Cell Rep Med.* 2023;4(1):100858.

30

APP (Advanced Practice Provider) Integration and Utilization in Reproductive Medicine

Carol Lesser and Keith Blauer

Advanced Practice Providers or "APPs" refer to non-physician medical providers with advanced degrees and training enabling them to work collaboratively with physician and nurse colleagues in the delivery of patient care. This group includes nurse practitioners, nurse midwives, and physician assistants.

APPs diagnose and manage medical conditions, including prescribing medications within their scope of practice, which is governed by education, certification, and state licensing laws. As the national demand for reproductive medicine care continues to rise without a proportionate increase in Reproductive Endocrinology and Infertility physicians (REIs) to care for these patients, many reproductive medicine centers have turned to the incorporation of APPs into the delivery of reproductive medicine. Their inclusion is designed to shorten patient wait times for appointments and treatments while providing valuable support to patients, physicians, nurses, and other staff. In October 2022, Senapati et al. asserted in the *New England Journal of Medicine* (NEJM) that APPs with the appropriate training in reproductive medicine and supervision, should be utilized within an REI practice to streamline and increase practice productivity.[1]

It is worth mentioning that the term "midlevel provider" and "physician extender" have been replaced with APP in recognition of the significant and collaborative role of this group of professionals who want to be viewed with parity. Attention to current nomenclature reflects the changing role of the APP and demonstrates recognition for their important contribution to the patient-care team.

Boston IVF hired its first advanced practice provider over three decades ago. This model has proven to be both cost and time efficient, encouraging all staff to work to the full extent of their education, training, and experience. The incorporation of APPs for specific visits has contributed to practice growth across our centers. Physicians have more time to concentrate on aspects of patient care requiring their specific skills and training, with the confidence that patients are receiving quality medical care for other visits. Patients and support staff appreciate having another trained professional to turn to for assistance as needed, which can help prevent unnecessary frustration when access to one's physician is limited.

The APP role is continually evolving to keep pace with the ever-changing needs of both infertility patients as well as physician and nursing colleagues. Reflecting the increasing complexity of the assisted reproductive technology (ART) field and patient needs, responsibilities and skill set have expanded significantly over time. We will delineate the APP role and responsibilities as they currently stand at Boston IVF. While APPs function in all US states, the scope of practice is defined by varying state laws and regulations. It is important to understand what your state permits as you define the role of the APP in your practice or center and to periodically check for updates in scope of practice.

While nurse practitioners, physician assistants, and nurse midwives have different training and maintenance of certification requirements, the similarities between APPs outweigh the differences. Our experience is that they function equally after their training is completed.[2, 3]

 DOI: 10.1201/9781003460275-30

APP Consults

1. At Boston IVF, routine initial consults are assigned to APPs. Most of these visits are via Zoom. Typical initial consults include individuals or couples with primary or secondary infertility; single patients or same sex couples requesting third-party reproduction techniques such as donor insemination, the use of an egg donor, and/or gestational surrogate; and women and individuals who request egg-freezing. This also includes couples electing to defer parenthood, requesting embryo-freezing.
2. APPs see women individuals with ovulatory dysfunction such as PCOS (Polycystic Ovary Syndrome) and patients with previously diagnosed infertility conditions such as tubal occlusion, endometriosis, or male factor who need completion of basic testing. At Boston IVF, APP initial consults usually exclude second or third opinions, surgical consults, emergent oncology patients or couples/individuals with known complex medical conditions, although these exclusions may be revisited on a case-by-case basis or needs. Yet some practices might opt to assign these initial patients to the APP to expedite entry into a particular practice.
3. During these visits, the APP collects a comprehensive patient history, reviews and summarizes previous testing, and orders clinically indicated fertility tests and procedures. Patients then schedule a follow-up visit with their physician to discuss their results and treatment options. This enables the physician to initiate treatment more efficiently, with a completed basic battery of medical tests. The expectation is that all testing will be completed within one menstrual cycle or its equivalent.
4. APPs conduct what Boston IVF calls return to care visits, typically after the delivery of a child or a break in treatment as when patients are seeking assistance for another pregnancy or resuming prior treatment following a pause in treatment. APPs can order interval or outstanding labs or testing that may be needed before treatment can be reinitiated. It is important to note that Massachusetts has an insurance mandate and requires testing such as ovarian reserve/uterine cavity evaluation to be updated periodically in order to obtain insurance coverage.
5. APPs are responsible for early pregnancy management including initial and repeat prenatal visits. This includes successful and failed pregnancies. Urgent slots are allocated to the APP schedule on a daily basis to accommodate emergent visits. These visits include pain or bleeding in early pregnancy, abnormally rising hCG levels, or ovarian hyperstimulation (OHSS) related complaints. APPs counsel patients on missed abortions, ectopic pregnancies, and pregnancies of unknown location (PUL). Caring for routine pregnancies combined with coordination of the management of pregnancy loss is a routine part of their daily responsibilities. This includes communication with the patient's care team to develop a follow-up plan or overseeing management of Methotrexate or Mifepristone/Misoprostol administration. Providing a summary of the infertility evaluation and treatment received to the referring OB/GYN is a part of the transition to OB care and is part of an APP responsibility.
6. APPs lend ongoing support to the nursing team. This includes reviewing patient emails or phone calls and addressing their concerns or questions. If a patient has a treatment-related issue, the APP can intervene when the physician's preferred management is well understood. APPs help train new nursing personnel and remain available to lend support to nursing as needed. APPs can provide educational lectures to the nursing and support staff on topics of interest.
7. APPs can function as effective ambassadors for their practices by performing outreach opportunities in the form of lunch-and-learns or other meetups with local OB/GYNs. The goal is to develop collaborative relationships with colleagues who can refer patients for ART or infertility care with the intention of referring them back to their OB as soon as possible.
8. Review of patient labs in our electronic medical record (EMR) system is divided among APPs and physicians. At Boston IVF, physicians typically review all in-cycle monitoring labs that require medication and dosing decisions that same day. APPs review all pre-cycle labs and

baseline serum and ultrasound results to determine if a patient can initiate her planned treatment cycle after reviewing her baseline serum and/or ultrasound results. This varies from center to center, as some APPs make in-cycle decisions routinely.

APPs Responsibilities

Review of Test Results

APPs make recommendations on abnormal tests based on company policy and/or a written set of physician preferences. It is prudent for each clinic to produce standard operating procedures (SOPs) and agreed-upon policies for routine clinical care. This allows for standardization, maximizes efficiency, and reduces error. In addition, it allows for easy transition of care as well as cross-coverage in staff during vacation/leave or holidays. To facilitate this, each physician provides a detailed list of their preferred management of common lab abnormalities. This includes management of subclinical hypothyroidism, abnormal glucose levels, hyperprolactinemia, or abnormal hematology results. Each physician states their preferences while able to make revisions over time. APPs follow these guidelines when addressing abnormal results and know when to manage an issue or refer to the PCP (primary care practitioners) or OB/GYN. APPs are responsible for keeping their key physician preference lists up to date. They can:

- Forward results to physicians in the case of complex decision-making.
- Approve baseline labs for cycle start or defer to physician for a decision on abnormal labs.
- Interpret anovulatory labs and make recommendations to initiate treatment or offer medications to initiate a withdrawal bleed when appropriate.
- APPs review semen analysis reports and adjunct sperm tests reported daily, including IUI prep results.

Review of Paper or Prior Records

Electronic medical records and labs that precede the patient's initial visit or were sent after initiation of care is another APP responsibility. This can include copious lengthy records from prior reproductive medicine centers for those who have moved or are seeking a second or third opinion. APPs condense and summarize the salient aspects of the patient's prior medical workup and treatments for physician consideration in devising a treatment plan while avoiding unnecessary retesting. Physicians meeting with patients then have the advantage of a comprehensive review of their prior treatments and tests.

While Boston IVF has not integrated the following functions into their APP defined role, other ART practices have. In certain states and in other practices, APPs can:

- Manage ovulation induction, ovulation enhancement/superovulation cycles with IUI/timed intercourse (TIC), and donor sperm cycles
- Office hysteroscopy
- Baseline and follicular ultrasound scans, especially when dedicated ultrasonographers are not available
- Early pregnancy ultrasound scans

APPs perform routine procedures including:

- Saline sonograms (SIS or SSG)
- Hysterosalpingogram-contrast sonography (HyCoSy)
- Hysterosalpingogram (HSG)
- Endometrial biopsy

- ERA biopsy
- Uterine plasma rich protein (PRP) infusion
- Intrauterine insemination (IUI) when a tenaculum is required/prior history of difficult catheter placement
- Physical exams for egg donors, gestational carriers (GCAR) and for both female and male patients for clinical trials
- Basic pelvic floor therapy for patients with vaginismus who are unable to complete their workup

Challenges Facing Integration of the APP into the Reproductive Medicine Care Team

As demand for ART services and the complexity of reproductive medicine continues to grow exponentially, IVF centers face challenges in attracting experienced nurses and APPs to join their team, especially those with prior training and expertise in REI. Unlike physician colleagues who complete lengthy REI fellowship training and must demonstrate competency through board completion, APPs and RNs learn entirely on the job. The learning curve has steepened in recent years and the loss of qualified individuals during and post the Covid pandemic has left centers trying to fill open positions, often in competition with other centers.

In addition to the challenges of attracting and retaining experienced nurses and APPs to reproductive medicine centers, there are also challenges in integrating them into the care team. One of the challenges is the steep learning curve for new hires who lack prior experience in reproductive endocrinology and infertility (REI). This puts a burden on the existing APP team, who already have busy patient panels and little time for training.

To address this issue, the American Society for Reproductive Medicine (ASRM) and the Nurses Professional Group (NPG) are working together to develop standardized policies and training competencies for APPs in reproductive medicine. The goal is to provide both didactic and hands-on training for common procedures. Once these training modules are developed, REI centers will be encouraged to require their staff to complete the courses and demonstrate competency in designated areas.

Another effort to improve the training and preparation of nurses and APPs in reproductive medicine is the revival of the voluntary certification course in basic REI nursing by the National Certification Corporation (NCC). This course, now called Reproductive Health and Infertility, would provide entry-level RNs and APPs with a basic core competency module and a certification exam. ASRM also offers an ASRM Nurse Certificate Course, which many practices require as part of their orientation program.

The physician and APP task force will produce a practice document for ASRM and develop practice guidelines, competencies, and educational materials to help APPs gain the necessary skills for their role. Their goal is to develop standardized policies and training competencies for APPs in reproductive medicine that will address both didactic and hands-on training needs for common procedures.

This may include ultrasound training from the American Institute of Ultrasound in Medicine (AIUM). Once training modules have been developed, centers will be encouraged to strongly recommend or require their staff to complete the courses and/or demonstrate competency in the designated areas.

These changes aim to improve the training and preparedness of IVF nurses and APPs. The proposed guidelines will represent a significant improvement in how APPs are prepared and trained for their vital role with the intention of attracting more qualified individuals to the field.

With better trained and prepared IVF nurses and APPs, the care provided will be of a higher caliber which will continue to improve and will hopefully lead to happier and more satisfied staff and patients.

The integration of APPs into reproductive medicine centers has proven to be beneficial in streamlining patient care, reducing wait times, and providing valuable support to the care team. With the ongoing efforts to improve training and standardize practices, the role of APPs in reproductive medicine will continue to evolve and contribute to the growth and success of reproductive medicine centers.[4, 5]

Key Points

- Advanced Practice Providers (APPs) are non-physician medical providers with advanced degrees and training who collaborate with physicians and nurses in patient-care delivery.
- APPs in reproductive medicine centers help shorten patient wait times and provide valuable support to patients, physicians, nurses, and staff.
- The role of APPs in reproductive medicine is continuously evolving to meet the changing needs of infertility patients and colleagues.
- Challenges in integrating APPs into reproductive medicine centers include attracting experienced nurses and APPs to the field and addressing the steep learning curve for new hires.
- Efforts are being made to develop standardized policies, training competencies, and certification courses for APPs in reproductive medicine.
- The goal is to improve the training and preparedness of nurses and APPs in reproductive medicine to enhance patient care and satisfaction.

Resources

The American Society for Reproductive Medicine (ASRM) offers educational and training modules that can be beneficial for APPs working in the field of infertility. While specific modules may vary over time, here are some examples of educational resources provided by ASRM:

Annual Meeting: ASRM organizes an annual meeting that brings together professionals in reproductive medicine. APPs can attend sessions, workshops, and presentations to enhance their understanding of infertility management, reproductive health, and related topics.

Online Learning: ASRM offers a variety of online learning opportunities, including webinars, eLearning, and courses on various topics related to reproductive medicine. These resources can help APPs expand their knowledge and stay updated with the latest advancements in the field.

Practice Committee Documents: ASRM publishes practice guidelines, committee opinions, and other documents that provide evidence-based recommendations and best practices in reproductive medicine. APPs can utilize these resources to enhance their clinical decision-making and patient care.

Publications: ASRM publishes scientific journals, newsletters, and other publications that cover a wide range of reproductive medicine topics. APPs can access these resources to stay informed about the latest research and clinical developments in infertility management.

It is important to regularly check the ASRM website for updates on available educational resources and training opportunities tailored specifically for APPs in infertility. Additionally, there is an Annual IVF Nurses Congress for nurses and APPs in reproductive medicine called StartART with online educational activities provided between conferences.

REFERENCES

1. Senapati S, Tuomala RE. Advanced practice providers in reproductive medicine: integrating roles in an evolving specialty. *N Engl J Med*. 2022;387(15):1449–1451.
2. Senapati S, Layman LC. The role of the advanced practice provider in reproductive endocrinology and infertility. *Fertil Steril*. 2018;110(6):947–949.
3. Senapati S et al. Impact of nurse practitioners on patient care in reproductive endocrinology and infertility practices. *Fertil Steril*. 2017;107(1):129–133.

4. Fogleman C, Bunting J. The role of nurse practitioners in reproductive endocrinology and infertility practices. *J Nurse Pract*. 2016;12(10):e437–e442.
5. Layman LC et al. The role of advanced practice providers in reproductive endocrinology and infertility practices in the United States: a survey of the Society for Reproductive Endocrinology and Infertility. *Fertil Steril*. 2016;105(5):1197–1202.e1.

31

Integrating Quality Management into a Fertility Practice

Michael M. Alper, Quetrell D. Heyward, and Alan S. Penzias

What is a Quality Management System (QMS), and what does it have to do with an infertility practice? If you have never heard the term QMS, you are not alone. We did not have a clue of what it meant initially, and we certainly had no idea of its relevance to medicine. The purpose of this chapter is not to give a detailed analysis of a QMS, but rather to understand how it relates (in simple terms) to what we do every day in our practice of medicine.

The underlying purpose of a QMS is simple— *say what you do and do what you say.* A QMS provides the tools to clearly delineate what everyone's responsibility is within your organization. It gets down to the core of your corporate essence—what you are about, why you do what you do, how you do it, and how you can do things better. The system is derived from the organization itself and not something imposed from the outside. Therefore, part of the fun of developing a QMS is the creation of it. Sure, it is work, but it can also be worthwhile, as we hope to explain in this chapter.

Why Is Quality Management Important?

Let us illustrate an example for the need of a QMS. We visited a highly respected *in vitro* fertilization (IVF) practice in the northeastern United States and asked the medical director what protocol they followed to replace frozen embryos. He precisely and carefully reviewed their technique to accomplish this. We then asked him for a written summary so we could discuss his technique with our colleagues back in Boston. After shuffling through his files, he came up with an over-photocopied and illegible summary of the protocol. He apologized and commented that "most of what we do is in our heads." So, what is wrong with this picture? How are residents, fellows, and new colleagues supposed to learn existing protocols at this IVF center? How do the nurses know what is expected of them? How can one keep track of changes in the protocol to observe subsequent changes in outcome? Documentation is the cornerstone of a QMS, and this example illustrates the dire need for a QMS in any infertility practice.

IVF centers are complex organizations. They involve the integration of many specialized professionals including physicians, nurses, scientists, administrators, and others. In fact, they are "mini-hospitals," and the different entities must work together to make the organization succeed (Figure 31.1). They must also be effective communicators given a change in one area can quickly affect other areas. If this were to occur without adequate communication, the organization runs the risk of ruin. A QMS assures that the infrastructure is set for all of the players in the organization to communicate and achieve common goals. Failure of an organization to function adequately may result in potentially serious errors at the very worst or corporate dysfunction at the very least.

DOI: 10.1201/9781003460275-31

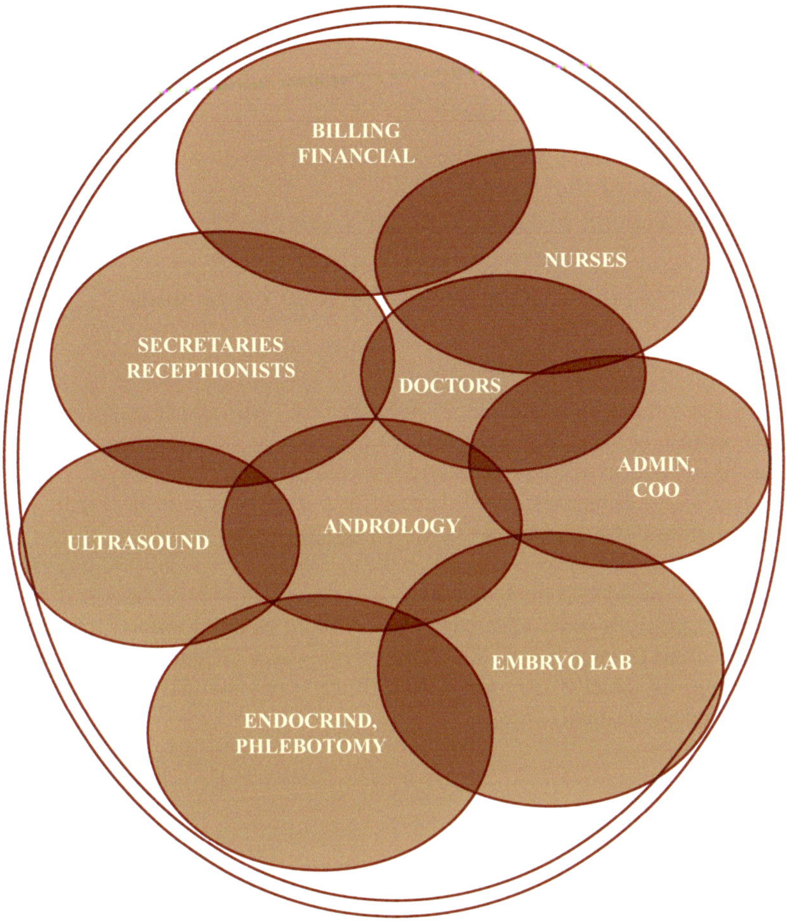

FIGURE 31.1 The IVF team must be a coordinated effort of many disciplines that must all communicate with one another.

ISO—an Example of a Quality Management System

The International Standard Organization, known as "ISO," is the most recognized standard for a QMS. This is a global organization with regional extensions in most countries to represent the international standard and ensure certain benchmarks are being met by businesses worldwide. For example, the steps for constructing hardware such as a bolt need to be standardized so that a particular sized bolt from Company A could replace another from Company B; and these standards exist for several thousand products to keep some degree of uniformity. Moreover, an ISO also functions to develop manufacturing standards. For instance, if you are designing an aircraft for Boeing and want to install a particular aircraft part, you would purchase it only from a manufacturer that was ISO-certified. That way, you can guarantee that quality control, environmental management, and occupational health standards, among others, are being satisfied. Similarly, ISO standards exist for service industries, also known as "ISO-9001" standards, which can be applied to many facets of the healthcare industry including IVF centers.

With regard to becoming ISO-certified, there are multiple steps that must be taken (Figure 31.2). First, one should understand the standards that must be met. Typically, consultants with QMS experience work with the organization to comprehend and apply said standards. The time needed for this process varies with the organization and its size but typically takes several months. Next, the consultant must work with the employees to develop a QM system according to ISO standards and implement it to ensure adequate

How to get ISO-certified:

1. Know the ISO standard
2. Document a quality management system
3. Implement the system
4. Be surveyed (assessed) by an accredited registrar
5. Be issued a Certificate of Conformity
6. Be listed in the Register of Certified Companies

FIGURE 31.2 Steps required for ISO certification.

functionality. A survey is then conducted and, if successful, the certificate of conformity is issued. Last, following initial certification, it is important to remember that an annual inspection from an outside certification body must occur to maintain the ISO certification.

The ISO standard requirements are clearly laid out in a 23-page document (Figure 31.3), which is readily available from the ISO organizations such as ASQ (American Society for Quality). These must be applied to the particular entity of interest.

We have interpreted how an ISO improves the day-to-day operations of an organization in the following sections to make them more understandable. A more detailed account can be found in the references at the end of the chapter, but the main areas of assistance include: (1) documentation, (2) nonconformance tracking, (3) process approach, (4) staff expectations, (5) innovation, (6) leadership, (7) communication, and (8) customer focus.

Documentation

Before implementing a QMS at Boston IVF, we asked all employees to collect every single document that they have seen in the organization, regardless of its age. These included protocols, handouts, and marketing materials, amongst others. To our astonishment, we uncovered close to 3,000 documents by the end of the process, including many variations of the same document!

A QMS requires a company to organize and maintain its documents. These documents need to be clearly identified and assigned to someone in the organization to control. Furthermore, any and all revisions must be authorized and recorded, and all employees must know where to find the latest versions. It may sound simple, but it requires considerable effort to recognize which items within these documents are important and revamp/revise outdated materials. This exercise of identifying and managing an organization's documents is an important part of "cleaning house," and results in a more structured approach, which we can attest to from personal experience.

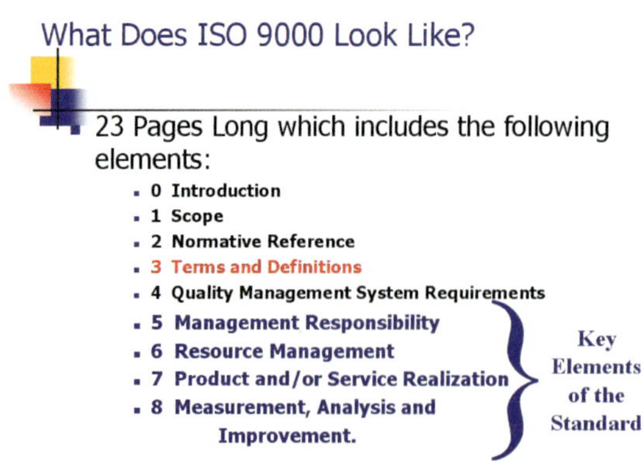

FIGURE 31.3 Key elements required for ISO certification.

Nevertheless, documentation goes well beyond collecting and categorizing materials. Virtually everything that occurs within an organization that involves a process should be recorded. What should happen when a potential patient calls requesting information? How are patient complaints handled? All of these instructions and more should be clearly laid out for employees.

Non-conformances

As technology continues to progress, the complexities of what organizations can do by harnessing technology will also continue to advance, and with these advancements comes an increased risk of "non-conformances." In general, non-conformances describe a failure to comply with an accepted standard or protocol, which can be seen in many different industries. In healthcare, for instance, non-conformances can be seen when a provider fails to perform the customary workup to diagnose a condition or when a standard treatment is not utilized for said condition or diagnosis.

An integral part of a QMS is the documentation of non-conformances. Similar to the aforementioned definition, the ISO defines a non-conformance as the "non-fulfillment of a requirement," i.e. any problem, error, or deviation from protocol, and requires that non-conformances be documented as well as any subsequent follow-up or corrective action. This is commonly done via an electronic database, but regardless of the method, it is important to approach these non-conformances to prevent any potential mishaps from occurring within the organization. Whether it is preventing a plane crash in the aviation industry or preventing a major clinical error in the healthcare industry, tracking non-conformances within a QMS can have a major impact on an organization's operational excellence.

Process Approach

So often in life and business, we make decisions based on emotions rather than facts. However, a QMS helps an organization eliminate this idea of emotionally-driven decision-making and focus on using an analysis of truths to solve problems. Sure, gut feelings are important, but tackling both major and minor corporate decisions requires a methodological approach and careful exploration. For example, what happens if an employee has an idea for improving a procedure? He or she may tell their supervisor, but the idea could die if not carefully evaluated. Consequently, there needs to be a system in place for suggestions to be heard and investigated, which leads us to this idea of process improvement. Another simple but widely applicable example is ordering materials. Who can order what in the organization? Is there a process that exists for purchasing that covers all departments? These concepts must be well thought-out and comprehensively documented for all processes in order for employees to clearly understand how things are done within the organization.

Staff Expectations

It is typical for employees to want to succeed at their work. Experience dictates that when an employee fails to perform well, it is commonly the result of a supervisor's failure to clearly delineate said employee's expectations or their failure to provide the adequate training and tools that the employee requires to perform their job effectively.

Therefore, it is vital that a clear job description with set responsibilities be presented to the employee. Additionally, we often fall short when training staff on how to accomplish what we expect of them given training does not start and end at orientation. Many companies fail to realize that training should be seamlessly incorporated at regular intervals during an employee's lifespan with the organization to ensure that certain operational standards continue to be met. A QMS can help with this as it requires organizations to clearly identify how staff training and competency is managed. After all, a company's greatest asset is its employees, and it is imperative both for the employee and the organization that performance is continuously measured and accountability is clearly delineated.

Innovation

A fundamental requirement of a QMS system is to foster continual improvement. There is rarely a task in any organization that cannot be done better. So, how does one foster the notion that constant innovation is critical for the future of any company? This corporate personality trait starts from the top to the bottom of the company. Every employee with an idea for improvement must be encouraged to share their ideas and know the steps to take when presenting their suggestions. After all, it is the employees on the front line who often know how to make their jobs more effective or efficient.

Leadership

The mission of any organization needs to be developed and followed. For that to occur, management must exhibit leadership. However, in many schools and healthcare institutions, physicians receive no formal leadership training. In fact, it is uncommon for physicians who spend most of their career learning how to care for individual patients to also have the skills to motivate and lead an organization. These skills are typically developed in business (as opposed to medical) schools. In the fertility setting, in particular, several physicians commonly practice under one roof; nonetheless, a common frustration among clinics is bringing the group together to develop common practice patterns. It actually is not hard to accomplish this, but there needs to be an individual or individuals assigned to drive this process.

While experiential leadership training is a common way to gain crucial management skills, other methods can also be effective, and plenty of books have been written on the skills required to be a leader. Some of these abilities include, amongst others, good communication, positive energy, a belief in people, a balanced lifestyle, and a willingness to continually learn. Leaders create an environment centered on purpose and direction. They forge an atmosphere where people are fully involved in achieving the organization's objectives, and a QMS can aid in establishing these management responsibilities.

Communication

Proper communication, both within the IVF center and with the outside world, is of paramount importance. In fact, miscommunication can result in significant medical errors which are costly and can negatively impact the reputation of the center.

Like many other clinical practices, IVF centers involve many disciplines, and a change in any one of these career fields can have an effect on others. For example, if a physician decides to routinely order three additional blood tests during their IVF cycles, then nursing, phlebotomy, billing, and other physicians must all be aware of the change. However, how do these changes in procedure get communicated and followed? Furthermore, are these changes discussed among the center at large to determine whether general practices should be adjusted?

As one of the primary clinical decision-makers in a practice, physicians are often perceived as having their own way of doing things and unwilling to change to develop a more uniform method of treatment. This is not the case, though, when physicians have an outlet to discuss and debate their views. Consequently, there must be an effective process through meetings, discussions, or even retreats away from the office to review clinical matters and discuss protocols.

Nevertheless, the key to delivering optimal service to our patients is through effective communication not only with each other within the organization but with patients as well. Do patients have trouble speaking to the nurse? Is voicemail preventing a patient from having the human touch? Frustration from the inability of our patients to speak to the clinical staff in a timely manner is a frequently a distressing issue for them.

Customer Focus

A quality management system re-focuses the organization on improving quality, but quality is not a vague concept or dream. If it cannot be measured, then it cannot be considered quality. The organization must be able to quantify and measure performance, and customer satisfaction is that performance-measuring tool that determines the ultimate success of an IVF center. Nevertheless, in order to measure customer satisfaction and determine the path to success, we must first discover the identity of our customer.

So, who are our customers? Certainly, our patients are our primary customer, and in order for us to know we are excelling, we must ask them. Our product is not a baby but the resolution of infertility. Some patients leave our IVF centers with a baby but are dissatisfied with their experience. On the contrary, we have many patients without success who are extremely appreciative of our efforts in helping them deal with and resolve their fertility issues. Therefore, our business is to provide a service, not a product. Since we cannot control whether that service will ultimately be successful in achieving a pregnancy, we must direct our efforts to helping our patient population build their families by whichever means, or if not possible, resolving those goals and comforting them in their adjustment to a child-free future.

During this process, we should not ask ourselves how we are doing at treating our patients, but instead we should ask the patients. How can we do this, you ask? Well, the best method is to survey them and follow those responses over time. These surveys must analyze all areas of the organization and must be detailed enough to uncover deficiencies. Sometimes the results are surprising, but you'll never know what they are until you ask the customer and find out.

Nevertheless, we must also realize that an IVF center has many customers beyond the patients. We have relationships with pharmacies, pharmaceutical companies, vendors, and insurance companies. These entities are also our customers and must be managed as well. Furthermore, it should never be forgotten that our employees are our internal customers. No company is effective with unhappy employees; therefore, one must realize that the employees are one of the best marketing tools a company has, and they must also be satisfied to project the positive, excellent service provided by the organization at large.

Key Points

1. A Quality Management System (QMS) is a system that assists an organization in documenting employee responsibilities, processes, procedures, and other activities to track quality metrics and encourage future improvements.
2. The International Standard Organization (ISO) is the most recognized standard of a QMS and a global organization that ensures certain benchmarks are being met by businesses worldwide.
3. The ISO supports a company in excelling in multiple areas such as (1) documentation, (2) non-conformance tracking, (3) process approach, (4) staff expectations, (5) innovation, (6) leadership, (7) communication, and (8) customer focus.

BIBLIOGRAPHY

1. Alper MM et al. Is your IVF program good? *Hum Reprod.* 2002;17(1):8–10.
2. Alper MM. Experience with ISO quality control in assisted reproductive technology. *Fertil Steril.* 2013;100(6):1503–1508.
3. ASQ [internet]: http://www.asq.org/.
4. Carson BE et al. *Quality management systems for assisted reproductive technology.* ISO 9001:2000). CRC Press, London, 2004.
5. Keck C. *Quality management in assisted reproduction.* KAP CZ, Brno, 2003.
6. Sakkas D et al. Types and frequency of non-conformances in an IVF laboratory. *Hum Reprod.* 2018;33(12): 2196–2204.

32

Promoting Your Practice: The Use of Social Media

Theo LoPreste

In the ever-evolving landscape of fertility healthcare, mastering the nuances of various social media platforms is essential. Each platform offers unique features that, when leveraged correctly, can significantly enhance a fertility center's ability to connect with current patients, build a supportive online community, and drive new patient volume. This chapter delves into the critical role social media plays in the fertility treatment sector, examining its benefits and strategic applications.

Benefits of Social Media for a Fertility Center

Social media has become an indispensable tool for a fertility center, enhancing patient engagement, leveraging team knowledge, and offering personalized experiences. This section explores the multifaceted benefits, highlighting how social media can transform patient interactions and establish a center as a local market leader.

Enhanced Patient Engagement

Social media platforms provide direct communication channels between physicians and patients, facilitating immediate interactions and responses. Fertility centers can use these platforms to answer questions, provide updates, and offer support, creating a more engaged and informed patient base. This level of engagement helps build trust and loyalty, as patients feel more connected to their healthcare providers.

Leveraging of Team Knowledge

A fertility center can position itself as a leader in the local market by leveraging its collective team knowledge on social media. By sharing expert insights, addressing common fertility concerns, and offering detailed explanations of treatments, the center can demonstrate its expertise. This approach not only attracts current patients but also builds trust and credibility with future patients, enhancing the center's reputation. Additionally, it empowers people with knowledge and reduces anxiety related to fertility treatments.

Personalized Patient Experiences

Social media allows fertility centers to attract future patients by sharing personalized content like testimonials and success stories. This approach builds trust, demonstrates expertise, and addresses potential patients' specific concerns, making the center appear more relatable and supportive. By showcasing real-world outcomes and creating an empathetic online presence, centers can effectively engage with prospective patients, enhancing their likelihood of choosing a practice for their fertility needs.

DOI: 10.1201/9781003460275-32

Expanded Reach and Awareness

Social media enables fertility centers to significantly expand their reach and raise awareness about fertility issues and treatments. By utilizing targeted ads and sharing valuable content, centers can attract a broader audience, including individuals who may not yet be considering treatment. This increased visibility helps to educate the public, reduce stigma around fertility challenges, and positions the center as a proactive and inclusive healthcare provider.

Types of Social Media Posts

Understanding diverse types of social media posts is crucial for maximizing outreach and engagement. Fertility centers can strategically use various posts to attract and retain patients. Here are the primary types of social media posts and their effective uses.

Organic Posts

Organic posts are unpaid content shared on a center's social media profile, including valuable information, photos, videos, and graphics. For fertility centers, these might feature behind-the-scenes looks, educational content about fertility treatments, patient testimonials, and staff introductions. Creating a regular cadence of organic posts helps build a loyal following and establishes the center as a trustworthy information source.

Example: A post sharing a success story of a couple who recently had a baby through IVF at the center, accompanied by a heartfelt message from the center's staff.

Boosted Posts

Boosted posts on Facebook and Instagram are regular posts that the center promotes for a fee to reach a broader audience. This increases visibility beyond immediate followers and is ideal for promoting events like webinars or recent blog posts.

Example: Boosting a post about an upcoming online seminar on fertility treatments to reach individuals who might benefit from the information but do not follow the center's page.

Sponsored Posts

Sponsored posts are advertisements created to appear as part of a user's feed. These posts can be highly targeted to reach potential patients and are particularly effective for increasing center awareness.

Example: A sponsored post targeting women aged 30–40 in a specific area, highlighting a special event or encouraging viewers to schedule an appointment.

Co-Sponsored Posts

Co-sponsored posts are collaborations between two organizations or influencers, combining audiences for mutual benefit. Partnering with relevant health organizations, wellness brands, or influencers can amplify reach and credibility.

Example: A co-sponsored post with a health influencer sharing their fertility journey, highlighting a special event hosted by the center.

Video Content

Videos are highly engaging and can include live streams, recorded sessions, or animated infographics. They are essential for explaining complex procedures, sharing patient stories, or offering virtual tours of the center.

Example: A live Q&A session on social media with a fertility specialist, allowing viewers to ask questions in real-time or use of an "IVF 101" pre-recorded educational video.

User-Generated Content

User-generated content involves sharing posts created by patients, such as testimonials, photos, or videos of their experiences. This content provides authentic insights and builds trust.

Example: Reposting a photo shared by a former patient holding their newborn, thanking the center for their support throughout the fertility journey.

Infographics and Educational Posts

Infographics and educational posts simplify complex information, making it easily digestible. These posts are valuable for raising awareness and educating the audience about fertility and health.

Example: An infographic explaining the various stages of the egg freezing process, making it easier for potential patients to understand what to expect.

By strategically using these types of social media posts, fertility centers can effectively engage with their audience, build trust, and attract new patients. Each type of post serves a unique purpose, ensuring comprehensive coverage and maximum impact.

The Crucial Role of a Content Calendar for Social Media Accounts

A content calendar is vital for maintaining a consistent, engaging, and trustworthy social media presence for fertility centers. It ensures strategic planning, high-quality content variety, and efficient resource management. By implementing a well-structured content calendar, centers can maximize their social media impact and solidify their leadership in the field.

Ensures Consistency

Consistency is key in maintaining an engaging and trustworthy social media presence. A content calendar helps fertility centers plan and schedule posts in advance, ensuring that content is consistently shared across all platforms. This regular posting schedule keeps the audience engaged and aware of the center's ongoing activities and updates.

Facilitates Strategic Planning

A content calendar allows centers to strategically plan their content around important dates, events, and campaigns. This includes awareness days, health observances, and center-specific events such as webinars or patient appreciation days. By aligning content with these key dates, centers can maximize engagement and relevance, making their posts more impactful.

Maintains Quality and Variety

Planning content in advance ensures that a variety of high-quality posts are shared. A well-thought-out calendar includes a mix of educational posts, patient testimonials, promotional content, and interactive posts such as Q&A sessions. This variety keeps the audience engaged and caters to different interests and needs, enhancing the overall social media experience.

Promotes Efficient Resource Management

A content calendar allows for better resource management by distributing content creation efforts over time. This prevents last-minute rushes and ensures that each piece of content is well-researched, well-crafted, and aligns with the center's goals. It also allows for the involvement of different team members in the content creation process.

Key Points:

Overall, a content calendar is a crucial tool for fertility centers looking to maintain a robust and effective social media presence. It ensures consistency, allows for strategic planning, maintains quality and variety, and optimizes resource management. By implementing a well-structured content calendar, fertility centers can maximize their social media impact, attract and retain patients, and solidify their position as leaders in their field.

Platform-Specific Strategies

Effective social media marketing for a fertility center hinges on understanding your audience. This knowledge shapes content and ensures that both organic and paid ads resonate with the target demographic. By leveraging analytics, centers can refine their strategies, optimize ad spend, and achieve impactful, cost-effective marketing outcomes.

Facebook: Fostering Community and Support

Strengths: Ideal for community building, hosting live Q&A events, and sharing detailed information. It has a large user base and supports various content types (text, images, videos, links).

Weaknesses: Geared towards an older demographic. Organic reach has declined, necessitating paid advertisements to reach a broader audience.

Despite its strengths in community building and content sharing, Facebook has encountered challenges, particularly with its declining organic reach. Recent data suggest that organic posts on Facebook now reach only about 5.5% of a page's followers,[1] compelling businesses, including healthcare providers, to increasingly rely on paid advertisements to ensure broader content visibility.

Instagram: Visual Storytelling and Inspiration

Strengths: Perfect for visual storytelling and engagement. High engagement among younger demographics, particularly millennials and Gen Z. Supports various content types (images, videos, stories).

Weaknesses: Algorithm changes can affect content visibility. Competition is high among visually focused content creators.

Instagram's visual nature makes it an ideal platform for fertility centers to share visually appealing content. Centers can leverage the power of storytelling through impactful images, carousel posts, and Instagram Stories. Success stories, staff spotlights, and behind-the-scenes glimpses can humanize the center and create a connection with the audience. However, it's important to note that algorithm changes on Instagram can impact content visibility,[2] and the platform's high competition among visually focused content creators require centers to continuously refine their content strategy to maintain engagement.

YouTube: In-Depth Educational Content and Webinars

Strengths: Ideal for long-form, educational content. High searchability and can reach a global audience.

Weaknesses: Requires more effort to produce high-quality videos. Competition is high, requiring strong SEO strategies to stand out.

YouTube's visual and long-form content format makes it an ideal platform for fertility centers to share in-depth educational content. Centers can create informative videos on various fertility treatments, procedures, and patient experiences. Webinars, virtual tours of the center, and interviews with fertility experts can all find a home on YouTube. According to a 2023 report, YouTube has over 2.5 billion monthly active users, highlighting its immense popularity and potential for reaching a vast audience. It is also the second-most popular search engine after Google.[5] However, producing high-quality videos requires more effort, and centers may face competition from other content creators on the platform, necessitating strong SEO strategies to ensure their videos stand out and reach their target audience effectively.

TikTok: Engaging Through Short-Form Video Content

Strengths: Explosive growth and popularity among younger demographics. Highly engaging short-form video format. Supports creativity and authenticity.

Weaknesses: Limited content length may challenge conveying complex information. Algorithm changes can impact content visibility. Additionally, the future of TikTok remains uncertain due to political concerns surrounding its ownership and data privacy issues.[3]

While TikTok may seem unconventional for healthcare professionals, its engaging short-form video format can be leveraged to share behind-the-scenes content, debunk myths about fertility treatments, and provide quick fertility tips. TikTok's algorithm favors creativity and authenticity, allowing fertility professionals to showcase their human side and connect with a broader audience. However, the limited content length may challenge conveying complex information, and algorithm changes on TikTok can impact content visibility, requiring centers to adapt their strategies accordingly.

X (Formerly Twitter): Real-Time Engagement and Thought Leadership

Strengths: Real-time engagement and direct communication with followers. Ideal for sharing breaking news, research findings, and center updates.

Weaknesses: Limited character count can be restrictive for conveying detailed information. Less visual focus compared to other platforms.

X's algorithm prioritizes trending topics and highly engaging content, which can make it challenging for niche and specialized content such as fertility treatments to gain visibility. Tweets on this topic may get lost in the fast-paced and cluttered X feed. Overall, while X can be a useful tool for general awareness, it may not be the most effective medium for reaching and engaging individuals who are seeking detailed, supportive, and confidential information about fertility treatments.

LinkedIn: Professional Networking and Thought Leadership

Strengths: Excellent for professional networking and detailed content. Attracts a professional audience and is ideal for B2B engagement.

Weaknesses: Limited to professional content, which may not engage all patient demographics. Slower engagement growth compared to other platforms.

LinkedIn, focused on professional networking, lets fertility professionals showcase expertise and establish thought leadership. Centers can share research, provide ground-breaking insights, and participate in professional discussions. Publishing long-form articles provides in-depth information for a professional audience. However, LinkedIn's slower engagement may require supplementing with visually engaging content on other platforms.[4]

Understanding Your Audience and Leveraging Analytics

Knowing Your Audience

To create impactful social media content, a fertility center must first have a deep understanding of its audience. This includes demographic details such as age, gender, location, and marital status, as well as psychographic insights like interests, behaviors, and challenges related to fertility. By knowing your audience, you can tailor your messages to address their specific needs and concerns.

For instance, a fertility center targeting women aged 30–40 might focus on content related to advanced maternal age, the benefits of early fertility testing, and detailed explanations of various fertility treatments. This targeted approach ensures that the content is relevant and engaging, increasing the likelihood of patient recruitment.

Importance of Analytics

Analytics are crucial for measuring social media strategy effectiveness. Platforms like Facebook, Instagram, and others offer tools to track engagement rates, click-through rates, and audience demographics. Regular analysis helps determine which content resonates with which demographics and allows for strategy adjustments. For instance, if videos about patient success stories get higher engagement than images, more videos can be prioritized. Analytics also refine paid ad targeting, optimizing ad spend, and enhancing marketing efficiency.

Cost-Effectiveness

Understanding your audience and utilizing analytics also contribute to cost-effectiveness. Social media marketing can be more affordable than traditional advertising methods, but only if resources are allocated wisely. By targeting ads precisely and creating content that resonates with the audience, a fertility center can achieve high engagement and conversion rates without overspending.

Tips for Managing a Fertility Center's Social Media Page

Understanding the expectations of both current and future patients is crucial for fertility centers to create a meaningful and impactful social media presence. By focusing on providing reliable information, emotional support, engaging content, and responsive communication, centers can foster stronger connections with their patient community.

Prioritize Educational Content

Educational posts help social media users make informed decisions and feel more confident about their treatment choices. Detailed explanations of fertility treatments, live Q&A's, pre-recorded webinars, and more, help reduce anxiety and misinformation.

Visualize

Engaging content, including videos, infographics, and images, is highly effective in capturing user interest. Visual content that explains complex medical procedures, showcases center facilities, or shares patient success stories can enhance understanding and retention of information.

Create a Supportive Environment

Social media offers a platform for users to connect and share their family-building experiences. Both current and future patients value the emotional support they receive through social media interactions. Encouraging the sharing of personal stories and testimonials, while also providing content that addresses the emotional aspects of infertility and family building, fosters a supportive environment.

Showcase Diversity and Promote Inclusion

Highlighting the diverse backgrounds and experiences of both patients and staff fosters an inclusive and welcoming environment. Representation in social media content helps individuals from different cultures, family structures, gender identities, and sexual orientations feel seen, respected, and valued. By intentionally incorporating diverse voices and experiences, fertility clinics can create a supportive community that reflects the varied journeys to parenthood and ensures that all individuals feel included in their care.

Spotlight Patient Testimonials and Success Stories

Prospective and current patients find inspiration and hope in the success stories of others. Sharing patient testimonials and success stories can significantly boost the morale of those considering or undergoing treatment.

Highlight Center Reviews and Feedback

Profile followers want to know about others' care experiences. Reviews and feedback from fellow patients can provide insights and help prospective patients make informed decisions.

Ensure Timely Responses to Questions and Comments

Prompt responses from centers on social media are crucial in building user trust and satisfaction. Centers should have dedicated personnel to monitor their social media channels and ensure that questions or comments are answered promptly.

Respond to Negative Feedback

Addressing negative feedback or concerns transparently and professionally is crucial. Patients appreciate it when centers acknowledge issues and take steps to resolve them. Deleting poor reviews can harm the legitimacy of the center's social media presence and show a lack of respect for patient feedback. Instead, centers should respond respectfully and constructively to negative reviews. They should acknowledge the experience of the reviewer and outline, if possible, what action can be taken to ensure future patients have a better experience. This approach helps maintain a positive online reputation and builds trust with the patient community.

Protect Privacy

One of the paramount concerns for patients is the protection of their privacy. Centers must ensure that they are HIPAA compliant when sharing patient information or testimonials on social media. Obtaining explicit consent from patients before posting their stories or images is essential. Carefully analyze all photos taken in the center before posting to ensure computer screens, paperwork, and other material do not display personal patient information.

Social Media Strategies for Fertility Doctors

A robust social media presence can enhance a fertility doctor's visibility and practice. This section explores the benefits, potential pitfalls, and considerations for establishing and maintaining a social media presence.

Benefits of a Social Media Presence

Visibility and Reach

Social media platforms such as Facebook, Instagram, TikTok, LinkedIn, and X have millions of active users. By maintaining a social media presence, fertility doctors can reach a broader audience beyond their immediate geographical location. This increased visibility can attract potential patients who are seeking fertility treatments and looking for trusted healthcare providers.

Patient Education

Patients often turn to the internet for health-related information. Fertility doctors can use social media to share accurate, evidence-based information about fertility treatments, success rates, and new advancements in the field. This not only educates patients but also positions the doctor as a knowledgeable and reliable source of information.

Trust and Credibility

A well-maintained social media page can enhance a doctor's credibility. Sharing patient testimonials, success stories, and behind-the-scenes content can humanize the doctor and build trust. According to a study co-authored by researchers at Reproductive Medicine Associates of New Jersey, 79.9% of patients felt that social media provided a benefit to their experience while at their fertility center.[6]

Direct Engagement with Patients

Social media allows for real-time interaction with patients. Doctors can answer questions, provide support, and offer personalized advice through comments and direct messages. This level of engagement can strengthen the patient–doctor relationship and improve patient satisfaction.

Community Building

Creating a supportive online community can help patients feel less isolated in their fertility journey. Doctors can facilitate this by creating private groups where patients can share their experiences, ask questions, and offer support to one another.

Challenges of a Social Media Presence

Inconsistent Posting

Inconsistent posting can make a doctor appear disengaged and unreliable. A well-structured content plan ensures consistency, strengthens credibility, and builds patient trust.

Ensuring Brand Consistency

Maintaining brand consistency—adhering to colors, fonts, and design elements—can be challenging across platforms. Without strict adherence to a style guide, branding may become inconsistent, diminishing the doctor/clinic's professional image and hindering trust and recognition.

Patients Seeking Medical Advice

Some patients report urgent concerns via social media, expecting immediate help instead of contacting their doctor (through the clinic/patient portal) or dialing 911. Doctors should post disclaimers and diligently monitor messages to redirect emergencies appropriately.

Privacy Risks

Patients may share personal health details publicly, unaware of privacy risks. Public responses can violate HIPAA. Doctors must educate patients on secure communication, moderate content, and enforce privacy policies.

Unrealistic Response Expectations

Many users expect instant replies from clinics and/or doctors. Delays can cause frustration and negative feedback. Setting response time expectations and balancing engagement with time limitations is essential.

Misinformation and Patient Frustration

False claims about treatments and success rates spread quickly. Patients may also express frustrations about costs or clinic policies. Doctors should provide accurate information, maintain professionalism, and direct complex concerns to a care coordinator.

Why It's OK for a Doctor to Not Have a Social Media Profile

Time and Resource Constraints

Maintaining a social media presence demands significant time, effort, and resources. For doctors with busy practices, it may not be feasible to effectively manage a personal social media page. Instead, contributing to the center's social media page can have a more substantial impact, leveraging shared resources and collective efforts.

Professional Boundaries

Some doctors may prefer to maintain strict professional boundaries and avoid the potential risks associated with social media, such as privacy breaches or negative interactions.

Focus on Other Channels

Doctors can still engage and educate patients through other means, such as live Q&A's, pre-recorded educational videos on YouTube, and more.

Key Points

- **A Strategic Content Plan Maximizes Impact:** A well-structured content calendar ensures consistency, quality, and variety in social media posts. By planning around key events, patient testimonials, and educational topics, fertility centers can maintain a strong online presence and effectively manage resources to optimize engagement and outreach.
- **Platform-Specific Strategies Improve Reach and Effectiveness:** Different social media platforms serve distinct purposes—Instagram is ideal for visual storytelling; YouTube provides in-depth education; TikTok engages through short-form videos; and although past its prime, Facebook can still be beneficial for community-building. Understanding platform strengths and tailoring content accordingly ensures better audience connection and maximizes impact.
- **Leveraging Analytics and Audience Insights Enhances Marketing Efficiency:** Data-driven decision-making is crucial for refining social media strategies. By analyzing engagement metrics, fertility centers can identify which types of content resonate with their audience, improve targeting for paid ads, and allocate marketing resources more effectively to maximize return on investment.
- **Managing Social Media Responsibly Ensures Compliance and Credibility:** Fertility centers must ensure timely and professional responses to user inquiries and handle negative feedback transparently. Clear social media policies help protect patient privacy, maintain professional boundaries, and prevent misinformation, reinforcing the center's reputation as a trusted healthcare provider.
- **A Style Guide Strengthens Brand Identity and Patient Trust:** Maintaining brand consistency across social media is crucial for credibility and recognition. A style guide ensures all content—whether text, images, or videos—follows uniform branding elements such as tone, colors, and fonts. This consistency reinforces the center's professionalism, strengthens patient trust, and makes content recognizable, ensuring a cohesive and polished digital presence.
- **Maximizing Impact through Shared Social Media Efforts:** Maintaining a personal social media presence requires significant time and effort, which may not be feasible for doctors with demanding practices. Instead, contributing to the center's official social media platforms can be a more efficient and effective way to engage with patients, share expertise, and uphold the clinic's messaging. By leveraging shared resources and collective efforts, doctors can still build visibility and trust without the burden of managing an individual page.

REFERENCES

1. Hootsuite. Social Media Benchmarks: Q4 2023 Data & Tips [internet], 2024: https://blog.hootsuite.com/social-media-benchmarks/
2. Sprout Social. The Instagram algorithm: how it works and strategies for 2024 [internet], 2023: https://sproutsocial.com/insights/instagram-algorithm/
3. Freking K. House passes a bill that could lead to a TikTok ban if Chinese owner refuses to sell. Associated Press [internet], 2024: https://apnews.com/article/tiktok-ban-house-vote-china-national-security-8fa7258fae1a4902d344c9d978d58a37
4. Swipe Insight. LinkedIn Engagement and Reach Plummet: Key Metrics Show Significant Decline [internet], 2024: https://web.swipeinsight.app/posts/linkedin-engagement-and-reach-plummet-key-metrics-show-significant-decline-6378
5. Oberlo. 10 YouTube Stats Every Marketer Should Know in 2023 [internet], 2023: https://www.oberlo.com/blog/youtube-statistics)
6. Broughton DE et al. Social media in the REI clinic: what do patients want? *J Assist Reprod Genet.* 2018;35(7):1259–1263.

33

The True ART: How to Deliver the Best Patient Care

David L. Stern

The journey through fertility treatment is an emotional process, demanding not just medical expertise but also compassionate and effective patient care. In many cases, something that seems so natural (the ability to have a child), the woman is faced with month after month of failure. Many women go to their annual OBGYN appointment and are asked if they need a refill of their contraceptive. There is rarely a discussion with the doctor about family planning (meaning, when to have children), but the subliminal message the patient receives is that they are so fertile, they need to actively prevent a pregnancy by taking some form of contraception. This creates an artificial expectation that when the woman *is* ready to have a child, all she needs to do is stop taking her contraception and she'll get pregnant. Many patients who end up at a fertility center have experienced the frustration of feeling let down by their bodies. It is a similar situation for men, who rarely undergo testing (many men don't go to an annual checkup, and if they do, they are not having a semen analysis). Often a couple will come to a fertility center and the male partners will never have done a simple semen analysis to confirm that his sperm are normal. In our society, often fertility is a female problem.

In this chapter, we explore the intricacies of providing the best patient care, which includes engaging patients, utilizing customer relationship management (CRM) to enhance clinic–patient interactions, communicating effectively, educating patients on diverse treatment options, introducing innovative patient education platforms, providing clarity on insurance coverage, and the potential need for multiple treatment cycles.

Patient Engagement: The Heart of Comprehensive Care

Patient engagement lies at the core of delivering exceptional care in fertility centers. It extends beyond the clinical realm, encompassing the emotional and informational support that patients require throughout their fertility journey. Engaged patients are not just passive recipients of medical services; they are active participants in their care, making informed decisions and feeling a sense of partnership with their healthcare providers.

Establishing trust is foundational to patient engagement. Fertility centers must prioritize building strong, empathetic relationships with patients. This involves active listening, understanding individual needs, and demonstrating genuine compassion. When patients feel heard and understood, they are more likely to engage actively in their care and openly communicate their concerns. Fertility treatment is not "cookie-cutter" medicine and needs to be individualized based on the patient diagnosis. Building trust starts with a clinical review of the patient's test results and subsequent diagnosis. An individualized treatment plan should then be discussed with the patient which incorporates the pros and cons of different treatment options. By spending time during the initial and follow-up visits with the patient, this helps to build trust and confidence in the fertility center, physician, and clinical team.

DOI: 10.1201/9781003460275-33

The Role of Communication

Effective communication is a cornerstone of patient engagement. Fertility centers should foster open lines of communication that go beyond the clinical setting. Regular updates, clear explanations of treatment plans, and responsiveness to patient inquiries contribute to a positive patient experience. This two-way communication not only provides information but also ensures that patients feel valued and involved in their care. Communication begins from the first phone call, even before there is a patient relationship. Having a centralized call center can help to streamline this communication with prospective patients and initiate the step of customer relationship management (CRM) systems. Once the individual or couple becomes a patient, having a clear understanding of who are the right individuals to contact within the practice provides clarity and sets the right level of expectation. Investing in a call center for existing patients for general questions is one way to distribute the workload among center staff. Oftentimes, nurses are asked questions that are not clinical in nature and could be addressed by someone else in the practice. One way to utilize technology is to have a chat-bot or FAQ section on a patient portal or a secure patient website. This allows for "real-time" interaction and meets the needs of the patient while reducing their stress during a cycle. Patients in fertility centers are used to having their questions answered quickly. Our society is built on a real-time engagement model where it's easy to Google an answer to a question. Patients expect the same level of communication and will be frustrated if they feel that they are not getting a rapid response from staff.

Utilizing Technology for Engagement

In the rapidly evolving landscape of healthcare, the integration of technology has become integral to improving patient satisfaction. Implementing patient portals, mobile apps, and other digital platforms provide patients with convenient access to information and communication with their healthcare team. These tools facilitate real-time updates, appointment scheduling, and access to educational resources, enhancing the overall patient participation.

Implementing user-friendly patient portals allows individuals to access their medical records, schedule appointments, and communicate securely with healthcare providers. This not only promotes convenience but also empowers patients to take an active role in managing their health. Utilizing secure messaging systems enables quick and confidential communication between patients and healthcare providers. This real-time communication channel facilitates prompt responses to patient inquiries, appointment reminders, and the efficient handling of non-emergency medical concerns.

Since the COVID pandemic, telemedicine has become a convenient way for patients to interact with their physicians and healthcare providers. This is particularly beneficial for follow-up appointments, enhancing accessibility and flexibility for patients.

Automated appointment reminders, delivered via SMS, email, or mobile apps, reduce the likelihood of missed appointments. This not only improves scheduling efficiency but also demonstrates the medical practice's commitment to patient convenience.

Personalizing Engagement

In busy fertility centers, often patients can "feel like a number." When they come in for cycle monitoring (blood testing and ultrasounds), they are surrounded by many other patients in the waiting room. This can serve as a deterrent for patients, and often they feel like their care is not personalized, due to the high volume of patients. Recognizing the diversity of patient needs, fertility centers should adopt a personalized approach to engagement. Boston IVF's approach is to create physician-centric teams, where the physician is surrounded by a nurse, medical assistant, financial counselor, and administrative assistant. The patient has a defined team that knows them and is helping them navigate the fertility treatment journey. The physician will make all of the treatment decisions for that patient, and the dedicated team member will be the one to convey the instructions to the patient. Personalized engagement demonstrates a commitment to treating each patient as a unique individual with unique needs.

Involving Patients in Decision-Making

Engaged patients actively participate in decision-making regarding their fertility treatments. Fertility centers should encourage shared decision-making, involving patients in discussions about treatment options, potential risks, and expected outcomes. Many patients will research center success rates on the SART or CDC website. These statistics provide an overview of all the patients within a certain age category (<35, 35–37, 38–40, >40), but the mistake many patients make is not understanding that each patient is different. A younger patient may have a hormone profile of an older patient, and therefore, not fall into the success rate of a younger patient. Utilizing technology can allow fertility centers to collect data and share with patients the likelihood of similar patients (diagnosis, age, hormone, etc.) to become pregnant. This type of tool can be helpful to show the difference in an IVF treatment versus an IUI treatment in terms of success. Fertility patients are optimists. They believe, going into their first IVF cycle, that they will be successful—no matter what the odds. Shifting the clinical conversation to a patient's "cumulative success rate" versus the individual cycle success rate will better set expectations of the overall chance of success with continued treatment in the event of a failed cycle. Crafting these conversations around hope will increase control at the patient level and likely result in higher retention rates/lower dropout rates in the event of an unsuccessful cycle. This collaborative approach empowers patients to make choices aligned with their values and preferences, fostering a sense of ownership in their fertility journey.

Emotional Support as a Pillar of Engagement

Recognizing the emotional challenges associated with fertility treatments, fertility centers that offer emotional support, either through third-party companies or as part of an in-house offering, can help patients navigate this difficult journey. This includes not only acknowledging the emotional aspects of the journey but also offering counseling services, support groups, and resources for coping with the psychological toll. Emotional support is a crucial element of patient engagement, ensuring that patients feel cared for beyond the clinical procedures and can be a point of differentiation from other fertility centers.

Understanding the psychological burden on patients is critical in understanding the needs of infertile patients, as this patient burden can often result in discontinuation of treatment. In a systematic review of reasons and predictors of discontinuation of treatment of 22 studies, which included 21,453 patients[1] —the most common reasons included:

- Postponement of treatment (39%)
- Physical or psychological burden (19%)
- Relational and personal problems (17%)
- Treatment rejection (13%)
- Organizational (12%)
- Clinic issues (8%)

In 2015, Lande et al conducted a survey among 134 couples and showed that the top reason for treatment termination included the psychological burden of treatment, and in particular, that these patients lost hope.[2]

In 2011, Van Empel et al conducted a study among 925 patients and 227 physicians that showed, while pregnancy rates were most important to physicians, patient-centered care was most important to patients.[3] Further, the study revealed that a lack of patient-centered care was the most cited reason for switching clinics. The evidence here would suggest a disconnect between physician priority and patient priority; perhaps failing to meet the patient's needs results in patients switching clinics, which can lead to a loss of business and a possible opportunity for success with those patients.

Leveraging Customer Relationship Management (CRM)

Implementing a robust CRM system is instrumental in fostering patient engagement. CRM allows fertility centers to track patient interactions, preferences, and communication history. This data empowers healthcare providers to personalize their approach, providing a more tailored and empathetic experience for patients.

Utilizing CRM data, fertility centers can personalize communication with patients. This could include sending targeted informational materials, reminders for appointments, and even recognizing important milestones in the patient's fertility journey. Personalized interactions demonstrate a commitment to understanding and addressing individual patient needs. Tracking dropouts is another advantage of utilizing CRM data and a way for fertility centers to identify patients who have not come in for appointments or not made follow-up appointments. Personalized communication can then offer Q&A with a staff member to see if there are questions that can be addressed to bring them back in for an appointment and potential treatment.

Feedback and Continuous Quality Improvement (CQI)

An essential aspect of patient engagement is soliciting and utilizing patient feedback. Fertility centers should actively seek input from patients about their experiences, preferences, and suggestions for improvement. Utilizing patient satisfaction surveys through digital channels allows medical practices to collect actionable patient evaluation. This information provides insights into patient involvement, allowing for prompt identification of areas for improvement and acknowledgment of successful practices. This feedback loop allows for continuous improvement in services, demonstrating responsiveness to patient needs, and enhancing overall patient satisfaction. It can also serve as an opportunity to have patients share their positive interactions with others via social media and other online review sites. Actively engaging with patients on social media and monitoring online reviews contributes to a transparent and responsive image. Addressing concerns, expressing gratitude for positive responses, and providing timely responses demonstrate the practice's commitment to patient satisfaction and continuous improvement. For internal team building, recognizing staff through appreciation bonuses (gift card) rewards behaviors of providing excellent care. During the annual Boston Globe “Salute to Nurses,” we ask patients to share their stories of how our nursing team has provided support for their treatment journey. In 2023 over 70 patients shared stories, which was the highest number of patient stories from any type of medical provider in the Boston area.

At Boston IVF, we measure patient satisfaction through our customer relationship management platform and incorporate the patient responses into a monthly Continuous Quality Improvement (CQI)/Risk Management meeting for review. Our goal is to achieve a ≥95% overall patient satisfaction score.

Examples of survey questions include:

- Facility questions
    - On a scale of 0–10, please rate the facility's comfortability.
    - On a scale of 0–10, please rate the facility's cleanliness.
    - The facility had adequate parking available. (Agree/Disagree)
    - The waiting room had adequate seating available. (Agree/Disagree)
- Reception questions
    - I found the receptionist to be friendly and courteous. (Agree/Disagree)
    - I found the receptionist to be helpful and informative. (Agree/Disagree)
    - Please leave any additional feedback you have regarding your experience with the receptionist.
- Provider questions
    - I left my consultation feeling fully informed. (Agree/Disagree)
    - I felt confident and comfortable with my provider. (Agree/Disagree)

    - My provider portrayed professionalism and care during my visit. (Agree/Disagree)
    - My provider made me feel like an individual and not just a number. (Agree/Disagree)
    - How likely are you to recommend this provider to a friend/family member seeking assistance with infertility?
    - Please leave any additional feedback regarding your experience with your provider.
- Financial Coordinator Questions
    - Did you meet with a financial coordinator? (Yes/No)
    - I had no issues setting up an appointment with a financial coordinator. (Agree/Disagree)
    - I found my financial coordinator to be helpful and informative. (Agree/Disagree)
    - I found my financial coordinator to be kind and courteous. (Agree/Disagree)
    - Please leave any additional feedback regarding your experience with a financial coordinator.
- Overall experience question
    - On a scale of 0 to 10, please rate your overall experience with Boston IVF.

We conduct monthly meetings to review the results of the patient survey as well as to review other opportunities for improvement. We take patient feedback very seriously and have invested in having a patient advocate who addresses patient complaints. When we receive a patient complaint, we do an internal investigation to better understand the root cause of the complaint and what steps were taken that may have impacted the patient negatively. This includes our patient advocate speaking with all of those involved (patient, physician, nurse, lab, or others as needed) to understand the issue in a more encompassing manner.

The CQI committee consists of an interdepartmental group of employees ranging from the senior management team to medical directors and laboratory management staff. It is an integrated, continuous effort to measure, monitor, and improve patient safety and the performance of infertility and assisted reproductive technology (ART) services.

The goals of the CQI Committee are to:

- Support the organization's mission and strategic plan.
- Systematically plan, monitor performance, analyze current performance, and improve and sustain improvements in processes and outcomes of patient care through interdisciplinary teams, clinical service, department activities, and peer review.
- Minimize or reduce opportunities for an adverse impact on patients and staff.
- Develop performance measures consistent with the organizational strategic plan.
- Measure the organization's key outcomes, activities, and processes to support safety, improvement, innovation, and learning.
- Integrate organization-wide performance improvement activities.
- Promote interdepartmental and interdisciplinary communication with an integrated approach to problem solving.
- Develop an environment that encourages and empowers staff to identify and address issues through the performance improvement process.
- Support compliance with accreditation standards and regulatory agency requirements.

Fostering a Community of Support

Beyond individual engagement, fertility centers can foster a sense of community among patients. Support groups, online forums, and events that bring patients together create a supportive network where individuals can share experiences, offer encouragement, and build connections. This community-oriented approach contributes to a more resilient and empowered patient population. Patient advocacy groups, such as RESOLVE, can be a way to show support for the patients that we treat.

Effective Communication Strategies

Patients vary in their preferred communication channels. Fertility centers should adopt a multichannel approach, incorporating email, phone calls, and secure messaging platforms. This ensures that information reaches patients in a timely and accessible manner, catering to their individual preferences. In the realm of fertility treatment, timely communication is crucial. Patients appreciate clear and prompt updates regarding their treatment progress, test results, and any changes in the plan. Fertility centers should establish communication protocols to ensure patients are always well-informed. Educating patients on fertility treatment options requires a personalized approach. Fertility centers should assess each patient's understanding, preferences, and concerns, tailoring educational materials accordingly. This ensures that patients make informed decisions aligned with their values and expectations.

While patients expect to be successful on their first cycle, many patients require more than one treatment cycle to have a child. Even in the best IVF centers, the success rates are not 100% (healthy young women [under 35], 40–50% can expect to become pregnant over a three-month period).[4] As a women ages, her chances of becoming pregnant declines. Even with ART treatment, success rates vary significantly by age. Fertility treatment is a journey that may require multiple cycles to achieve success. Fertility centers should educate patients about the realistic expectations of the process, emphasizing that success may take time. Managing expectations from the beginning helps patients mentally and emotionally prepare for potential challenges and increases overall satisfaction with the care they receive.

The Role of Technology in Communication

Integrating technology can streamline communication processes. Implementing secure patient portals or mobile apps allows patients to access information conveniently and communicate with their healthcare team. Technology not only enhances efficiency but also empowers patients to actively participate in their care. The EngagedMD patient education platform offers a cutting-edge solution for delivering personalized and interactive educational content. Fertility centers can leverage this platform to provide patients with in-depth information about various treatment options, potential outcomes, and the overall fertility journey. The platform facilitates self-paced learning, empowering patients to navigate their fertility choices with confidence.

Fertility centers should not view patient education as a one-time event but as an ongoing process. Regular workshops, webinars, and access to resources through platforms like EngagedMD can keep patients informed at every stage of their fertility treatment. This continuous education fosters a sense of empowerment and partnership between patients and healthcare providers.

Understanding Insurance Coverage

Unfortunately, infertility is not designated as a disease at a national level. As a result, each state decides if insurance companies are required to cover patients undergoing infertility treatment. As of Spring 2025, 21 states plus D.C. have passed fertility insurance coverage laws; 15 of those laws include IVF coverage and 17 of those cover fertility preservation for iatrogenic (medically-induced) infertility[5] (Figure 33.1).

The complexities of insurance coverage can be overwhelming for patients. Fertility centers should initiate comprehensive education programs to help patients understand their insurance plans. This involves clarifying which treatments may be covered and what expenses may be considered out-of-pocket. In many cases, the patient will be responsible for attaining the correct prior approvals required by the insurance company for treatment coverage. This approval process can be long (2–4 weeks) and sometimes frustrating. It is important to set realistic expectations for patients so that they understand what their coverage includes (out-of-pocket maximums, testing requirements, lifetime maximum coverage, etc.). Dedicated financial counselors play a crucial role in helping patients navigate the financial aspects of fertility treatments. Offering one-on-one consultations ensures that patients receive personalized guidance based on their insurance plans and financial situations. This personalized approach can alleviate financial concerns and contribute to a more positive patient experience.

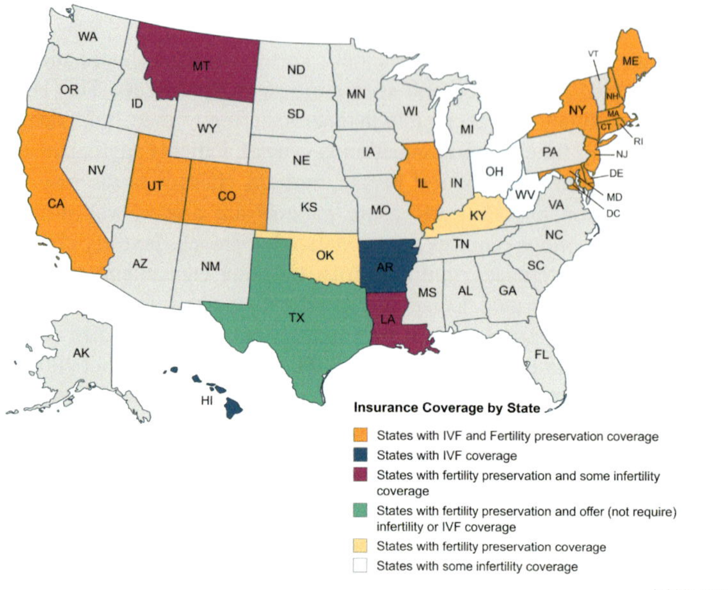

FIGURE 33.1 Insurance coverage by state (from ref. 5 with permission).

Establishing clear financial policies is paramount to helping patients understand the potential costs associated with fertility treatments. Fertility centers should provide transparent information about fees, payment plans, and any additional expenses. This transparency enables patients to plan for the financial aspects of their fertility journey. There are several third-party companies (such as LendingClub, CapexMD, Ally) that offer financing for patients undergoing fertility treatment. These financing programs can provide real-time approval and different financing options (APR and length of loan). In working with a third-party company, IVF centers offer the flexibility to patients to pay for treatment over an extended period of time, and the IVF center is paid right away.

There are also IVF centers that offer multicycle or guarantee-type programs to reduce the burden of paying for multiple cycles one at time. Many patients may require more than one treatment cycle, and these types of programs offer a savings to patients.

Ancillary Services for Holistic Care

Role of Acupuncture

Ancillary services such as acupuncture can complement fertility treatments. Research suggests that acupuncture may help reduce stress, improve blood flow to the reproductive organs, and enhance the overall success of fertility treatments. Offering acupuncture services as part of a comprehensive care plan demonstrates a commitment to holistic patient well-being.

Dietary Support

Nutrition plays a crucial role in fertility, and dietary support can be a valuable adjunct to medical interventions. Fertility centers can collaborate with nutritionists to provide tailored dietary guidance that supports optimal reproductive health. This holistic approach recognizes the interconnectedness of physical and emotional well-being during the fertility journey.

Key Points

- **Patient Engagement and Communication**: The emotional aspect of fertility treatments requires compassionate care alongside medical expertise. Fertility centers must build strong, empathetic relationships with patients through active listening, personalized treatment plans, and clear communication. This includes regular updates, easy access to information, and responsiveness to patient inquiries.
- **Technology Integration**: Using patient portals, mobile apps, and telemedicine enhances communication and convenience, allowing patients to access medical records, schedule appointments, and receive updates. Real-time interaction tools like chat-bots or FAQs can reduce patient stress during treatment cycles.
- **Personalized Care**: Due to high patient volumes, fertility centers should provide a personalized approach, where each patient has a dedicated team that understands their unique needs. This builds trust and encourages patient involvement in treatment decisions.
- **Emotional Support and Coping**: Offering emotional support, including counseling and support groups, is crucial to help patients manage the psychological burden of fertility treatments. Acknowledging these challenges and providing support can prevent treatment discontinuation.
- **Utilizing CRM for Engagement**: Fertility centers can use Customer Relationship Management (CRM) systems to track patient interactions and preferences, tailoring communication to individual needs. This improves patient experience, boosts satisfaction, and enhances retention by addressing concerns proactively.

REFERENCES

1. Gameiro S et al. Why do patients discontinue fertility treatment? A systematic review of reasons and predictors of discontinuation in fertility treatment. *Human Reprod Update* 2012;18:652–69.
2. Lande Y et al. Why do couples discontinue unlimited free IVF treatments? *Gynecol Endocrinol* 2015;31(3):233–6.
3. van Empel Dancet EA et al. Physicians underestimate the importance of patient-centeredness to patients: a discrete choice experiment in fertility care. *Human Reprod* 2011;26(3):584–93.
4. ASRM. Reproductive Facts [internet]: www.reproductivefacts.org/.
5. RESOLVE: The National Infertility Association [internet]: https://resolve.org/learn/financial-resources-for-family-building/insurance-coverage/insurance-coverage-by-state/.

Index

Q

R

S